Concise

Histology

LESLIE P. GARTNER, PhD

Professor of Anatomy (*Retired*)
Department of Biomedical Sciences
Baltimore College of Dental Surgery
Dental School
University of Maryland
Baltimore, Maryland

JAMES L. HIATT, PhD

Professor Emeritus
Department of Biomedical Sciences
Baltimore College of Dental Surgery
Dental School
University of Maryland
Baltimore, Maryland

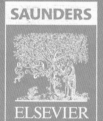

SAUNDERS

ELSEVIER

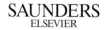

1600 John F. Kennedy Boulevard
Suite 1800
Philadelphia, PA 19103-2899

CONCISE HISTOLOGY

ISBN: 978-0-7020-3114-4

Library of Congress Cataloging-in-Publication Data

Gartner, Leslie P.
    Concise histology / Leslie P. Gartner, James L. Hiatt.—1st ed.
        p. ; cm.
    Based on: Color textbook of histology / Leslie P. Gartner, James L. Hiatt. 3rd ed. c2007.
    Includes index.
    ISBN 978-0-7020-3114-4
    1. Histology.   I. Hiatt, James L.,—   II. Gartner, Leslie P., 1943—Color textbook of histology.
III. Title.
    [DNLM: 1. Histology—Atlases.   QS 517 G244c 2011]
    QM551.G366 2011
    611'.018—dc22

                                                                        2010013017

Acquisitions Editor: Kate Dimock
Developmental Editor: Barbara Cicalese

Design Direction: Lou Forgione
Electronic Media Manager: Carol Emery

Working together to grow
libraries in developing countries

www.elsevier.com | www.bookaid.org | www.sabre.org

ELSEVIER | BOOK AID International | Sabre Foundation

Printed in China

Last digit is the print number: 9   8   7   6   5   4   3   2   1

To my wife, Roseann;
my daughter, Jennifer;
and my mother, Mary
LPG

To my grandchildren,
Nathan David,
James Mallary,
Hanna Elisabeth,
Alexandra Renate,
Eric James,
and Elise Victoria
JLH

Once again, we are gratified to release a new histology textbook, one that is based on the third edition of our *Color Textbook of Histology*, a well-established textbook not only in its original language but also in several other languages.

In the past three decades, histology has evolved from the purely descriptive science of microscopic anatomy to a composite study integrating functional anatomy with both molecular and cell biology. This new textbook is designed in an unusual manner in that each even-numbered page tells the story in words and the facing odd-numbered page illustrates the textual story by beautiful four-color illustrations that are borrowed from the third edition of our *Color Textbook of Histology*. Therefore, each set of facing pages may be thought of as individual learning units. To demonstrate the relevance of the information presented to the health professions, almost every *learning unit* is reinforced by clinical considerations pertinent to the topic. Students and faculty alike will, no doubt, note the absence of photomicrographs and electron micrographs in *Concise Histology*. We made a deliberate decision to exclude that material from the hard copy and to place it, instead, on the Student Consult website that is associated with this book. We did that to reduce the size of the book, thereby making life easier for the student who has to learn material that a decade ago was taught in 16 weeks and currently is done so in perhaps half that time. Student Consult houses not only all the illustrations located on the right side of the facing pages of the book but also 150 photomicrographs and electron micrographs, identified by chapter, with appropriate examination questions and the answers to those questions so that the student can test his or her ability not only to recognize the organs/tissues/cells in question but also their functional characteristics. Included on Student Consult are clinical scenarios with appropriate USMLE I-type questions that not only further demonstrate the relevance of histology to the health sciences but also prepare medical students for the histology component of the boards. The designs of the hard copy of this textbook, as well as that of the ancillary web-based material, intend to highlight the essential concepts underlying our presentation of histology, namely that there is a close relationship between structure and function.

Although we have made every effort to present a complete and accurate account of the subject matter, we realize that there are omissions and errors in any undertaking of this magnitude. Therefore, we continue to encourage and welcome suggestions, advice, and criticism that will facilitate the improvement of future editions of this textbook.

Leslie P. Gartner
James L. Hiatt

Acknowledgments

Histology is a visual subject; therefore, excellent graphic illustrations are imperative. For that we are indebted to Todd Smith for his careful attention to detail in revising and creating new illustrations. We also thank our many colleagues from around the world and their publishers who generously permitted us to borrow illustrative materials.

Finally, our thanks go to the project team at Elsevier for all their help, namely Kate Dimock, Barbara Cicalese, Lou Forgione, and Carol Emery. We also thank Linnea Hermanson for her painstaking effort in the production of this text book.

Contents

1   Introduction to Histology 2

2   Cytoplasm 8

3   Nucleus 26

4   Extracellular Matrix 40

5   Epithelium and Glands 48

6   Connective Tissue 62

7   Cartilage and Bone 74

8   Muscle 94

9   Nervous Tissue 108

10 Blood and Hematopoiesis 132

11 Circulatory System 152

12 Lymphoid (Immune) System 168

13 Endocrine System 188

14 Integument 204

15 Respiratory System 218

16 Digestive System: Oral Cavity 230

17 Digestive System: Alimentary Canal 238

18 Digestive System: Glands 250

19 Urinary System 260

20 Female Reproductive System 272

21 Male Reproductive System 286

22 Special Senses 304

Index 325

Concise Histology

1 INTRODUCTION TO HISTOLOGY

Histology is a study of the tissues of animals and plants, but the *Concise Histology* deals only with mammalian tissues, specifically, that of *Homo sapiens*. In addition to the structure of the tissues, cells, organs, and organ systems compose the theme of this textbook—hence, a better term for the subject matter presented in this book is *microscopic anatomy*. It is well known by the reader of this book that the body is a conglomerate of:

- Cells
- **Extracellular matrix (ECM)**, in which the cells are embedded
- **Extracellular fluid** that percolates through the ECM to bring nutrients, oxygen, and signaling molecules to the cells and to take waste products, carbon dioxide, still more signaling molecules, hormones, and pharmacologic agents away from the cells
  - The extracellular fluid is derived from blood plasma and released into the ECM at the arterial side of capillary beds, and most of the fluid is returned to the blood plasma at the venous ends of capillary beds.
  - The remainder of the extracellular fluid enters the lower pressure lymphatic system of vessels to be returned to the bloodstream at the junction of the internal jugular vein and subclavian vein of the right and left sides.

Modern textbooks of histology discuss not only the microscopic morphology of the body, but also its function. The subject matter of this book also invokes cell biology, physiology, molecular biology, biochemistry, gross anatomy, embryology, and even a modicum of clinical medicine in the form of *Clinical Considerations*. It is hoped that the study of histology will illuminate for the reader the interrelationship of **structure** and **function**. Before all this could be realized, however, techniques had to be developed to permit the visualization of cells and tissues that, although dead, present an accurate representation of the living appearance.

> **KEY WORDS**
> - **Light microscopy**
> - **Immunocytochemistry**
> - **Autoradiography**
> - **Confocal microscopy**
> - **Transmission electron microscopy**
> - **Scanning electron microscopy**

Light Microscopy

TISSUE PREPARATION

A small block of tissue, harvested from an anesthetized or newly dead subject:

1. Is **fixed**, usually with neutral buffered formalin that is treated in such a manner that the proteins in the tissue are rapidly cross-linked so that they remain in the same place where they were while the subject was alive.
2. Once fixed, is **dehydrated** in a graded series of alcohols
3. Immersed in xylene, which makes the tissue transparent.
4. To be able to view thin sections of the tissue under a microscope, the tissue has to be **embedded** in melted paraffin that infiltrates the tissue. The tissue is placed into a small receptacle and allowed to cool, forming a **paraffin block** containing the tissue.
5. Sliced into 5- to 10-µm thin **sections** using a microtome whose very sharp blade is capable of slicing thin increments of tissue from the block.
6. The sections are transferred to adhesive-coated glass slides, the paraffin is removed from the section by a xylene bath, and the tissue is **rehydrated** by the use of a graded series of alcohols (reversed in order when dehydration took place).
7. The rehydrated sections are **stained** with various water-soluble dyes (Table 1.1); **hematoxylin and eosin (H&E)** are the most common stains used in normal histologic preparations. Hematoxylin stains the acid components of cells and tissues a bluish color, and eosin stains the basic components of cells and tissues a pinkish color.

Modern light microscopes use a series of lenses arranged to provide the maximum magnification with the greatest clarity. Because more than one lens is used, this is known as a **compound microscope** (Fig. 1.1).

Table 1.1 COMMON HISTOLOGIC STAINS AND REACTIONS

Reagent	Result
Hematoxylin	*Blue*—nucleus; acidic regions of the cytoplasm; cartilage matrix
Eosin	*Pink*—basic regions of the cytoplasm; collagen fibers
Masson's trichrome	*Dark blue*—nuclei
	Red—muscle, keratin, cytoplasm
	Light blue—mucinogen, collagen
Orcein elastic stain	*Brown*—elastic fibers
Weigert's elastic stain	*Blue*—elastic fibers
Silver stain	*Black*—reticular fibers
Iron hematoxylin	*Black*—striations of muscle, nuclei, erythrocytes
Periodic acid–Schiff	*Magenta*—glycogen and carbohydrate-rich molecules
Wright's and Giemsa*	*Pink*—erythrocytes, eosinophil stains
	Blue—cytoplasm of monocytes of blood cells and lymphocytes

*Used for granules differential staining of blood cells.

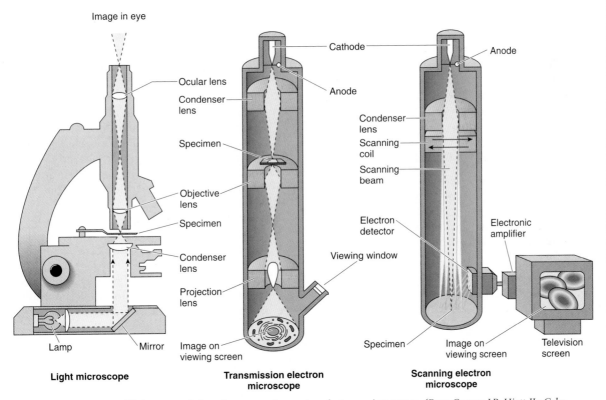

Figure 1.1 Comparison of light, transmission electron, and scanning electron microscopes. *(From Gartner LP, Hiatt JL: Color Textbook of Histology, 3rd ed. Philadelphia, Saunders, 2007, p 4.)*

TISSUE PREPARATION (cont.)

A high-intensity lightbulb provides the light, which is focused on the specimen from below by a **condenser lens**. The light that passes through the specimen is gathered by one of the **objective lenses** that sits on a rotatable turret, allowing a change in magnification from low to medium to high, and an oil lens, which in conventional microscopes magnifies the image 4, 10, 20, 40, and 100 times. The first three are dry lenses, whereas the oil lens uses immersion oil to act as an interface between the glass of the slide and the glass of the objective lens. The light from the objective lens is gathered by the **ocular lens**, usually 10 times, for final magnification of 40, 100, 200, 400, and 1000 times, and the image is focused on the retina.

INTERPRETATION OF MICROSCOPIC SECTIONS

Histologic sections are two-dimensional planes cut from a three-dimensional structure. Initially, it is difficult for the student to reconcile the image seen in the microscope with the tissue or organ from which it was harvested. A simple demonstration of a coiled tube sectioned at various angles (Fig. 1.2) is instructive in learning how to reconstruct the three-dimensional morphology from viewing a series of two-dimensional sections.

ADVANCED VISUALIZATION PROCEDURES

Various techniques were developed to use the microscope in elucidating functional aspects of the cells, tissues, and organs being studied. The most commonly used techniques are histochemistry (and cytochemistry), immunocytochemistry, and autoradiography.

- **Histochemistry** and **cytochemistry** use chemical reactions, enzymatic processes, and physicochemical processes that not only stain the tissue, but also permit the localization of extracellular and intracellular macromolecules of interest.
  - One of the most used histochemical methods is the periodic acid–Schiff (PAS) reagent, which stains glycogen and molecules rich in carbohydrates a purplish-red color. By treating consecutive sections with the enzyme amylase, to digest glycogen, the absence of the purplish-red color indicates that glycogen was present at that particular location.
  - Other histochemical and cytochemical techniques can localize enzymes; however, it is not the enzyme that is visualized, but the presence of the reaction product that precipitated as a colored compound at the site of the reaction.
- **Immunocytochemistry** provides a more accurate localization of a particular macromolecule than does histochemistry or cytochemistry.
  - This is a more complex method, however, because it involves the development of an antibody against the macromolecule of interest in the **direct method**, or
  - Development of an antibody against a primary antibody in the **indirect method** (Fig. 1.3) and labeling the developed antibody with a fluorescing label, such as rhodamine or fluorescein. The indirect method is more sensitive and more accurate than the direct method because more fluorescent labeled antibodies bind to the primary antibody than in the direct method. Additionally, most of the time, primary antibodies are more expensive and more limited in their availability.
  - Immunocytochemistry can also be applied to electron microscopy by attaching the heavy metal ferritin instead of a fluorescent label.
- The method of **autoradiography** uses a radioactive isotope (usually tritium, ^3H), which is integrated into the molecule that is being investigated.
  - If one wishes to follow the synthesis of a particular protein, tritiated amino acid is fed into the system, and specimens are harvested at defined periods.
  - Sections are processed in a normal fashion, but instead of a coverslip, photographic emulsion is placed on the section, and the slide is stored in the dark for many weeks.
  - The emulsion is developed and fixed as if it were a photographic plate, and a coverslip is placed over the section.
  - Microscopic examination displays the presence of silver grains over the regions where the isotope labeled molecule was located.
  - A method of autoradiography has been developed for electron microscopy.

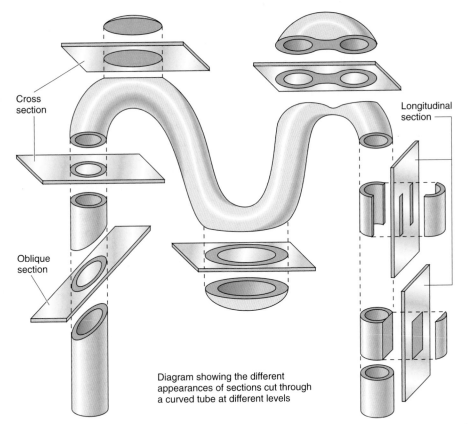

Cross section

Longitudinal section

Oblique section

Diagram showing the different appearances of sections cut through a curved tube at different levels

Figure 1.2 Two-dimensional views of a three-dimensional tube sectioned in various planes. *(From Gartner LP, Hiatt JL: Color Textbook of Histology, 3rd ed. Philadelphia, Saunders, 2007, p 4.)*

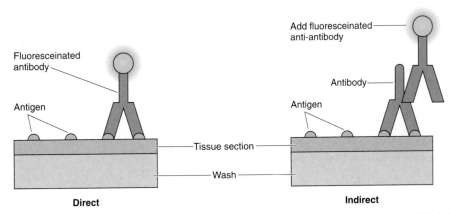

Fluoresceinated antibody

Antigen

Add fluoresceinated anti-antibody

Antibody

Antigen

Tissue section

Wash

Direct

Indirect

Figure 1.3 Direct and indirect methods of immunocytochemistry. *Left,* An antibody against an antigen was labeled with a fluorescent dye and viewed with a fluorescent microscope. Fluorescence occurs only over the location of the labeled antibody. *Right,* Fluorescent labeled antibodies were prepared against an antibody that reacts with a particular antigen. When viewed with a fluorescent microscope, the fluorescence represents the location of the antibody that reacts with the antigen. *(From Gartner LP, Hiatt JL: Color Textbook of Histology, 3rd ed. Philadelphia, Saunders, 2007, p 5.)*

Confocal Microscopy

Confocal microscopy uses a laser beam that is focused on the specimen impregnated with fluorescent dyes; the impinging laser beam that passes through a dichroic mirror excites the dyes, which then fluoresce (Fig. 1.4).

- The beam of laser light passes through a pinhole that is computer controlled so that the beam scans along the surface of the specimen, and the fluorescence originates as the specimen is being scanned.
- The emitted fluorescent light is captured as it passes through the pinhole in a direction opposite from that of the laser light. Each emitted light represents only a single point on the specimen being scanned.
- The emitted light is captured by a photomultiplier tube; as each pixel is gathered, the pixels are compiled by a computer into an image of the specimen.
- Because each scan observes only a very thin plane within the specimen, multiple passes at different levels may be used to construct a three-dimensional image of the specimen.

Electron Microscopy

Electron microscopes use a beam of electrons instead of photons as their light source, and, instead of glass lenses, they use electromagnets to spread and focus the electron beam (Fig. 1.5).

- The **resolution** of a microscope depends on the wavelength of the light source, and the wavelength of an electron beam is far shorter than that of visible light; the resolution of an electron beam is about 1000 times greater than that of visible light. The resolving power of a compound light microscope is about 200 nm, whereas that of a transmission electron microscope is 0.2 nm, providing a magnification of 150,000 times, which permits the visualization of a single macromolecule such as myosin.

- There are two types of electron microscopy: transmission electron microscopy (TEM) and scanning electron microscopy (SEM).
  - As the name implies, **TEM** (see Fig. 1.3, right) requires the electrons to pass through a very thinly sliced specimen that was treated with a heavy metal stain (e.g., lead phosphate or uranyl acetate) and hit a phosphorescent plate, which absorbs the electron and gives off a point of light whose intensity is a function of the electron's kinetic energy. As the electron interacts with the specimen, it loses some of its kinetic energy, and the more heavy metal is absorbed by a particular region of the specimen, the more energy the electron loses. In this fashion, the resultant image consists of points of light of different intensities ranging from light to dark gray. The image can be captured by placing an electron-sensitive photographic plate in the place of the phosphorescent plate. The photographic plate can be developed in the normal fashion, and the plate can be printed as a black-and-white photograph.
  - **SEM** (see Fig. 1.5) does not require the electrons to pass through the specimen. Instead, the surface of the specimen is bombarded with electrons and the resulting image is a three-dimensional representation of the specimen. To achieve this, the specimen is coated with a heavy metal, such as gold or palladium. As the electron beam bombards the surface of the specimen, the heavy metal coating scatters some of the electrons (**backscatter electrons**), whereas some of the impinging electrons cause the ejection of the heavy metal's electrons (**secondary electrons**). Backscatter and secondary electrons are captured by electron detectors and are interpreted as a three-dimensional image that is projected onto a monitor. The digitized image can be saved as a file and printed as a photograph.

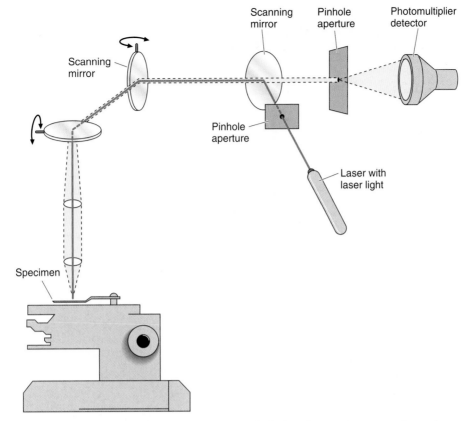

Figure 1.4 Confocal microscope displaying the pinhole through which the laser beam enters to scan the specimen and the path of the fluorescent light that subsequently is emitted by the specimen to be captured by the photomultiplier detector. *(From Gartner LP, Hiatt JL: Color Textbook of Histology, 3rd ed. Philadelphia, Saunders, 2007, p 8.)*

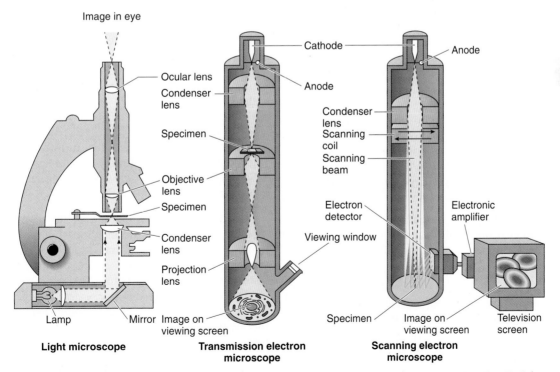

Figure 1.5 Comparison of light, transmission electron, and scanning electron microscopes. *(From Gartner LP, Hiatt JL: Color Textbook of Histology, 3rd ed. Philadelphia, Saunders, 2007, p 4.)*

2 CYTOPLASM

Complex organisms are composed of **cells** and **extracellular materials**. Although there are more than 200 types of cells that constitute these organisms, each with various functions, the cells and the extracellular matrix are categorized into the four basic **tissues**: epithelium, connective tissue, muscle, and nervous tissue. Tissues form organs, and combinations of **organs** form **organ systems**.

Generally, a cell is a membrane-bound structure filled with **protoplasm** that may be categorized into two components, the **cytoplasm** and the **karyoplasms** (Fig. 2.1).

> **KEY WORDS**
> - **Cell**
> - **Ion channels**
> - **Carrier proteins**
> - **Organelles**
> - **Protein synthesis**
> - **Membrane trafficking**
> - **Cytoskeleton**
> - **Inclusions**

- **Karyoplasm** constitutes the **nucleus** and is surrounded by the **nuclear envelope**.
- This chapter discusses the cell membrane and the cytoplasm of a generalized cell.
  - The main substance of the cytoplasm is the **cytosol**, a fluid suspension in which the inorganic and organic chemicals, macromolecules, pigments, crystals, and **organelles** are dissolved or suspended.
  - The cytosol is surrounded by a semipermeable, lipid bilayer **cell membrane** (**plasmalemma**, **plasma membrane**) in which proteins are embedded.

Cell Membrane (Plasmalemma, Plasma Membrane)

The **cell membrane** is approximately 7 to 8 nm in thickness and is composed of a lipid bilayer comprising amphipathic phospholipids, cholesterol, and embedded or attached proteins (Fig. 2.2). Viewed with the electron microscope, the plasmalemma appears to have two dense layers:

- An **inner** (cytoplasmic) **leaflet**
- An **outer leaflet**, which sandwich between them an intermediate clear, hydrophobic, layer

This tripartite structure is known as a **unit membrane** and forms not only the cell membrane, but also all other membranous structures of the cell. In the average membrane, the protein components constitute approximately 50% by weight. The arrangement of the phospholipid molecules is such that:

- The hydrophilic polar heads face the periphery, forming the extracellular and intracellular surfaces.

- The hydrophobic fatty acid chains of the two facing phospholipid sheets (inner and outer leaflets) project toward the center of the membrane, forming the intermediate clear layer.

Cholesterol is usually tucked away among the fatty acid tails of the phospholipid molecules. When the cell membrane is frozen and then fractured, it cleaves preferentially along the hydrophobic clear layer, making the two internal surfaces of the leaflets visible (Fig. 2.3).

- The surface of the inner leaflet (closest to the protoplasm) is the **P-face**.
- The surface of the outer leaflet (closer to the extracellular space) is known as the **E-face**.

Proteins of the cell membrane are **integral proteins** or **peripheral proteins**. Integral proteins are:

- **Transmembrane proteins**, in that they occupy the entire thickness of the membrane, and they extend into the cytoplasm and into the extracellular space
- **Peripheral proteins** that are not embedded into the membrane; instead, they adhere either to the cytoplasmic or to the extracellular surface of the membrane. During freeze fracture, more proteins remain attached to the P-face than to the E-face.
- The extracellular surface of the cell membrane, which may have a **glycocalyx** (cell coat), composed of carbohydrates that form **glycoproteins** or **glycolipids**, depending on whether they form bonds with the integral proteins or with the phospholipids

The **integral** and **peripheral proteins** have some mobility in the two-dimensional phospholipid membrane and resemble a mosaic that is constantly changing. The movements of these proteins are restricted, and the membrane representation that used to be called the *fluid mosaic model* is now known as the **modified fluid mosaic model**. Regions of the membrane are slightly thickened because they possess a rich concentration of glycosphingolipids and cholesterol surrounding a cluster of membrane proteins. These specialized regions, **lipid rafts**, function in cell signaling.

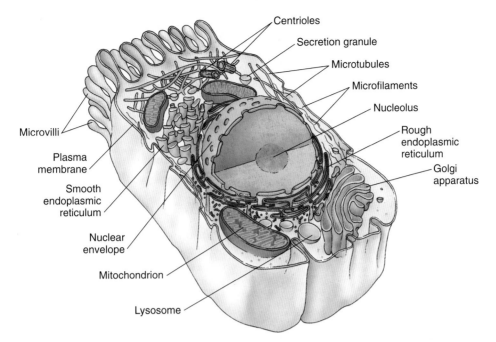

Figure 2.1 A generalized cell and its organelles. *(From Gartner LP, Hiatt JL: Color Textbook of Histology, 3rd ed. Philadelphia, Saunders, 2007, p 14.)*

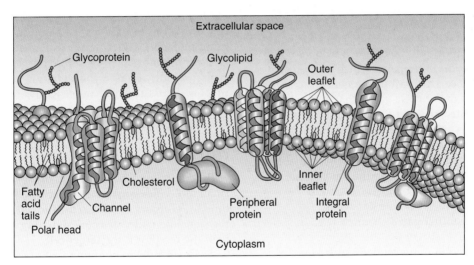

Figure 2.2 Fluid mosaic model of the cell membrane. *(From Gartner LP, Hiatt JL: Color Textbook of Histology, 3rd ed. Philadelphia, Saunders, 2007, p 16.)*

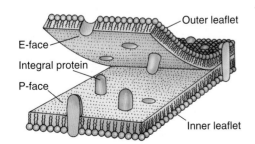

Figure 2.3 The E-face and the P-face of the plasma membrane. *(From Gartner LP, Hiatt JL: Color Textbook of Histology, 3rd ed. Philadelphia, Saunders, 2007, p 16.)*

MEMBRANE TRANSPORT PROTEINS

The plasmalemma is permeable to nonpolar molecules, such as oxygen, and uncharged polar molecules, such as water and glycerol, and these may cross the membrane by simple diffusion following a concentration gradient. Ions and small polar molecules require assistance, however, from certain multipass integral proteins, known as **membrane transport proteins**, which function in the transfer of these substances across the cell membrane.

- If the process does not require energy, the transfer across the plasmalemma is **passive transport**.
- If the process requires the expenditure of energy, it is known as **active transport** (Fig. 2.4).

Membrane transport proteins are of two types: **channel proteins** and **carrier proteins**.

- **Channel proteins** participate only in passive transport because they do not have the ability to use the expenditure of energy to work against a concentration gradient.
    - To be able to accomplish their function, channel proteins are folded in such a fashion that they provide hydrophilic **ion channels** across the cell membrane.
    - Most of these channels can control the entry of substances into their lumen by possessing barriers, known as **gates**, which block their entrance or exit. Various mechanisms control the opening of these **gated channels**.
- **Voltage-gated channels**, such as Na^+ channels of nerve fibers, are opened when the membrane is depolarized (see Chapter 9).
- **Ligand-gated channels** open when a signaling molecule (ligand) binds to the ion channel. Some ligand-gated channels respond to neurotransmitters and are known as **neurotransmitter-gated** channels (e.g., in skeletal muscle).
- Others respond to nucleotides, such as cyclic adenosine monophosphate (cAMP) or cyclic guanosine monophosphate (cGMP), and are referred to as **nucleotide-gated channels** (e.g., in rods of the retina).
- **Mechanically gated channels** respond to physical contact for opening, as in the bending of the stereocilia of the hair cells of the inner ear.
- **G protein–gated ion channels**, such as the acetylcholine receptors of cardiac muscle cells, require the activation of a G protein before the gate can be opened.
    - **Ungated channels** are always open. K^+ **leak channels** are the most common ungated channels, and these are responsible for the maintenance of the resting potentials of nerve cells. **Aquaporins**, channels designed for the transport of H_2O, are also ungated channels.
- **Carrier proteins** are multipass proteins; however, they have the ability not only to be passive conduits that allow material to pass down a concentration gradient, but also to use adenosine triphosphate (ATP)–driven mechanisms to transport material *against* a concentration gradient. They also differ from ion channels because they have internal binding sites for the ions or molecules that they are designed to transfer. The transport may be of one molecule or ion in a single direction (**uniport**), or coupled—that is, two different ones in the:
    - Same direction (**symport**) or
    - Opposite direction (**antiport**)

The most common example of carrier proteins is the Na^+-K^+ pump that uses Na^+,K^+-**ATPase** to cotransport three sodium ions against a concentration gradient out of the cell and two potassium ions into the cell. Some carrier proteins use the intracellular and extracellular Na^+ concentration differential as a force to drive the movement of some ions or small molecules or both against a concentration gradient. This process, performed by coupled carrier proteins, is known as **secondary active transport**, and glucose and Na^+ are frequently cotransported in this manner.

CELL SIGNALING

Cells communicate with each other by releasing small molecules (**signaling molecules, ligands**) that bind to **receptors** of other cells. The cell that releases the signaling molecule is the **signaling cell**. The cell with the receptor is the **target cell**.

Frequently the roles of these cells may be reversed because often the communication is bidirectional. The receptors may be located on the cell membrane, and the ligand in this case is a **polar molecule**. If the receptor is intracellular or intranuclear, the ligand may be a **nonpolar, hydrophobic molecule** (e.g., steroid hormone), or the receptor on the cell surface **transduces** the signal by the activation of an intracellular **second messenger system** (e.g., G protein–linked receptors).

A Passive Transport

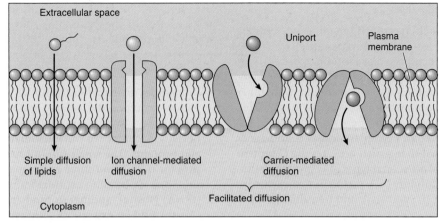

B Active Transport

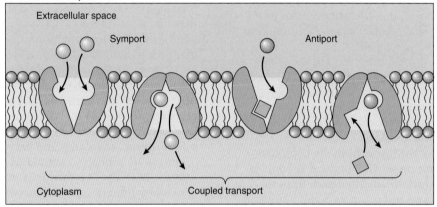

Figure 2.4 Types of transport. **A,** Passive transport that does not require the input of energy. **B,** Active transport is an energy-requiring mechanism. *(From Gartner LP, Hiatt JL: Color Textbook of Histology, 3rd ed. Philadelphia, Saunders, 2007, p 18.)*

CLINICAL CONSIDERATIONS

The amino acid cystine is removed from the lumen of the renal proximal tubule by a carrier protein. Some individuals who inherited two copies of the same mutation, one from each parent, that forms defective cysteine carrier proteins have a condition known as **cystinuria**. These individuals have a high enough concentration of this amino acid in their urine to form cystine stones. Cystinuria manifests between age 10 and 30 years, and the condition is responsible for recurrent kidney stones. Diagnosis is made on the basis of microscopic examination of the urine showing the presence of cystine crystals and by urinalysis showing abnormal levels of cystine. The condition can be very painful, but in many cases increased fluid intake dilutes the urine sufficiently to prevent the formation of stones.

G Protein–Linked Receptors and Secondary Messengers of the Cell

G protein–linked receptors (guanine nucleotide–binding proteins) are transmembrane proteins whose extracytoplasmic aspects have binding sites for specific signaling molecules (ligands), and their cytoplasmic aspect is bound to a **G protein** on the inner leaflet of the plasmalemma. When the signaling molecule binds to the extracytoplasmic moiety of the receptor, the receptor's cytoplasmic aspect undergoes a conformational change that activates the G protein (Fig. 2.5). There are several types of G proteins: stimulatory (G_s), inhibitory (G_i), pertussin-toxin sensitive and insensitive (G_o and G_{Bq}), and transducin (G_t).

- G_s **proteins** are trimeric in that they are composed of α, β, and γ subunits. They are usually inactive, and in the inactive state they have a guanosine diphosphate (GDP) bound to their cytoplasmic aspect.
- When the G_s protein is activated, it exchanges its GDP for a guanosine triphosphate (GTP); the α subunit dissociates from the other two components and contacts adenylate cyclase, activating it to catalyze the transformation of cytoplasmic ATP to **cAMP**.
- Uncoupling of the ligand from the G protein–linked receptor causes **GTP** of the α subunit to be dephosphorylated and to detach from the adenylate cyclase and rejoin its β and γ subunits.
- cAMP, one of the secondary messengers of cells, activates **A kinase**, which initiates the eliciting of a specific response from the cell.
- In other cells, cAMP enters the nucleus and activates **CRE-binding protein**, which binds to regulatory regions of genes, known as **CREs** (cAMP response elements), which permit the transcription of that particular gene effecting the specific response from the cell.

Protein Synthetic Machinery of the Cell

A major function of most cells is the synthesis of proteins either for use by the cell itself or to be exported for use elsewhere in the body. Protein synthesis has:

- An intranuclear component, **transcription**, that is, the synthesis of a **messenger RNA (mRNA)** molecule, and
- **Translation**, the cytoplasmic component, which entails the assembly of the correct amino acid sequence, based on the nucleotide template of the mRNA to form the specific protein

The cytoplasmic component of protein synthesis uses ribosomes only if the protein to be formed is released free in the cytosol or ribosomes and the rough endoplasmic reticulum (RER) (Fig. 2.6) if the protein is to be packaged for storage within the cell or to be released into the extracellular space.

- **Ribosomes** are small (12 nm × 25 nm), bipartite particles composed of a large and a small subunit. Each subunit, manufactured in the nucleus, is composed of **ribosomal RNA (rRNA)** and **proteins**. The small subunit has binding sites for mRNA and three additional binding sites: one for binding peptidyl transfer RNA (tRNA) (**P-site**), another to bind aminoacyl tRNA (**A-site**), and an exit site (**E-site**) where the empty tRNA leaves the ribosome. The large subunit binds to the small subunit and has special rRNA that acts as an enzyme, known as **ribozyme**, which catalyzes the formation of peptide bonds that permit amino acids to bond to each other.
- There are two types of **endoplasmic reticulum (ER)**: smooth endoplasmic reticulum (SER) and RER. Although the former is not involved in protein synthesis, for the sake of completeness, its structure is discussed here.
  - **SER** consists of tubules and flat vesicles whose lumina are probably continuous with those of the RER. The SER functions in lipid and steroid synthesis, glycogen metabolism, and detoxification of noxious substances, and in muscle as an intracellular storage site for calcium.
  - **RER** functions in the synthesis of proteins that are destined to be packaged either for storage within the cell or for release into the extracellular space. It is composed of flattened, interconnected vesicles, and its cytoplasmic surface is studded with ribosomes and polysomes that are actively translating mRNA and forming protein. The RER possesses the integral proteins **signal recognition particle receptor** (docking protein), **ribophorins** I and II, and **translocators**, proteins that bind ribosomes to the RER and open as a pore through which nascent proteins can enter the cisternal (luminal) aspect of the RER. The cisternal aspect of the RER membrane houses the enzyme **signal peptidase** and **dolichol phosphate**, which functions in N-glycosylation. The cisterna of the RER is continuous with the perinuclear cistern of the nuclear envelope.

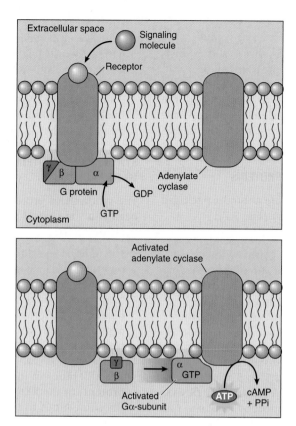

Figure 2.5 G protein–linked receptor. PPi, inorganic pyrophosphate. *(From Gartner LP, Hiatt JL: Color Textbook of Histology, 3rd ed. Philadelphia, Saunders, 2007, p 21.)*

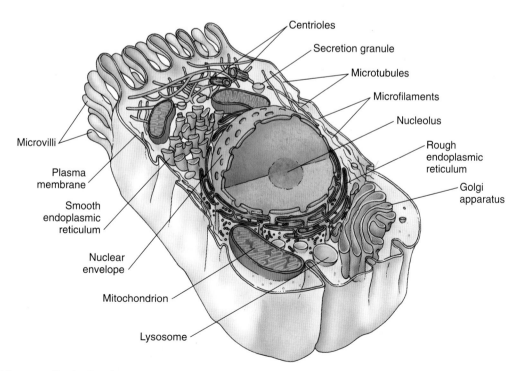

Figure 2.6 A generalized cell and its organelles. *(From Gartner LP, Hiatt JL: Color Textbook of Histology, 3rd ed. Philadelphia, Saunders, 2007, p 14.)*

Protein Synthesis

The process of protein synthesis always begins when an mRNA is bound to a ribosome in the cytosol and, if the protein is not to be packaged, is then finished in the cytosol. If the protein is to be packaged, the mRNA contains the code for a **signal peptide** whose translation is the signal to move the ribosome-mRNA complex to the RER.

SYNTHESIS OF NONPACKAGED PROTEINS

The synthesis of proteins that are not to be packaged occurs in the following manner (Fig. 2.7):

- An mRNA leaves the nucleus through a nuclear pore complex (see Chapter 3), enters the cytosol, and binds a small ribosomal subunit, whose **P-site** is occupied by a methionine-bearing **initiator tRNA**. The **anticodon** of the tRNA matches the **codon** of the mRNA, aligning the system in the proper position. A large ribosomal subunit joins the complex, and translation begins as the ribosome moves the distance of a single codon along the mRNA in a 5′ to 3′ direction.
- An amino acid bearing tRNA (**aminoacyl tRNA**), if it possesses the correct anticodon, binds to the **A-site** of the small ribosomal subunit, and its amino acids form a peptide bond with the methionine in the P-site. The methionine is released by the tRNA located on the P-site, and the tRNA of the A-site now has two amino acids attached to it (methionine and the newly arrived amino acid). The empty tRNA moves from the P-site to the **E-site**, and the tRNA loaded with the two amino acids moves to the P-site. Finally, the entire ribosome moves the distance of a single codon along the mRNA in a 5′ to 3′ direction.
- A new acylated tRNA possessing the correct anticodon attaches to the A-site. It picks up the two amino acids from the t-RNA at the P-site and now has three amino acids attached to it. The tRNA at the E-site is ejected, and the empty tRNA at the P-site moves to the now vacant E-site. The tRNA with its three amino acids moves from the A-site to the P-site, and the entire ribosome moves the distance of a single codon in a 5′ to 3′ direction. A new acylated tRNA possessing the correct anticodon occupies the now vacant A-site.
- As this process continues, new small ribosomal subunits attach to the 5′ end of the mRNA; in this manner, several ribosomes are translating the same mRNA simultaneously. A single mRNA strand with several ribosomes is referred to as a **polysome**.

- The process of new acylated tRNA is added to the sequence until the **stop codon** is reached, which signals that the last amino acid of the protein has been incorporated into the nascent protein chain. The last empty tRNA is released at the E-site, no new tRNAs occupy the A-site, and the small and large ribosomal subunits dissociate from the mRNA.

SYNTHESIS OF PROTEINS THAT ARE TO BE PACKAGED

The synthesis of proteins to be packaged (Fig. 2.8) begins in the cytosol in the same fashion as previously described.

- The peptide chain that is formed is the **signal peptide** that is recognized by the **signal recognition particle (SRP)**, a molecule composed of protein and RNA that is freely floating in the cytosol. SRP binds to the signal peptide, protein synthesis ceases, and the ribosome-mRNA-SRP complex moves to the RER.
- The SRP binds to the **SRP receptor (docking protein)** of the RER membrane, and the ribosome binds to **translocator proteins**— integral proteins—of the RER membrane. As the binding occurs, the SRP is released; translation continues, and the base of the translocator opens up, forming a **pore** into the RER cistern. The nascent protein enters the RER lumen through the pore.
- The signal peptide is cleaved off by the enzyme signal peptidase, and some of the elongating proteins are **N-glycosylated** by dolichol phosphate present in the luminal aspect of the RER membrane. This process is assisted by the RER-specific proteins ribophorin I and ribophorin II in the RER membrane. The process of translation is finished when the stop codon is reached.
- The newly synthesized protein is released into the RER cistern, where it is modified further and folded in the proper fashion in the presence of chaperones.
- The completed proteins are packaged into **transfer vesicles** to leave the RER and be transported to the **Golgi apparatus** for further modification and final packaging.
- **Misfolded proteins** are retrotranslocated through a translocator that is similar to the one that they used to enter the ER during synthesis. When in the cytoplasm, they are ubiquitylated and destroyed by proteasomes.

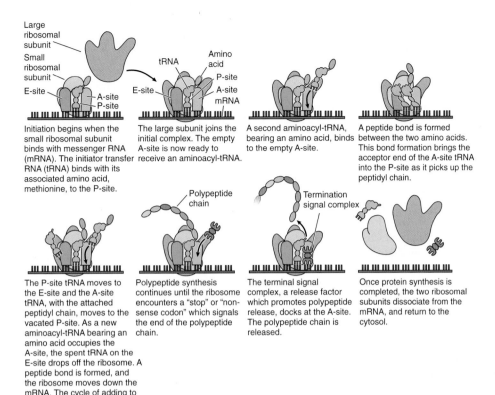

Initiation begins when the small ribosomal subunit binds with messenger RNA (mRNA). The initiator transfer RNA (tRNA) binds with its associated amino acid, methionine, to the P-site.

The large subunit joins the initial complex. The empty A-site is now ready to receive an aminoacyl-tRNA.

A second aminoacyl-tRNA, bearing an amino acid, binds to the empty A-site.

A peptide bond is formed between the two amino acids. This bond formation brings the acceptor end of the A-site tRNA into the P-site as it picks up the peptidyl chain.

The P-site tRNA moves to the E-site and the A-site tRNA, with the attached peptidyl chain, moves to the vacated P-site. As a new aminoacyl-tRNA bearing an amino acid occupies the A-site, the spent tRNA on the E-site drops off the ribosome. A peptide bond is formed, and the ribosome moves down the mRNA. The cycle of adding to the forming protein chain continues.

Polypeptide synthesis continues until the ribosome encounters a "stop" or "non-sense codon" which signals the end of the polypeptide chain.

The terminal signal complex, a release factor which promotes polypeptide release, docks at the A-site. The polypeptide chain is released.

Once protein synthesis is completed, the two ribosomal subunits dissociate from the mRNA, and return to the cytosol.

Figure 2.7 Synthesis of proteins that are not to be packaged occurs in the cytosol. *(From Gartner LP, Hiatt JL: Color Textbook of Histology, 3rd ed. Philadelphia, Saunders, 2007, p 26.)*

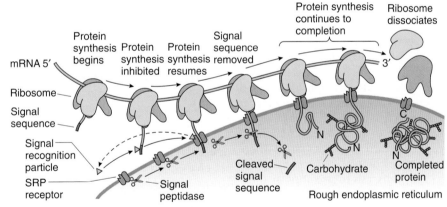

Figure 2.8 Synthesis of proteins that are to be packaged occurs on the RER surface. *(From Gartner LP, Hiatt JL: Color Textbook of Histology, 3rd ed. Philadelphia, Saunders, 2007, p 27.)*

CLINICAL CONSIDERATIONS

The amino acid sequence of a protein determines its primary structure. A minor alteration of the primary structure usually does not affect the functionality of the protein; however, there are cases where a point mutation—that is, the substitution of a single amino acid for another—makes a major difference in the ability of that protein to perform its intended function. An example of such a deleterious point mutation occurs in hemoglobin, where the normally present glutamine in the sixth position of the β-chain is exchanged for valine, a condition known as **sickle cell anemia**. During low oxygen tension, such as after strenuous exercise, the modified β-chain causes the erythrocytes to become disfigured so that they appear sickle-shaped, and their ability to ferry oxygen is much reduced. These defective red blood cells are prone to fragmentation because they lose their normal pliability.

Golgi Apparatus

The **Golgi apparatus (Golgi complex)** is composed of clusters of preferentially oriented tubules and a series of flattened, convex membrane-bound vesicles stacked one above the other, where each vesicle resembles an uncut pita bread with a central lumen, the **cistern** (Fig. 2.9). A cell may have one to several Golgi complexes, each of which has a:

- Convex entry face near the nucleus, known as the *cis*-Golgi network (CGN)
- *Cis*-face, where newly synthesized proteins from the RER enter the Golgi complex
- Concave exit face, oriented toward the cell membrane, known as the *trans*-face
- One to several **intermediate faces**, interposed between the *cis*-face and *trans*-face
- Complex of vesicles and tubules, known as the **vesicular-tubular cluster** (VTC, formerly ERGIC), located between the transitional region of the RER and the *cis*-Golgi network
- In association with the *trans*-face is another cluster of vesicles, the *trans*-Golgi network (TGN)

The functions of the Golgi complex include carbohydrate synthesis and the modification and sorting of proteins.

Protein Trafficking

Vesicles ferrying material (e.g., proteins or carbohydrates) from one organelle to another or between regions of the same organelle are known as **transport vesicles**, and the material they transport is referred to as **cargo**. Transport vesicles possess a protein coat (known as **coated vesicles**) on their cytosolic aspect that permits the vesicle to bud off and adhere to these organelles and to reach the proper target. There are three major types of proteinaceous coats (with some subtypes) that cells use to accomplish these goals:

- **Coatomer I (COP I)**
- **Coatomer II (COP II)**
- **Clathrin**

These coats ensure that the correct material becomes the cargo and that the membrane is formed into a vesicle of correct size and shape. Each coat is used to encourage a specific type of transport (Fig. 2.10). As the coated vesicle reaches the membrane of its target organelle, it loses its coat and fuses with the target membrane. The ability of the vesicle and the target membrane to recognize each other depends on **SNARE proteins** (soluble attachment receptor N-ethylmaleimide sensitive fusion proteins) and a group of GTPases specializing in target recognition known as **Rabs**. SNAREs allow binding only of the correct vesicle with the intended target. The initial docking of the vesicle is mediated in part by the Rabs protein. At the cell membrane, there are SNARE-rich regions, known as **porosomes**, where vesicles dock to deliver their contents into the extracellular space.

Proteins leave the **transitional ER**, a region of the RER that is devoid of ribosomes, packaged in small **transport vesicles** whose membrane, derived from the RER, is covered by COP II (see Fig. 2.10). These COP II–coated vesicles travel to the vesicular-tubular cluster, lose their COP II coat, and fuse with the VTC. The delivered cargo is examined, and if it contains an escaped ER resident protein that protein is returned to the ER via COP I–coated vesicles (**retrograde transport**), and the remaining, correct cargo is passed to the Golgi apparatus also in COP I–coated vesicles (**anterograde transport**). The proteins are passed to the various faces of the Golgi apparatus—again probably via COP I–coated vesicles—where they are modified in each face and sent to the TGN for final packaging. The modified proteins are packaged in **clathrin-coated vesicles** or COP II–coated vesicles and are addressed to be sent to one of three places:

- The cell membrane, where they become inserted as membrane-bound proteins or where they fuse with the cell membrane to release their contents immediately into the extracellular space (**continuous exocytosis**)
- To be housed temporarily in the cytoplasm as storage (secretory) vesicles near the plasmalemma for eventual release of the cargo into the extracellular space (**discontinuous exocytosis**)
- Late endosomes to become incorporated into lysosomes

The process of discontinuous exocytosis requires a clathrin coat and is said to follow the **regulated pathway of secretory proteins**, whereas the process of continuous exocytosis requires COP II–coated vesicles and is said to follow the **constitutive pathway of secretory proteins**.

All of these protein-ferrying vesicles not only possess protein coats, but also have many membrane markers that allow them to be attached to microtubules and transported, by means of molecular motors, along these structures to their final destinations. The vesicles also possess markers that act as address labels, and the vesicles dock at their target by means of these molecules.

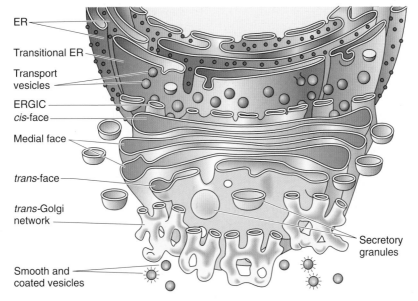

Figure 2.9 Rough endoplasmic reticulum and the Golgi complex. *(From Gartner LP, Hiatt JL: Color Textbook of Histology, 3rd ed. Philadelphia, Saunders, 2007, p 28.)*

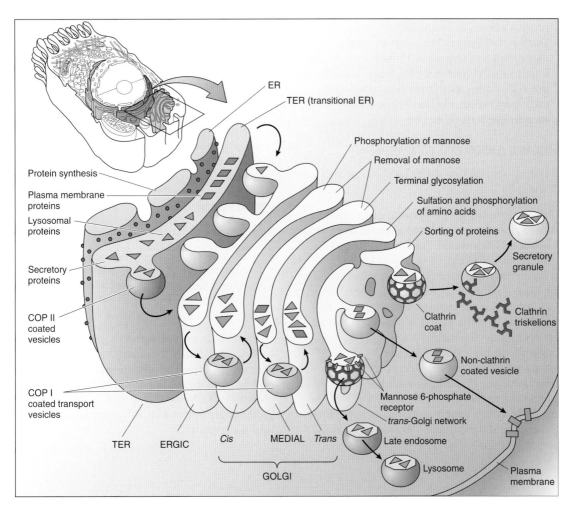

Figure 2.10 Protein trafficking through the Golgi complex and associated vesicles. *(From Gartner LP, Hiatt JL: Color Textbook of Histology, 3rd ed. Philadelphia, Saunders, 2007, p 30.)*

Membrane Trafficking

ENDOCYTOSIS: PHAGOSOMES AND PINOCYTOTIC VESICLES

The transfer of material from the extracellular space into the cytoplasm is known as **endocytosis**.

- Larger substances are **phagocytosed** into a vesicle known as a **phagosome**.
- Smaller molecules (**ligands**) are **pinocytosed** into a **pinocytotic vesicle**.
  - **Pinocytosis** is a carefully controlled process whereby the material to be engulfed is recognized via **cargo receptor proteins** located on the cell membrane that recognize the ligand extracellularly and clathrin intracellularly.
  - The ability to recognize and bind to clathrin molecules causes the formation of a pinocytic vesicle that may contain hundreds of ligand molecules.
  - Cells can also transfer material from the cytoplasm into the intercellular space, a process known as **exocytosis**.
  - During endocytosis, the plasmalemma loses membrane to the vesicles formed from it, and it gains the membranes of vesicles formed in the TGN during exocytosis. This continuous cycling of the membranes is known as **membrane trafficking** (Fig. 2.11).

ENDOSOMES (ENDOSOMAL COMPARTMENT)

Pinocytotic vesicles lose their clathrin coat and fuse with the:

- **Early endosome**, a membranous compartment located near the plasmalemma whose membrane possesses ATP-driven H^+ pumps that acidify its lumen to a pH of 6.0
- In some early endosomes, **recycling endosomes**, the ligand and its receptor are dissociated from each other, the receptor is returned to the cell membrane, and the ligand is either released into the cytoplasm or transferred to
- **Late endosomes**, another membranous compartment located at a deeper level within the cytoplasm. The H^+ pumps in the late endosomal membrane further acidify the lumen of this organelle, which continues to digest its luminal contents, and the partially degraded material is

transferred to lysosomes for complete degradation.

LYSOSOMES (ENDOLYSOSOMES)

Lysosomes are small, membrane-bound organelles housing dozens of hydrolytic enzymes that function at the low pH of 5.0, achieved by the presence of H^+ pumps in their membrane. Lysosomes degrade various substances whose useful components are released into the cytoplasm, whereas their indigestible substances remain enclosed by the lysosomal membrane, and the organelle becomes known as a **residual body**.

PEROXISOMES

Peroxisomes are similar to lysosomes in morphology, but they house many oxidative enzymes that are synthesized on free ribosomes and then transported into these organelles by the assistance of peroxisome-targeting signals that recognize dedicated membrane-bound receptors on the peroxisomal surface.

- The most prevalent enzyme in peroxisomes is **catalase**, which decomposes H_2O_2 into water and oxygen. This organelle also participates in lipid biosynthesis, especially of cholesterol; lipid catabolism by β-oxidation of long-chained fatty acids; and, in hepatocytes, bile acid formation.
- In the central nervous system, kidneys, testes, and heart, peroxisomes possess enzymes that participate in synthesis of **plasmalogen**, membrane phospholipids that protect cells against singlet oxygen.

PROTEASOMES

Proteasomes are small, barrel-shaped organelles that are responsible for:

- Degradation of proteins that are misfolded, damaged, denatured, or otherwise malformed
- Cleaving of antigenic proteins into smaller fragments known as **epitopes** (see Chapter 12)

Proteolysis via proteasomes is carefully managed by the cell through the energy-requiring attachment of multiple copies of **ubiquinone** to the candidate protein to form a **polyubiquinated protein**. The ubiquitin molecules and their degradation byproducts are released in an energy-requiring process into the cytosol.

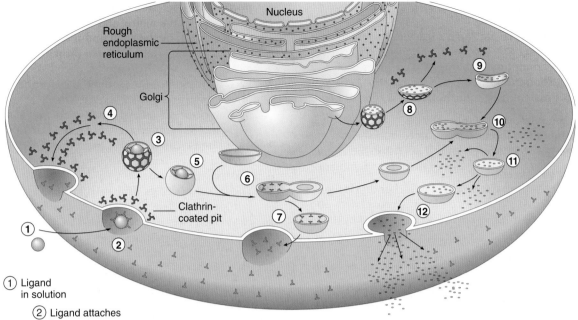

Figure 2.11 Endocytosis, endosomes, and lysosomes. CURL, compartment for uncoupling of receptor and ligand. *(From Gartner LP, Hiatt JL: Color Textbook of Histology, 3rd ed. Philadelphia, Saunders, 2007, p 33.)*

① Ligand
in solution

② Ligand attaches
to receptors

③ Clathrin-coated
endocytotic vesicle

④ Clathrin triskelions
recycle to plasma
membrane

⑤ Uncoated endocytotic
vesicle

⑥ Early endosome / recycling
endosome (CURL) pH ≅ 6.0

⑦ Recycling of receptors
to plasma membrane

⑧ Clathrin-coated vesicles
containing lysosomal hydrolases
or lysosomal membrane proteins

⑨ Late endosome
pH ≅ 5.5

⑩ Multivesicular body
(type of lysosome)

⑪ Degradation products
within residual body

⑫ Residual body fuses with cell membrane
and contents eliminated from cell

CLINICAL CONSIDERATIONS

Zellweger syndrome is a congenital, incurable, fatal disease of newborns; death occurs within 1 year after birth as a result of liver or respiratory failure or both. The disease is due to the inability of peroxisomes to incorporate peroxisomal enzymes because the requisite peroxisomal targeting signal receptors are missing from the membrane of the peroxisomes. This results in the inability of peroxisomes to perform β-oxidation of long-chain fatty acids to synthesize plasmalogens.

Mitochondria

Mitochondria are large organelles; some measure 7 μm long × 1 μm wide. The mean life span of a mitochondrion is about 10 days, after which the mitochondrion increases in length and then undergoes fission. Each mitochondrion is composed of a:

- Smooth outer membrane and
- Inner membrane that is folded into shelflike or tubelike structures, known as cristae, increasing greatly the surface area of the inner membrane

The principal function of mitochondria is the synthesis of **ATP** via a process known as **oxidative phosphorylation**. There are two spaces formed by the two membranes (Fig. 2.12B):

- **Intermembrane space**, located between the outer and inner membranes, and
- **Matrix (intercristal) space**, bounded by the inner membrane (see Fig. 2.12A), which houses the **matrix**, a viscous fluid with a high concentration of proteins, ribosomes, RNA, **circular DNA** (which codes for only 13 mitochondrial proteins), and dense granules of **phospholipoproteins**, known as **matrix granules**, which may have calcium-binding and magnesium-binding properties

The inner and outer membranes contact each other in regions, and here regulatory and transport proteins facilitate the movement of various molecules into and out of the mitochondrial spaces. The macromolecules targeted for the two mitochondrial membranes or the matrix use regions of the mitochondrial membranes where contact does not occur between them; however, these sites possess receptor molecules that recognize the targeted macromolecules.

- The **outer membrane** of the mitochondrion is smooth and quite permeable to small ions, and the presence of numerous **porins** permits the movement of H_2O across it. The content of the intermembrane space is very similar to the content of the cytosol.
- The folded inner membrane is rich in cardiolipins, phospholipids that possess four instead of two fatty acyl chains and greatly reduce the permeability of the inner membrane to protons and electrons. The inner membrane is also rich in the enzyme complex **ATP synthase**, which is responsible for the generation of ATP from ADP and inorganic phosphate.
  - ATP synthase is composed of two major portions, F_0 and F_1; the **F_0 portion** is mostly embedded in the inner membrane, and the **F_1**

portion (also referred to as the **head**) is suspended in the matrix and is connected to the F_0 portion by the **shaft** and is kept stationary by several additional proteins (see Fig. 2.12B).

- Each F_0 portion possesses three sites for the phosphorylation of ADP to ATP. The F_1 portion possesses a fixed outer sleeve and a freely movable inner sleeve composed of 10 to 14 subunits. The shaft also has a movable internal sleeve that extends into the F_0 portion and a fixed outer sleeve.
- The movable sleeves of the shaft and of the F_1 portion are together known as the **rotor**. The fixed outer sleeves are connected to the F_0 portion, and these three components are known as the **stator**.

The matrix contains the enzymes, which, using **pyruvate** generated from glycolysis and **fatty acids** generated from fats and transported into the mitochondrial matrix, convert them into **acetyl coenzyme A (CoA)**, whose acetyl moiety is used by the enzymes of the citric acid cycle to reduce oxidized nicotinamide adenine dinucleotide (NAD^+) to **NADH** and flavin adenine dinucleotide (FAD) to **$FADH_2$**. These reduced compounds accept high-energy electrons generated by the citric acid cycle and transfer them to a series of inner membrane integral proteins, known as the **electron transport chain** (Fig. 2.12C). The electron is passed along the chain, and its energy is used to transfer H^+ (i.e., protons) from the matrix into the intermembrane space. As the concentration of H^+ in the intermembrane space becomes greater than that of the matrix, the H^+ ions are driven back into the matrix by this concentration gradient, the **proton motive force**, and the only path open to them is through the ATP synthase.

The movement of protons down the rotor component of the ATP synthase causes it to rotate and rub against the stator, creating energy that is used by the three sites of the F_0 portion to phosphorylate ADP to the energy-rich compound ATP. Some of the ATP formed is used by the mitochondria, but most is transported into the cytosol for use by the cell.

Brown fat is especially abundant in animals that hibernate. The mitochondria of these lipocytes possess **thermogenins** instead of ATP synthase. Thermogenins have the ability to shunt protons from the intermembrane space into the matrix; however, oxidation in these cells is uncoupled from phosphorylation, and, instead of ATP, heat is generated by the proton motive force. The heat is used to bring the animal out of hibernation.

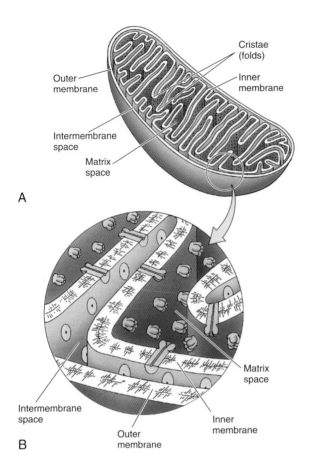

A

B

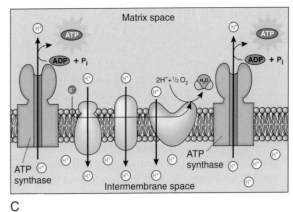

C

Figure 2.12 A, Three-dimensional view of a mitochondrion with shelflike cristae. **B,** Diagram of shelflike cristae at a higher magnification. **C,** Diagram of the electron transport chain and ATP synthase of the inner mitochondrial membrane. *(From Gartner LP, Hiatt JL: Color Textbook of Histology, 3rd ed. Philadelphia, Saunders, 2007, p 39.)*

CLINICAL CONSIDERATIONS

Mitochondrial myopathies are disorders that are inherited from the mother because all mitochondria of an individual are derived from the ovum. These infrequently occurring myopathies do not have a gender-related disposition. The prognosis depends on the muscle groups involved. Myopathy may be evidenced only as muscle weakness and tiring after exercise, but in severe cases it may be fatal. The disorder usually manifests by the end of the second decade of life. Common myopathies are Kearns-Sayre syndrome, myoclonus epilepsy, and mitochondrial encephalomyopathy. There are no known treatments for these diseases.

Inclusions and the Cytoskeleton

INCLUSIONS

Inclusions are nonliving elements of the cell that are freely present within the cytosol and are not membrane bound. The major inclusions are glycogen, lipids, pigments, and crystals.

- **Glycogen** is usually stored in the cytosol in the form of rosettes of β particles that are located in the vicinity of SER elements. These particles are used as an energy deposit that undergoes glycogenolysis to form glucose, which is converted to pyruvate for use in the citric acid cycle.
- **Lipids** are stored triglycerides that are catabolized into fatty acids that are fed into the citric acid cycle for the formation of pyruvate. Lipids are much more efficient storage forms of energy than glycogen because 1 g of lipid provides twice the amount of ATP as does 1 g of glycogen.
- Usually, **pigments** are not active metabolically, but may serve protective functions, such as **melanin** of the skin, which absorbs ultraviolet radiation and serves to protect DNA of epidermal cells from chromosomal damage. Melanin also assists the retina in its function of sight. Another pigment, **lipofuscin**, is probably formed from fusion of numerous residual bodies, the membrane bound structures that are undigestible remnants of lysosomal activity.
- **Crystals** are not usually present in mammalian cells, although Sertoli cells of the testis frequently contain crystals of **Charcot-Bottscher**, whose function, if any, is not understood.

CYTOSKELETON

The **cytoskeleton**, the three-dimensional structural framework of the cell, is composed of **microtubules**, **thin filaments**, and **intermediate filaments**. This framework not only functions in maintaining the morphologic integrity of the cell, but also permits cells to adhere to one another and to move along connective tissue elements, and facilitates exocytosis, endocytosis, and membrane trafficking within the cytosol. The cytoskeleton assists in the creation of compartments within the cell that localize intracellular enzyme systems so that specific biochemical reactions have a greater possibility of occurring.

- **Microtubules** are long, hollow-appearing, flexible, tubular structures, composed of α and β **tubulin** heterodimers (Fig. 2.13A). The tubulin

dimers are arranged in such a fashion that they form GTP-mediated linear assemblies known as **protofilaments**, and 13 of these protofilaments come together in a cylindrical array to form 25 nm–diameter microtubules whose hollow-appearing center is 15 nm in diameter. Each microtubule has a growing, **plus end** and a **minus end** that, unless embedded in a cloud of ring-shaped structures composed of γ tubulin molecules, would permit the shortening of the microtubule. The plus end is also stabilized by a removable **cap** that consists of specific microtubule-associated proteins (MAPs), which prevents the lengthening of the microtubule. It may be observed that microtubules have a specific polarity. Microtubules can become longer—a process known as **rescue**—or shorter—a process known as **catastrophe**—and this cyclic activity is referred to as **dynamic instability**.

- Additional MAPs act as molecular motor proteins, **kinesin** and **dynein**, that allow the microtubules to operate as cellular *highways* along which cargo is transported long distances toward either the plus end (kinesin) or the minus end (dynein).
- Still other MAPs act as spacers between microtubules; some, such as **MAP2**, keep the microtubules farther apart from each other, whereas others, such as **tau**, permit microtubules to be bundled closer to each other.
- Usually, the minus ends of most microtubules of a cell originate from the same region of the cell, known as the **centrosome**, or the **microtubule organizing center** (MTOC) of the cell. Microtubules sustain cell morphology, assist in intracellular transport, form the mitotic and meiotic spindle apparatus, form the cores of cilia and flagella, and form **centrioles** and **basal bodies**.
- **Centrioles** are small, cylindrical structures composed of two pairs of nine triplet microtubules where the two centrioles are arranged perpendicular to each other (Fig. 2.13D). During the S-phase of the cell cycle, each component of the pair replicates itself. Centrioles form the centrosome and, during cell division, act as nucleation sites of the spindle apparatus. They also form the basal bodies that direct the development of cilia and flagella.

A Microtubule

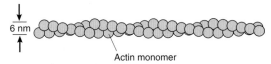

Cross section **Longitudinal view**

α Tubulin
β Tubulin
Tubulin dimers (heterodimers)
(+) End
5 nm
25 nm

B Thin filaments (actin)

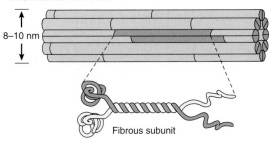

6 nm

Actin monomer

C Intermediate filaments

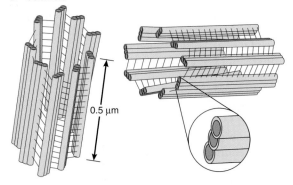

8–10 nm

Fibrous subunit

D Centriole

0.5 μm

Figure 2.13 Three-dimensional diagrams of the various components of the cytoskeleton. **A,** Microtubule. **B,** Thin filament. **C,** Intermediate filament. **D,** Centriole. *(From Gartner LP, Hiatt JL: Color Textbook of Histology, 3rd ed. Philadelphia, Saunders, 2007, p 43.)*

CLINICAL CONSIDERATIONS

GLYCOGEN STORAGE DISORDERS

Some individuals have glycogen storage disorders as a result of their inability to degrade glycogen, resulting in excess accumulation of this substance in the cells. There are three classifications of this disease: (1) hepatic, (2) myopathic, and (3) miscellaneous. The lack or malfunction of one of the enzymes responsible for the degradation is responsible for these disorders.

MELANIN CONDITIONS

Individuals who are unable to manufacture melanin, usually because of a genetic mutation involving the enzyme tyrosinase, have very light skin coloration and red eyes. This individuals have **albinism**. Individuals who produce more than the normal amount of melanin have darker than normal skin and exhibit scalelike patches of dark coloration. These individuals have a condition known as lamellar ichthyosis. Still other individuals may not possess melanocytes, the cells that manufacture melanin. These individuals have a condition known as vitiligo.

CYTOSKELETON (cont.)

- **Thin filaments** (**microfilaments**) are composed of **G-actin** monomers that have assembled (a process requiring ATP) in a polarized fashion into two chains of **F-actin** filaments coiled around each other, forming a 6-nm-thick filament (see Fig. 2.14B). Actin in its monomeric and filamentous forms constitutes approximately 15% of the protein content of most cells, making it one of the most abundant intracellular proteins. Similar to microtubules, thin filaments have a **plus end** (**barbed** because of the presence of the myosin attachment site) and a **minus end** (**pointed** because of the absence of myosin attachment site). The lengthening of the filament occurs at a faster pace at the plus end.
  - When the thin filament achieves its required length, the two ends are capped by **capping proteins**, such as **gelsolin**, which stabilizes both ends of the filament by preventing further polymerization or depolymerization. Gelsolin has an additional role of cutting a thin filament in two and capping the severed ends.
  - Shortening of thin filaments can also occur by the action of **cofilin**, which induces depolymerization by the removal of G-actin monomers at the minus end. Lengthening of thin filaments requires the presence of a pool of G-actin monomers. These monomers are sequestered by thymosin within the cytosol, and the protein **profilin** facilitates the transfer of G-actin from thymosin to the plus end of the thin filament.
  - Branching of thin filaments is regulated by the protein complex, which functions in initiating the attachment of G-actin to an existing thin filament, and from that point on profilin increases the length of the branch. Thin filaments form associations with each other that have been categorized into contractile bundles, gel-like networks, and parallel bundles. Actin also participates in the establishment and maintenance of focal contacts of the cell whereby the cell attaches to the extracellular matrix.

- **Contractile bundles** are associated with myosin I through myosin IX, and function in the contractile process, in muscle contraction or the intracellular movement of cargo.
- **Gel-like networks** are associated with the protein **filamin** to form high-viscosity matrices such as those of the cell cortex.
- **Parallel bundles** are thin filaments associated with the proteins **villin** and **fimbrin**, which maintain the thin filaments in a parallel array, such as those of the core of microvilli and microspikes and in the terminal web.

- **Intermediate filaments**, ropelike structures 8 to 10 nm in diameter, form the framework of the cell, anchor the nucleus in its position, secure integral membrane proteins to the cytoskeleton, and react to extracellular matrix forces. Intermediate filaments (Fig. 2.14C) are composed of rodlike protein tetramers, eight of which form tightly bundled helices of protofilaments. Two protofilaments aggregate to form protofibrils, and four of these structures bind to each other to form an intermediate filament. There are about 40 categories of intermediate filaments depending on their polypeptide components and cellular distribution. The principal classes of intermediate filaments are keratins, desmin, vimentin, glial fibrillary acidic protein, neurofilaments, and nuclear lamins. **Intermediate filament binding proteins** attach to and bind intermediate filaments to assist in the formation of the three-dimensional cytoskeleton. The best known of these binding proteins are filaggrin, synemin, plectin, and plakins.
  - **Filaggrins** attach keratin filaments to each other to form them into bundles.
  - **Synemin binds desmin**, and **plectin** binds vimentin to form a three-dimensional framework in the cytosol.
  - **Plakins** attach keratin filaments to hemidesmosomes in epithelial cells and neurofilaments to thin filaments in dorsal ganglion neurons.

A   Microtubule

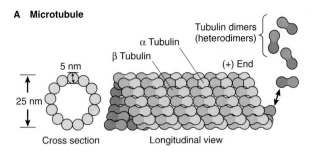

B   Thin filaments (actin)

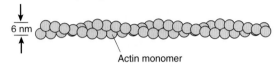

C   Intermediate filaments

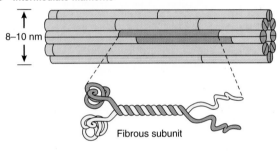

D   Centriole

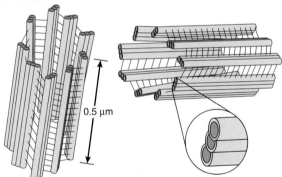

Figure 2.14 Three dimensional diagrams of the various components of the cytoskeleton. **A,** Microtubule. **B,** Thin filament. **C,** Intermediate filament. **D,** Centriole. *(From Gartner LP, Hiatt JL: Color Textbook of Histology, 3rd ed. Philadelphia, Saunders, 2007, p 43.)*

3 NUCLEUS

The largest organelle in the cell, the nucleus, not only contains most of the cell's DNA but also possesses the mechanisms for DNA and RNA synthesis. The nucleus contains three major components: **chromatin**, the cell's genetic material; **nucleolus**, where ribosomal RNA (rRNA) is synthesized, and ribosomal subunits are assembled; and **nucleoplasm**, a matrix containing various macromolecules and nuclear particles. The nucleus is surrounded by the nuclear envelope composed of two membranes. Although the nucleus may vary in shape, location, and number, in most cells it is centrally located and spherical in shape.

KEY WORDS
• **Nuclear pore complex**
• **Chromosomes**
• **Deoxyribonucleic acid (DNA)**
• **Ribonucleic acid (RNA)**
• **Cell cycle**
• **Mitosis**
• **Meiosis**
• **Apoptosis**

Nuclear Envelope

The nuclear envelope, composed of **inner** and **outer nuclear membranes** with an intervening perinuclear cisterna (10 to 30 nm in width) is perforated by **nuclear pores**, regions where the inner and outer nuclear membranes fuse with one another. Material is exchanged between the cytoplasm and the nucleus at these nuclear pores (Fig. 3.1).

- The 6-nm-thick **inner nuclear membrane** contacts the **nuclear lamina**, an interwoven meshwork of specialized intermediate filaments composed of **lamins A**, **B**, and **C**, located at the periphery in the nucleus. These lamins not only organize and support the perinuclear chromatin and the inner nuclear membrane, but they also assist in the reassembly of the nuclear envelope after cell division. Transmembrane proteins of the inner nuclear membrane, usually in association with matrix proteins, present contact sites for nuclear RNAs and chromosomes.
- The 6-nm-thick, ribosome-studded **outer nuclear membrane** is continuous with the rough endoplasmic reticulum, and its cytoplasmic surface is enmeshed in a network of **vimentin** (intermediate filaments).

NUCLEAR PORES AND NUCLEAR PORE COMPLEXES

Nuclear pores form where the outer and inner nuclear membranes fuse, permitting communication between the nucleus and the cytoplasm. Glycoproteins stud the periphery of each nuclear pore and participate in the formation of the **nuclear pore complex**. The **nuclear lamina** assists the nuclear pore complexes to communicate with each other in their function of permitting substances to traverse their pores.

- Three ringlike arrays of proteins, each displaying an eightfold symmetry and interconnected by vertical spokes and spanning both nuclear membranes, constitute a nuclear pore complex (100 to 125 nm in diameter).
- The three sets of rings layered above one another are named the *cytoplasmic ring, luminal spoke ring,* and *nuclear ring.* Additionally, there is a nuclear basket on the nuclear aspect of the pore complex (Fig. 3.2).
- Located on the rim of the cytoplasmic portion of the nuclear pore is the **cytoplasmic ring** composed of eight subunits, each possessing a cytoplasmic filament composed of a Ran-binding protein (GTP-binding protein) that assists in the import of materials from cytoplasm into nucleus.
- Another set of eight transmembrane proteins that project into the lumen of the pore and perinuclear cistern constitutes the **luminal spoke ring** (middle ring), whose central lumen is probably a gated channel that restricts passive diffusion. Other proteins associated with the complex assist in regulated transport through the nuclear pore complex.
- An oblong structure, the **transporter**, is occasionally observed to be occupying the central lumen. The transporter probably represents material that is being transported into or out of the nucleus.
- On the rim of the nucleoplasmic side of the pore complex is the **nuclear ring (nucleoplasmic ring)**, also composed of eight subunits. This innermost ring assists in the export of RNA into the cytoplasm.
- Suspended from the nuclear ring is the **nuclear basket**, a filamentous flexible basket-like structure, and a smaller **distal ring** that is attached to the distal portion of the nuclear basket.

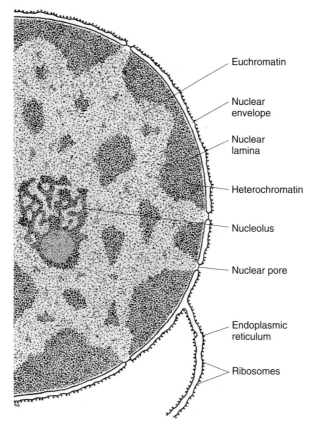

Figure 3.1 Diagram of a typical nucleus. *(From Gartner LP, Hiatt JL: Color Textbook of Histology, 3rd ed. Philadelphia, Saunders, 2007, p 52.)*

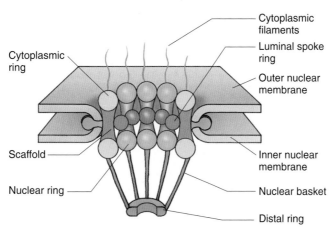

Figure 3.2 Nuclear pore complex. *(From Gartner LP, Hiatt JL: Color Textbook of Histology, 3rd ed. Philadelphia, Saunders, 2007, p 54.)*

Nuclear Pore Function

The open channel of the nuclear pore complex seems to be reduced by proteins of the complex so that substances larger than 11 nm cannot pass through the pore in either direction without being transported by the energy-requiring **receptor-mediated transport**.

- Signal sequences on the material to be transported must be recognized by receptors, **importins** and **exportins**, on the nuclear pore complex, and the regulation of the transport depends on Ran and nuclear pore complex–associated nucleoproteins.
- The importins possess **nuclear localization signals**.
- **Exportins** possess **nuclear export signals**.

Transport of protein subunits of ribosomes into the nucleus is an example of importin function, whereas transport of macromolecules such as RNA to the cytoplasm is an example of exportin function (Fig. 3.3).

Chromatin

The genetic material (**DNA**) of the cell resides in the nucleus as an integral part of the chromosomes, structures that are so tightly wound during mitosis that they can be observed with the light microscope, but at other times the chromosomes are unwound into thin chromatin strands.

- Most of the nuclear chromatin is partially unwound, is transcriptionally *inactive,* and is located at the periphery of the nucleus and is known as **heterochromatin**.
- Transcriptionally *active* chromatin, **euchromatin**, is completely unwound, exposing its 2-nm-wide string of DNA, wrapped around beads of nucleosomes, to be transcribed into RNA.
  - Each nucleosome is an octomer of proteins known as **histones** (H_2A, H_2B, H_3, and H_4) wrapped with two complete turns of DNA representing about 150 nucleotide pairs.
  - The **linker DNA** is about 200 base pairs that occupy the space between neighboring nucleosomes. Nucleosomes support the DNA strand and assist in regulating DNA replication, repair, and transcription.
  - Chromatin is packaged into 30-nm threads as helical coils of six nucleosomes per turn and bound with **histone H_1** (see Fig. 3.4).

CHROMOSOMES

As the cell prepares to undergo mitosis or meiosis, the chromatin fibers become extremely condensed forming chromosomes, reaching maximum condensation during metaphase (Fig. 3.4).

- Each species has its own specific number of chromosomes, referred to as its **genome** or total genetic makeup.
- The human genome is made up of 46 chromosomes: 23 homologous pairs of chromosomes, one set of the pair from each parent.
  - There are 22 pairs of somatic chromosomes (**autosomes**) and a single pair of **sex chromosomes**.
  - The single pair of female sex chromosomes is represented by two X chromosomes (**XX**), whereas the single pair of male sex chromosomes is represented by an X chromosome and a Y chromosome (**XY**).

Cytoplasm

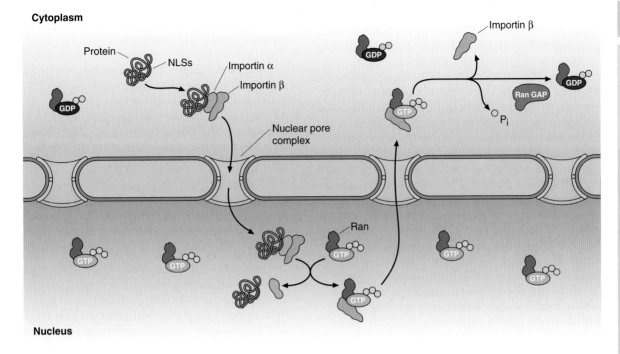

Figure 3.3 Role of Ran in nuclear import. GAP, GTPase-activating protein; GDP, guanosine diphosphate; NLSs, nuclear localization signals. *(From Gartner LP, Hiatt JL: Color Textbook of Histology, 3rd ed. Philadelphia, Saunders, 2007, p 54.)*

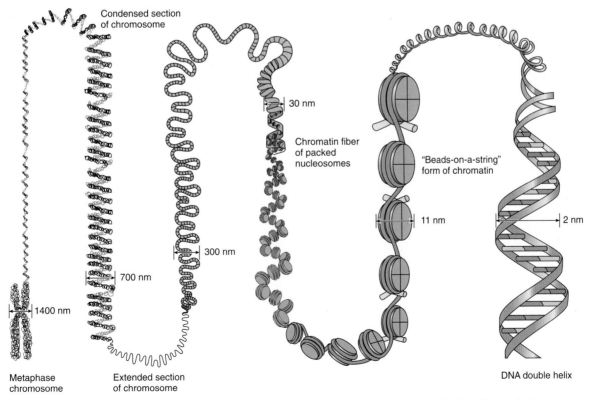

Figure 3.4 Chromatin packaging to form a chromosome. *(From Gartner LP, Hiatt JL: Color Textbook of Histology, 3rd ed. Philadelphia, Saunders, 2007, p 55.)*

DEOXYRIBONUCLEIC ACID AND RIBONUCLEIC ACID

Two types of nitrogenous bases, **purines** (adenine and guanine) and **pyrimidines** (cytosine and thymine), bound to two chains of deoxyribose sugar backbones constitute the **DNA molecule**, forming a linear sequence of nucleotides. Hydrogen bonds formed between facing complementary bases attach the two strands to each other to form the double helix.

The **RNA molecule** is similar to DNA, but instead of a double helix it is merely a single chain whose purines and pyrimidines are attached to a ribose sugar backbone (although in some RNA viruses it may be double chained). An additional difference is that one of the pyrimidine bases is **uracil** rather than thymine. The synthesis of RNA is called **transcription** because one of the DNA strands is used as a template, and a complementary chain of single-stranded RNA is the result. There are three different RNAs; the mode of transcription is the same for all three except that each type of RNA is synthesized by a specific RNA polymerase.

- **Messenger RNA (mRNA)**, catalyzed by RNA polymerase II, transports the genetic information transcribed from DNA that codes for a sequence of amino acids to the cytoplasm where protein synthesis occurs. The DNA molecule has transcribed to the RNA an exact copy of that particular region of the DNA molecule that constitutes one gene.
- **Transfer RNA (tRNA)**, catalyzed by RNA polymerase III, carries activated amino acids to the ribosome-mRNA complex so that protein synthesis can occur (see the section on protein synthesis in Chapter 2).
- **Ribosomal RNA (rRNA)**, catalyzed by RNA polymerase I, is synthesized in the nucleolus and is coupled to ribosomal proteins to be incorporated into the forming ribosomal subunits.

Transcription

Cofactors assist the enzyme, polymerase II, to unwind the DNA double helix two turns, thereby exposing the nucleotides of the DNA strands.

- One of the DNA strands is used by polymerase II as the template on which to assemble the complementary mRNA molecule.
- The DNA double helix continues to be unwound as transcription proceeds, and the same single strand of DNA continues to be used as the template for mRNA transcription.
- As more nucleotides are polymerized, the mRNA chain grows and finally becomes separated from the DNA template strand permitting the DNA double helix to reform (Fig. 3.5).

The transcribed RNA (primary transcript) molecule separated from the DNA molecule is termed a **precursor messenger RNA (pre-mRNA)** possessing coding elements (**exons**) and noncoding elements (**introns**).

- The noncoding introns must be removed so that the exons can be spliced together.
- The splicing requires that pre-mRNA molecules form complexes with nuclear processing proteins called **heterogeneous nuclear ribonucleoprotein particles (hnRNPs)**, and as splicing occurs the pre-mRNA molecule is reduced in length. Other processing is in effect during the splicing.
- This process involves complexes of five **small nuclear ribonucleoprotein particles (snRNPs)** and many other **non-snRNP splicing factors** that form the core of **splicosomes** that assist in this process to produce **messenger ribonucleoprotein (mRNP)**.
- When this task is completed and nuclear processing proteins are extracted, the remaining mRNA is ready to be transported through the nuclear pore complex and into the cytoplasm.

Although the intronic RNA segments stripped from the primary RNA strand represent a larger percent of the nuclear RNA than that in the spliced exons, it was believed that they had no function. More recent evidence indicates that these intronic RNA segments may perform regulatory functions in conjunction with regulatory proteins.

TRANSCRIPTION

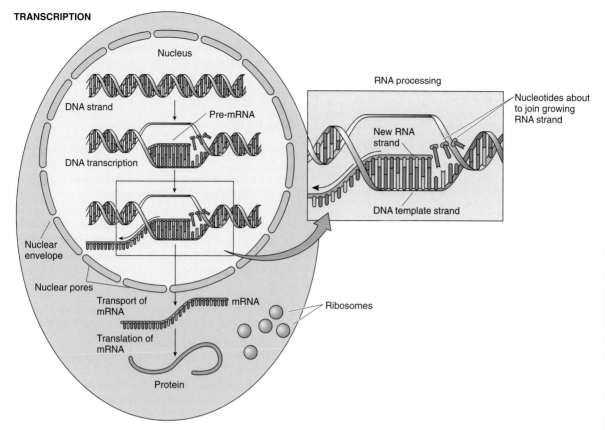

Figure 3.5 DNA transcription into mRNA. *(Modified from Alberts B, Bray D, Lewis J, et al: Molecular Biology of the Cell, 3rd ed. New York, Garland Publishing, 1994.)*

NUCLEOPLASM

The nucleoplasm is composed of interchromatin granules, perichromatin granules, snRNPs, and nuclear matrix (Fig. 3.6).

- **Interchromatin granules** (20 to 25 nm in diameter), found clustered among the chromatin material, contain RNPs and several enzymes, including adenosine triphosphatase (ATPase), guanosine triphosphatase (GTPase), β-glycerophosphatase, and nicotinamide adenine dinucleotide (NAD) pyrophosphatase. Their function is not understood.
- **Perichromatin granules** (30 to 50 nm in diameter), surrounded by a 25-nm-wide halo of unknown composition, are situated in the vicinity of the heterochromatin and consist of hnRNP-like molecules. Complexes of small RNAs and proteins, known as snRNPs, manipulate and transport hnRNP particles, which function in processing pre-mRNAs.

Nuclear Matrix

Structurally, the components of the nuclear matrix include fibrillar elements, residual nucleoli, residual RNP networks, and nuclear pore–nuclear lamina complex. A nucleoplasmic reticulum has been discovered more recently in the nuclear matrix that appears to be continuous with the endoplasmic reticulum of the cytoplasm and is believed to store calcium that is used within the nucleus. Additionally, inositol 1,4,5-triphosphate receptors, which regulate certain nuclear calcium signals, particularly signals involved with protein transport and transcription of certain genes, have been discovered in the nuclear matrix.

The nuclear matrix may be subdivided into different interacting compartments that enable the regulation of specific gene expression at particular moments of time, tRNA and mRNA transcription and processing, and the binding of various signaling molecules and viral agents.

NUCLEOLUS

The nucleolus, observed only during interphase, is a highly basophilic RNA and protein-rich structure present within the nucleus. Each nucleus contains a single nucleolus, although some cells house three or more nucleoli, and during mRNA synthesis the nucleoli enlarge in size and are associated with the portion of the chromosomes, the **nucleolus-associated chromatin**, whose DNA is being transcribed into mRNA or rRNA. The nucleolus presents four discernible regions:

- **Pale-staining fibrillar center**, characterized by the presence of the tips of chromosomes 13, 14, 15, 21, and 22 (in humans), representing the location of genes that code for rRNA
- **Pars fibrosa**, representing the transcription of nucleolar RNA
- **Pars granulosa**, the region of the nucleolus where ribosomal subunit assembly is occurring
- **Nucleolar matrix**, an arrangement of fibers that is responsible for maintaining the organization of the nucleolus

The nucleolus functions in assembling and organizing nonmitochondrial ribosomal subunits (Fig. 3.7), regulating certain processes of the cell cycle by sequestering or inactivating cyclic-dependent cyclases, facilitating the assembly of RNPs, assisting in the regulation of nuclear export, and perhaps participating in the regulation of the aging process.

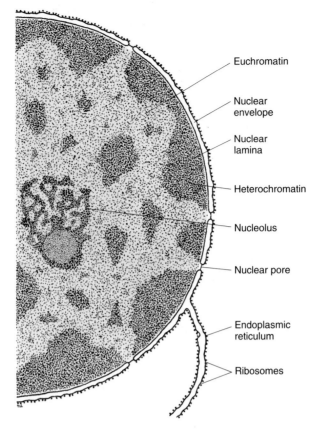

Figure 3.6 Nucleus. *(From Gartner LP, Hiatt JL: Color Textbook of Histology, 3rd ed. Philadelphia, Saunders, 2007, p 52.)*

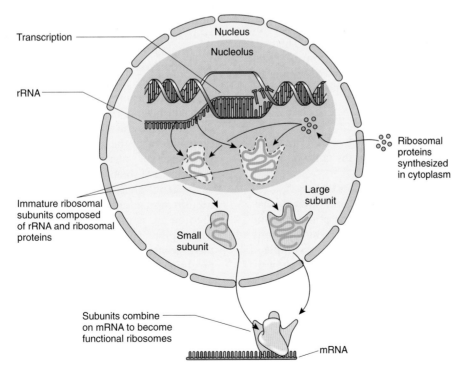

Figure 3.7 Ribosome formation. *(Modified from Alberts B, Bray D, Lewis J, et al: Molecular Biology of the Cell, 3rd ed. New York, Garland Publishing, 1994.)*

Cell Cycle

The **cell cycle**, a series of sequential cellular events in preparation for cell division, is composed of **interphase**, when the cell becomes larger and duplicates its genetic material, and **mitosis**, a process that results in the formation of two identical daughter cells. The cell cycle is usually described as beginning at the end of cell division when the cell is entering interphase (Fig. 3.8).

- Certain cells that are highly differentiated (e.g., muscle cells and neurons) cease to continue to go through mitosis and remain in a resting stage **G_0 (G zero) phase**.
- Other cells, such as peripheral lymphocytes, enter the **G_0 phase** temporarily and at a later time they may again enter the cell cycle.

Events such as mechanical forces, ischemia, or death of cells in a particular cell line may induce signaling cells to release growth factors that induce the expression of **proto-oncogenes**, which prompt the proliferative pathways of the cell. This process activates the release of a cascade of cytoplasmic **protein kinases** triggering a series of nuclear transcription factors regulating the expression of proto-oncogenes that result in cell division. Many cancers are the result of mutations in the proto-oncogenes that permit the uncontrolled proliferation of the mutated cell.

A group of proteins known as **cyclins**, by complexing with specific **cyclin-dependent kinases (CDKs)**, not only activate them, but also guide them to target proteins and, in that fashion, control the entry and advance of the cell through the cell cycle. There are three principal **checkpoints** where the control system can prevent the cell from entering or continuing the cell cycle. At each checkpoint, the cell may commit to finish the cell cycle, pause temporarily, or withdraw completely. These checkpoints are the:

- **Start/restriction point** in gap 1, which permits chromosome duplication and the entry into gap 2;
- **G_2/M checkpoint**, which initiates the condensation of chromosomes and other events necessary to permit the beginning of mitosis; and
- **Metaphase/anaphase checkpoint**, which permits the separation of sister chromatids, the completion of the M phase, and the process of cytokinesis.

The four classes of cyclins and the CDKs with which they complex are as follows:

- **G_1 cyclins**: Cyclin D, early in the G_1 phase, binds to CDK4 and to CDK6.
- **G_1/S cyclins**: Cyclin E is synthesized late in the G_1 phase and binds to CDK2. These three complexes, along with other intermediaries, permit the cell to enter and progress through the S phase.
- **S cyclins**: Cyclin A binds to CDK2 and CDK1 forming complexes that permit the cell to leave the S phase and enter the G_2 phase and induce the formation of cyclin B.
- **M cyclins**: Cyclin B binds to CDK1, and this complex allows the cell to leave the G_2 phase and enter the M phase.

When the functions of the cyclins have been completed, they are degraded to prevent their interference with the proper sequence of events.

INTERPHASE

Interphase is subdivided into three phases: **G_1 (gap) phase**, when the cell prepares to synthesize DNA; **S (synthetic) phase**, when DNA is replicated; and **G_2 phase**, when the cell prepares for the mitotic event (see Fig. 3.8).

- **G_1 phase**: At the conclusion of mitosis, the newly formed daughter cells enter the G_1 phase of the cell cycle, a stage characterized by the synthesis of the regulatory proteins necessary for DNA replication, the restoration of the nucleoli and of the original cell volume of the daughter cell, and the initiation of centriole duplication.
- **S phase**: The S phase is the synthetic phase where the genome is duplicated. At this point, the cell's normal complement of DNA has doubled from the normal (2n) to (4n) in preparation for the mitotic event.
- **G_2 phase**: The interval between the end of DNA synthesis and the beginning of mitosis is known as the gap 2 phase; during this phase, the RNA, tubulin, and additional proteins required for cell division are synthesized. Additionally, adenosine triphosphate (ATP) reserves are increased, and the newly synthesized DNA is checked for possible errors and, if present, corrected.

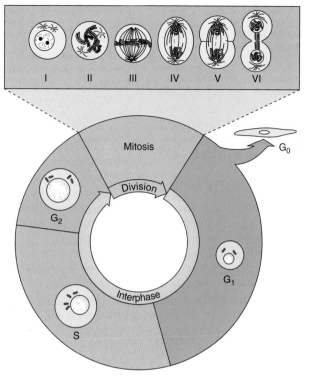

Figure 3.8 The cell cycle in an actively dividing cell. Nondividing cells such as neurons exit the cell cycle to enter the G_0 phase (resting phase). Other cells such as lymphocytes may return to the cell cycle. *(From Gartner LP, Hiatt JL: Color Textbook of Histology, 3rd ed. Philadelphia, Saunders, 2007, p 61.)*

CLINICAL CONSIDERATIONS

Cancer chemotherapy has been enhanced by a more complete understanding of the cell cycle and mitosis. Certain drugs can be employed at specific times to arrest cell proliferation by disrupting certain stages of the cell cycle. **Vincristine** disrupts the mitotic spindle arresting the cell in mitosis. **Colchicine**, a plant alkaloid, is used to produce the same effect and is used for individual chromosome studies and for karyotyping. **Methotrexate**, a drug that inhibits purine synthesis, and **5-fluorouracil**, a drug that inhibits pyrimidine synthesis, act during the S phase of the cell cycle, preventing cell division, and are used in chemotherapy treatment.

MITOSIS

Mitosis is the component of the cell cycle that follows the G_2 phase and results in the formation of two smaller but identical daughter cells from a single cell. The first event in this process is called **karyokinesis**, the division of the nuclear material, and is followed by **cytokinesis**, cytoplasmic division. Although the process of mitosis is a continuous one, for convenience of the student it is divided into five stages: **prophase**, **prometaphase**, **metaphase**, **anaphase**, and **telophase** (Fig. 3.9).

- The first phase of mitosis, **prophase**, is characterized by condensing chromosomes, the disappearance of the nucleolus, the beginning of the disruption of the nucleus, and the division of the **centrosome** into two halves migrating away from each other toward the opposite poles of the cell. Each half of the centrosome has a **centriole** and a **microtubule organizing center** (MOC). As the chromosomes, each composed of two **sister chromatids** held together at the **centromere** by **cohesin** (a chromatin binding protein), continue to condense, another MOC, the **kinetochore**, develops, and the formation of the **mitotic spindle apparatus** is initiated. This mitotic spindle apparatus is responsible for directing the sister chromatids in their migration to the opposing poles of the nucleus.
- During **prometaphase**, the nuclear envelope disappears secondary to the phosphorylation of the nuclear lamins. The chromosomes continue to condense and are randomly oriented within the cytoplasm. The mitotic spindle apparatus becomes defined by microtubules attached to the kinetochores, known as **mitotic spindle microtubules**, and polar microtubules that extend between the two centrosomes, known as **polar microtubules**. The former function in directing the chromosomes to their proper orientation, and the latter are believed to maintain the correct space between the two centrosomes.
- At **metaphase**, the maximally condensed chromosomes become aligned on the equatorial plate (**metaphase plate**) of the mitotic spindle in such a fashion that each chromatid lies parallel to the cell's equator.
- **Anaphase** begins when the cohesion proteins that attach the sister chromatids to each other at the centromere disappear, and the sister chromatids (chromosomes) start to be pulled apart. The chromosomes seem to play a passive role in the process of migration to the opposite poles of the cell. The **depolymerization** of the mitotic spindle microtubules in association with **dynein** is the responsible agent in the chromosome migration. During the latter part of anaphase, a **cleavage furrow** develops indicating that the plasmalemma is beginning to anticipate **cytokinesis**.
- By **telophase**, the chromosomes have reached the opposite poles of the cell, and the nuclear envelope is reformed because of the dephosphorylation of the nuclear lamins. The chromosomes begin to uncoil, and the **nucleolar organizing regions** of five pairs of chromosomes are unfolded.
  - Although **cytokinesis** (the division of the cytoplasm into two halves, forming two daughter cells) began during anaphase, it is completed in telophase.
  - As the cleavage furrow deepens in 360 degrees around the periphery of the cell, the cell resembles a dumbbell where the two spheres are very close to each other.
  - Eventually, only the **midbody**, the polar microtubules surrounded by a very thin rim of cytoplasm, connects the cytoplasm of the two daughter cells to each other.
  - Within each daughter cell, a **contractile ring**, composed of actin and myosin, is responsible for the constriction process, which is completed when the midbody's microtubules are depolymerized.
  - When the two daughter cells are completely separated from each other, the spindle apparatus also becomes depolymerized and cytokinesis is completed.
  - The two diploid (2n) daughter cells are identical to each other.

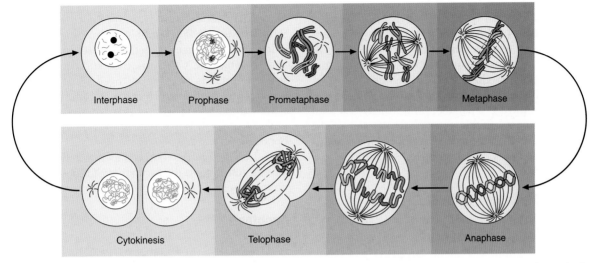

Figure 3.9 Stages of mitosis in a cell containing a diploid number of six chromosomes. *(From Gartner LP, Hiatt JL: Color Textbook of Histology, 3rd ed. Philadelphia, Saunders, 2007, p 64.)*

CLINICAL CONSIDERATIONS

Observations of a karyotype may indicate aneuploidy—an abnormal number of chromosomes. An example of this condition is in Down syndrome, in which the individual has an extra chromosome 21 (trisomy 21). Individuals with this condition exhibit stubby hands, mental retardation, a malformed heart, and many other congenital malformations. Klinefelter syndrome is an example of aneuploidy of the sex chromosomes. These individuals are males but possess an extra X chromosome (XXY). They exhibit the male phenotype, but do not develop secondary sex characteristics and are usually sterile. Individuals possessing less than the normal number of chromosomes exhibit monosomy. Turner syndrome (XO) is an example. These individuals are mentally retarded females exhibiting undeveloped ovaries and breasts and a small uterus.

Oncogenes are mutated forms of normal genes called **proto-oncogenes**, which code for proteins that control cell division. Proto-oncogenes exhibit four regulatory mechanisms of cell growth, including growth factors, growth factor receptors, signal transduction molecules, and nuclear transcription factors. Oncogenes may result from a viral infection or random genetic accidents. When present in a cell, oncogenes dominate genes over the normal proto-oncogene alleles, causing unregulated cell division and proliferation. Examples of cancer cells arising from oncogenes include **bladder cancer** and **acute myelogenous leukemia**. **Burkitt's lymphoma** develops from a proto-oncogene located on chromosome 8 that gets transformed onto chromosome 14, causing it to be detached from its normal regulatory element. Burkitt's lymphoma is endemic in some parts of Africa, affecting children and young adults; it affects the maxilla and mandible. Burkitt's lymphoma responds to chemotherapy.

MEIOSIS

Meiosis is a special type of cell division in which a single diploid (**2n**) cell produces four haploid (**1n**) germ cells. In females, one of the four haploid cells is known as an **ovum**, and the other three haploid cells are polar bodies that disintegrate. In males, the four haploid cells are **spermatozoa**. Meiosis—divided into two separate events, meiosis I and meiosis II—reduces the genetic complement of the germ cells, ensures genetic recombination by redistribution of genes, and introduces variability to the gene pool.

Meiosis I (Reductional Division)

During the cell cycle preceding meiosis, DNA in the germ cells is doubled to (**4n**) in the **S phase**, but the chromosome number remains at (**2n**) (Fig. 3.10).

- **Prophase I** is subdivided into the following five phases:
  - **Leptotene**: Chromosomes begin condensing.
  - **Zygotene**: Homologous chromosomes align in gene-to-gene register to form **synaptonemal complexes**.
  - **Pachytene**: Homologous chromosomes continue to condense; crossing-over sites (**chiasmata**) are formed between nonsister chromatids resulting in random exchange of genetic material.
  - **Diplotene**: Chromosomes continue to condense, followed by disjunction of the homologous pairs.
  - **Diakinesis**: As the chromosomes condense maximally, the synaptonemal complex disassembles, the nucleolus and the nuclear envelope disappear, and chromosomes are now free in the cytoplasm. A microtubule spindle begins to form.
- **Metaphase I**: Homologous chromosomes align in random order on the equatorial plate, ensuring a shuffling of the maternal and paternal chromosomes. Kinetochore microtubules attach to the kinetochores.
- **Anaphase I**: Homologous chromosomes, still composed of two sister chromatids, migrate to opposite poles.
- **Telophase I**: Telophase I of meiosis I is similar to telophase of mitosis. Chromosomes complete the migration to opposite poles, nuclei are reformed, and cytokinesis divides the one cell into two daughter cells, each with the (**1n**) number of chromosomes (23 chromosomes, but each composed of two chromatids, accounting for the (**2n**) amount of DNA) (see Fig. 3.10). The daughter cells now enter meiosis II.

Meiosis II (Equatorial Division)

The **equatorial division** is not preceded by another S phase. Meiosis II resembles mitosis and is subdivided into **prophase II**, **metaphase II**, **anaphase II**, and **telophase II**. Chromosomes, still composed of sister chromatids, become arranged along the equator, and attached kinetochore microtubules pull the sister chromatids apart and draw them to opposite poles of the cell. When the chromosomes reach the opposing poles, each daughter cell formed in meiosis I is subdivided into two new daughter cells via cytokinesis, resulting in the formation of four genetically unique haploid cells (Fig. 3.11).

Apoptosis

When cells die because they no longer receive nutrients or are exposed to sudden trauma, they undergo **necrosis**, a process that initiates an inflammatory response. Most cells kill themselves in a genetically determined manner, however, known as **apoptosis**, the best understood form of **programmed cell death**. Some cells undergo apoptosis because of specific environmental conditions, such as overcrowding; others undergo apoptosis because of their age; and others, such as virally transformed cells, are forced into apoptosis by cells of the immune system. During apoptosis, cells undergo morphologic changes: the cell shrinks, there is breakdown of the cytoskeleton, the nuclear envelope disassembles, and nuclear chromatin breaks up into fragments. These events are followed by the cell remnants becoming membrane-enclosed **apoptotic bodies** that are phagocytosed by macrophages. The process of apoptosis is regulated by **caspases**, proteolytic enzymes that act at particular aspartate residues of their target proteins. Each cell possesses the inactive form, **procaspases**, some of which become activated to form **initiator caspases**, which induce a cascade forming activated **executioner procaspases** and **target proteins** within the cell, initiating the morphological events listed earlier. Signals external to the cell activate membrane bound **death receptors**, which activate the caspase system to drive the cell into the **extrinsic pathway of apoptosis**. The **intrinsic pathway of apoptosis** is initiated by mitochondria that release cytochrome c into the cytosol. This molecule binds with **apoptotic procaspase-activating adaptor protein (Apaf1)**, which combines with other Apaf1 units to form a wheel-like **apoptosome** that induces a caspase cascade resulting in programmed cell death. Because the extrinsic pathway is unable to generate a sufficient caspase cascade by itself, it must activate the intrinsic pathway to induce a complete apoptosis cascade.

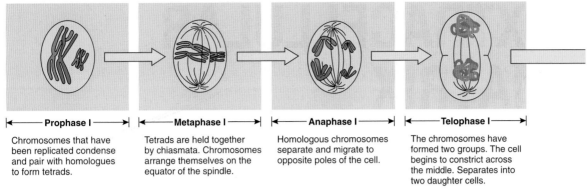

Figure 3.10 Stages of meiosis in a cell containing a diploid (2n) number of 4 chromosomes. Meiosis I. *(From Gartner LP, Hiatt JL: Color Textbook of Histology, 3rd ed. Philadelphia, Saunders, 2007, p 66.)*

Prophase I	Metaphase I	Anaphase I	Telophase I
Chromosomes that have been replicated condense and pair with homologues to form tetrads.	Tetrads are held together by chiasmata. Chromosomes arrange themselves on the equator of the spindle.	Homologous chromosomes separate and migrate to opposite poles of the cell.	The chromosomes have formed two groups. The cell begins to constrict across the middle. Separates into two daughter cells.

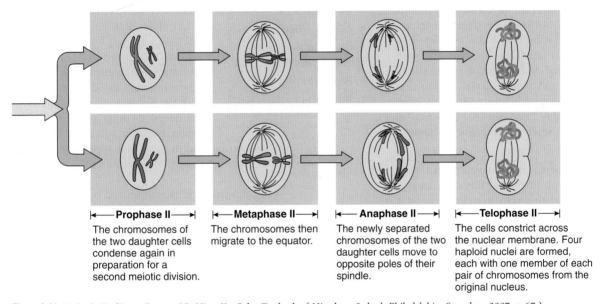

Prophase II	Metaphase II	Anaphase II	Telophase II
The chromosomes of the two daughter cells condense again in preparation for a second meiotic division.	The chromosomes then migrate to the equator.	The newly separated chromosomes of the two daughter cells move to opposite poles of their spindle.	The cells constrict across the nuclear membrane. Four haploid nuclei are formed, each with one member of each pair of chromosomes from the original nucleus.

Figure 3.11 Meiosis II. *(From Gartner LP, Hiatt JL: Color Textbook of Histology, 3rd ed. Philadelphia, Saunders, 2007, p 67.)*

CLINICAL CONSIDERATIONS

During meiosis I, when the homologous pairs of chromosomes normally separate and migrate to opposite poles (anaphase I), **nondisjunction** may occur—one daughter cell contains both homologous chromosomes resulting in 24 chromosomes, whereas the other daughter cell is totally without that chromosome, resulting in 22 chromosomes. At normal fertilization, one zygote has 47 chromosomes (trisomy), whereas the other zygote has 45 chromosomes (monosomy). Down syndrome is an example of trisomy 21. Nondisjunction occurs more frequently in chromosomes 8, 9, 13, 18, and 21, each producing unique characteristics. Nondisjunction occurs more frequently in women older than 35 years of age.

4 EXTRACELLULAR MATRIX

Cells with similar structural and functional characteristics assemble to form tissues that perform particular functions. The four tissues of the mammalian body are epithelium, connective tissue, muscular tissue, and nervous tissue. Each tissue is composed not only of cells, but also of nonliving material, the extracellular matrix (ECM), whose two components are ground substance and fibers (Fig. 4.1). ECM is manufactured by cells and delivered by them into the extracellular space and was believed to function only in the capacity of physical support. ECM has been shown, however, to have numerous additional responsibilities, such as:

> **KEY WORDS**
> - **Ground substance**
> - **Collagen**
> - **Collagen synthesis**
> - **Elastic fibers**
> - **Basement membrane**
> - **Basal lamina**
> - **Integrins**

- Influencing cell development, migration, mitosis, morphology, and function, and
- Permitting cells to migrate along it.

Fluid that escapes from blood vessels, known as extracellular fluid, carries nutrients, oxygen, and signaling molecules to the cells of the body, and the same fluid returns waste products, oxygen, and other cellular products to the bloodstream. Cells also leave the bloodstream and make their way through ECM to eliminate toxic elements, antigens, microorganisms, debris of dead cells, and other unwanted material located in ECM.

Ground Substance

Ground substance is a gel that consists of glycosaminoglycans (GAGs), proteoglycans, and glycoproteins.

- **GAGs** are long, unbranched, negatively charged polysaccharide chains composed of repeating units of disaccharides, one of which is always a **uronic acid** (iduronic acid or glucuronic acid) and the other an **amino sugar** (*N*-acetylglucosamine or *N*-acetylgalactosamine) (Table 4.1).
  - Their negative charge attracts Na$^+$ ions, which attract water molecules from the extracellular fluid, making all GAGs highly hydrated.

Because these macromolecules are usually attached to protein cores, they tend to be very closely packed, which makes them not only resist compression but also quite slippery.

- With the exception of **hyaluronic acid**, a massive GAG composed of more than 10,000 disaccharides, all GAGs are sulfated.
- The most common GAGs (keratan sulfate, chondroitin 4-sulfate, chondroitin 6-sulfate, heparan sulfate, heparin, and dermatan sulfate) are composed of approximately 300 disaccharides, are synthesized in the Golgi apparatus, and are covalently bound to a linear protein core.
- Hyaluronic acid is synthesized by the enzyme hyaluronan synthase on the cytoplasmic surface of the plasmalemma and is translocated into the extracellular space to become incorporated into ECM. A single hyaluronic acid molecule can be 20 µm long.
- **Proteoglycans** are very large macromolecules that are composed of a protein core to which sulfated GAGs are covalently bound (see Fig. 4.1). A proteoglycan resembles a *bottlebrush*, where the protein core is the wire stem and the GAGs comprise the bristles. These macromolecules vary in composition and in size:
  - **Decorin** is about 50 kDa with only a single GAG bound to its protein core, whereas
  - **Aggrecan**, with 200 GAGs, is 3 million Da.
- Because all of the GAGs are hydrated, each proteoglycan occupies a very large domain.
  - Many proteoglycans, such as aggrecan, are attached to hyaluronic acid, forming enormous proteoglycans. These macromolecules may be several hundred million daltons and possess a huge domain that is responsible for the gel state of the ground substance.
  - Functions of proteoglycans include resisting compression, binding signaling molecules and

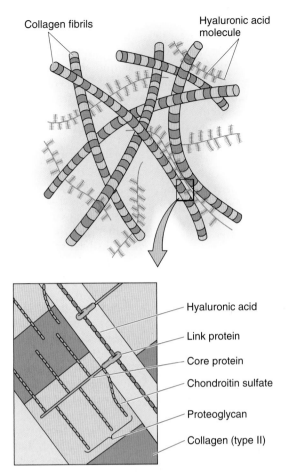

Figure 4.1 Diagrammatic representation of ECM. *Top,* Lower magnification showing the banded collagen fibers with the adherent proteoglycans. *Bottom,* GAGs attached to their protein core and the link proteins that attach them to hyaluronic acid, forming huge macromolecules that may be hundreds of million daltons in size. *(Adapted from Fawcett DW: Bloom and Fawcett's A Textbook of Histology, 11th ed. Philadelphia, Saunders, 1986.)*

Table 4.1 TYPES OF GLYCOSAMINOGLYCANS (GAGs)

GAG	Mass (Da)	Repeating Disaccharides	Location in Body
Hyaluronic acid	10^7–10^8	D-glucuronic acid-β-1,3-N-acetyl-D-glucosamine	Most connective tissue, synovial fluid, cartilage, dermis
Keratan sulfate I and II	10,000–30,000	Galactose-β-1,4-N-acetyl-D-glucosamine-6-SO_4	Cornea (keratan sulfate I), cartilage (keratan sulfate II)
Heparan sulfate	15,000–20,000	D-glucuronic acid-β-1,3-N-acetyl galactosamine L-iduronic acid-2 or -SO_4-β-1,3-N-acetyl-D-galactosamine	Blood vessels, lung, basal lamina
Heparin (90%) (10%)	15,000–20,000	L-iduronic acid-β-1,4-sulfo-D-glucosamine-6-SO_4 D-glucuronic acid-β-1,4-N-acetylglucosamine-6-SO_4	Mast cell granule, liver, lung, skin
Chondroitin 4-sulfate	10,000–30,000	D-glucuronic acid-β-1,3-N-acetylgalactosamine-6-SO_4	Cartilage, bone, cornea, blood vessels
Chondroitin 6-sulfate	10,000–30,000	D-glucuronic acid-β-1,3-N-acetylgalactosamine-6-SO_4	Cartilage, Wharton's jelly, blood vessels
Dermatan sulfate	10,000–30,000	L-iduronic acid-α-1,3-N-acetylglucosamine-4-SO_4	Heart valves, skin, blood vessels

Adapted from Gartner LP, Hiatt JL: Color Textbook of Histology, 3rd ed. Philadelphia, Saunders, 2007, p 71.

Ground Substance (cont.)

facilitating cell movement, impeding spread of infection, and assisting in the formation of collagen. When attached to the cell membrane, proteoglycans can assist in binding the cell to ECM and can act as a receptor molecule.

- **Glycoproteins** (**cell adhesive glycoproteins**) are large protein molecules with some carbohydrate moieties linked to them. They possess several binding domains that are specific for certain integrins and for ECM molecules, permitting the adherence of cells and elements of the ECM to each other. The best known glycoproteins are:
  - **Fibronectin**, a large V-shaped dimer of approximately 440,000 Da manufactured by connective tissue cells such as fibroblasts, has binding sites for numerous ECM components and for integrin molecules, facilitating the adhesion of cells to ECM. Plasma fibronectin, a soluble form of fibronectin, is present in blood where it aids in coagulation, phagocytosis, and wound healing.
  - **Laminin**, a very large epithelially produced glycoprotein (950,000 Da), consists of three polypeptide chains. It is almost always located on the epithelial aspect of the basal lamina and has binding sites for basal lamina components and for the integrins.
  - **Entactin** (**nidogen**), binds to laminin and type IV collagen, facilitating an adherence between laminin and the basal lamina.
  - **Tenascin** is a large glycoprotein (1700 kDa) composed of six polypeptides that resembles a spider with only six legs projecting outward from a central mass and has binding sites for fibronectin and syndecan, a transmembrane proteoglycan. It is usually limited to embryonic connective tissue, where it delineates pathways along which embryonic cells can migrate.
  - **Osteopontin** is localized to bone where it aids calcification and binds to osteoclast integrins.
  - **Chondronectin** and **osteonectin** resemble fibronectin but are present in cartilage and bone, respectively. They have binding sites for the cells of cartilage and bone and for the components of their particular ECMs.

Fibers

Historically, **collagen**, **reticular**, and **elastic fibers** have been described to constitute the **fibers** of ECM, although it is now known that reticular fibers are type II of collagen fibers.

Collagen, constituting about 25% of the proteins of the body, is inelastic, and in noncalcified connective tissue it resists tensile forces. Based on their amino acid sequences, there are about 25 different collagens, classified into three categories according to the manner in which they polymerize—fibril-forming, fibril-associated, and network-forming. Some authors also recognize collagen-like proteins.

- **Fibril-forming collagens** (the most common ones are types I, II, III, V, and XI) assemble into ropelike molecules that congregate to form flexible, cable-like structures, whose tensile strength exceeds that of stainless steel. Because they are white, they are also called **white fibers**.
- **Fibril-associated collagens** (types are IX and XII) are located on the surface of collagen fibrils and facilitate collagen fibrils to be bound to other collagen fibrils and to elements of ECM.
- **Network-forming collagens** (types IV and VII) do not form ropelike structures; instead they aggregate to form a feltlike meshwork that constitutes the major component of the lamina densa of the basal lamina (type IV) and anchoring fibrils (type VII) that aid in anchoring the basal lamina to the lamina reticularis of the connective tissue.
- **Collagen-like proteins** include type XVII, associated with hemidesmosomes, and type XVIII localized to the basal laminae of blood vessels.

STRUCTURE OF FIBRIL-FORMING COLLAGEN

Unstained collagen fibers are colorless when viewed under the microscope and are very long, but only about 10 μm in diameter. Viewed with the electron microscope, these fibers exhibit a characteristic 67-nm cross-banding and longitudinal striations indicating that they are formed by collections of thinner fibrils that are 10 to 300 nm in diameter. These thin fibrils are composed of tropocollagen:

- Many **tropocollagen** subunits are aligned head to toe and side by side.
- A tropocollagen molecule, 280 nm long and 1.5 nm in diameter, is composed of three **alpha chains** coiled about one another (Fig. 4.2).
- An alpha chain is composed of about 1000 amino acids; every third amino acid in the chain is **glycine**.
- The alpha chains are rich in **hydroxyproline** to hold the three alpha chains together; **hydroxylysine**, holding adjacent tropocollagen molecules to each other; and **proline**, which usually follows glycine.

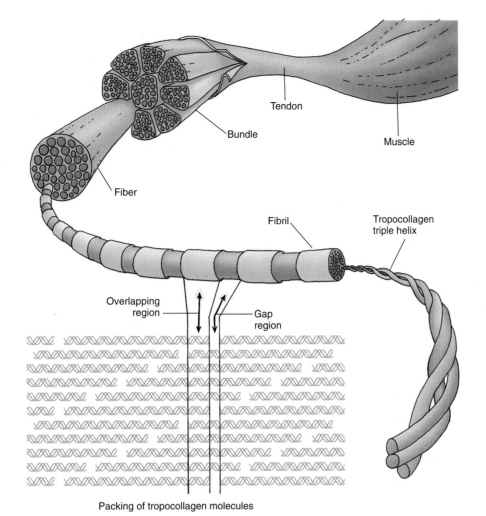

Figure 4.2 Components of type I collagen fiber. The arrangement of the gap and overlap regions of the adjoining tropocollagen molecules gives rise to the characteristic 67-nm cross-banding noted in electron micrographs. *(From Gartner LP, Hiatt JL: Color Textbook of Histology, 3rd ed. Philadelphia, Saunders, 2007, p 74.)*

CLINICAL CONSIDERATIONS

Collagenous colitis affects mostly middle-aged and elderly women, who present with loose, watery diarrhea with a relatively thick layer of acellular collagen just deep to the lining epithelium of the large intestine. Histologically, the epithelium of affected individuals is infiltrated by lymphocytes and neutrophils. The cause of collagenous colitis is unknown, although an autoimmune component has been postulated. The common treatment for this disease is administration of antidiarrheal or anti-inflammatory drugs or both. If infection is suspected, antibiotics may also alleviate the condition.

Alcoholic hepatitis is frequently accompanied by collagen deposition in the region of the central vein of the hepatic lobule. If the condition is not alleviated by the cessation of alcohol abuse, the patient may progress to a more serious state, **central hyaline sclerosis**, in which the inlet venule and the perivenular sinusoids are surrounded by a dense collagenous connective tissue, reducing blood flow and portal hypertension results. Patients with this disease present with fever, pain in the upper right quadrant of the abdomen, and jaundice; in 20% to 25% of cases, the condition may progress to liver failure and death.

Collagen Synthesis

Collagen is synthesized on the rough endoplasmic reticulum (RER) as individual **preprocollagen chains** coded for by individual mRNA molecules (Fig. 4.3).

- The amino and carboxyl terminals of these newly synthesized polypeptides possess extra propeptides.
- Within the RER cisterna, not only is the signal peptide removed, but also some of the proline and lysine residues are hydroxylated by peptidyl proline hydroxylase and peptidyl lysine hydroxylase, respectively.
- Additional post-translational modifications include selective glycosylation of some lysine residues.
- After the modifications, the three preprocollagen molecules use the propeptides to align with each other and form a tight helical configuration, but the propeptides do not wrap around each other.
- The three preprocollagen chains together are known as **procollagen,** which resembles a short rope with two frayed ends. The procollagen molecules do not adhere to each other, probably because of the propeptides, but leave the RER to enter the Golgi apparatus where oligosaccharides are added.
- They are packaged into coatomer protein (COP) I–coated vesicles and leave the *trans*-Golgi network and are transported out of the cell along the constitutive pathway.
- As the procollagen molecules are released into the extracellular space, their propeptides are cleaved by the membrane bound enzyme, **procollagen peptidase**, forming **tropocollagen** molecules (see Fig. 4.3).
- The absence of the propeptides permits the tropocollagen molecules to self-assemble and form type I collagen. The formation of type I collagen requires the presence of type XI collagen, which forms the core of type I collagen. Additionally, types III and V collagens are interspersed within the substance of the type I collagen fibrils. The alignment of the tropocollagen molecules and the shape of the collagen fiber that is being formed are determined by the cell that is synthesizing the collagen fiber.
- **Network-forming collagens** (types IV and VII) retain the propeptides of their procollagen molecules; they are unable to assemble into collagen fibers, and instead they form dimers that establish a feltlike meshwork.
- In some lymph nodes, the spleen, bone marrow, and thymus **reticular fibers** (type III collagen) are synthesized by specialized reticular cells that form a cellular sheath around these thin, branching, argyrophilic fibers to isolate them from their environment. In most other areas of the body, they are manufactured by fibroblasts or smooth muscle cells (in blood vessels) and Schwann cells (in peripheral nerves).

ELASTIC FIBERS

In contrast to collagen fibers, which are inelastic, **elastic fibers** may be stretched to 150% of their resting length, and when the tensile force is removed they return to their original length.

- **Elastic fibers**, also known as *yellow fibers* because of their color in their fresh state, are present in most noncalcified connective tissue elements of the body (manufactured by fibroblasts), and they are located in blood vessels (manufactured by smooth muscle cells) and elastic cartilage (synthesized by cartilage cells).
- These fibers may be present as very fine thin filaments, or they may be gathered into thick, coarse bundles. They are rarely visible in hematoxylin and eosin (H&E) dyed tissue sections, but become clearly evident with the use of special stains. Elastic fibers are composed of an amorphous elastin core surrounded by microfibrils (Fig. 4.4).
  - **Elastin** is a glycine-rich protein (72 kDa) that also has an abundance of alanine, lysine, proline, and valine, with a notable absence of hydroxylysine.
  - Four lysine molecules of different chains of this protein form highly deformable covalent bonds, known as **desmosine cross-links**, with each other. These desmosine cross-links provide the elasticity inherent to elastic fibers.
  - The **microfibrils** that surround the desmin core are composed of **fibrillin**, a 350-kDa glycoprotein.
  - During the synthesis of elastic fibers, the cell produces the microfibrils first and then deposits the amorphous elastin component into the region surrounded by the microfibrils.

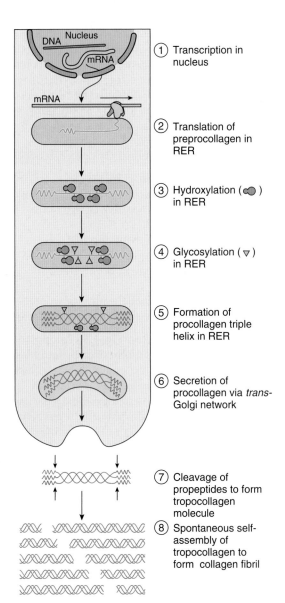

① Transcription in nucleus

② Translation of preprocollagen in RER

③ Hydroxylation (●) in RER

④ Glycosylation (▽) in RER

⑤ Formation of procollagen triple helix in RER

⑥ Secretion of procollagen via *trans*-Golgi network

⑦ Cleavage of propeptides to form tropocollagen molecule

⑧ Spontaneous self-assembly of tropocollagen to form collagen fibril

Figure 4.3 Type I collagen synthesis and assembly. Types III, V, and XI are not shown in this diagram. *(From Gartner LP, Hiatt JL: Color Textbook of Histology, 3rd ed. Philadelphia, Saunders, 2007, p 77.)*

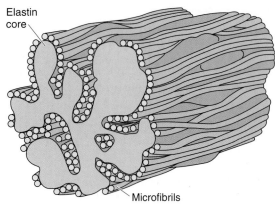

Figure 4.4 Elastic fiber. The amorphous elastin core is surrounded by microfibrils. *(From Gartner LP, Hiatt JL: Color Textbook of Histology, 3rd ed. Philadelphia, Saunders, 2007, p 80.)*

CLINICAL CONSIDERATIONS

Solar elastosis is a skin condition resulting from excess exposure to sun and ultraviolet rays in tanning salons. The sun-damaged skin is more wrinkled than normal, appears sagging, and looks and feels leathery. This condition is due to the damaged dermis, which has a decrease in collagen and increase in elastic fiber content. The elastic fibers lose some of their elasticity probably because their fibrillin components appear in disarray. This condition may progress to frank malignancy.

Scurvy is a condition that is due to the lack of vitamin C, a substance that is necessary for the hydroxylation of the proline moieties of preprocollagen. The paucity of hydroxyproline prevents tropocollagen molecules from assembling in a normal manner; tissues with a high turnover of collagen lead to loose teeth and bleeding gingivae. The consumption of vitamin C–rich foods corrects the problem.

Basement Membrane

Viewed with the light microscope, connective tissue and epithelium are always separated from each other by a narrow acellular zone, known as the **basement membrane**. On electron micrographs, the basement membrane can be seen to have two components:

- Very narrow, epithelially produced basal lamina
- Thicker, connective tissue–derived lamina reticularis (Fig. 4.5)

It is evident on electron micrographs that the **basal lamina** is also composed of two layers:

- A 50-nm-thick clear region, known as the **lamina lucida**, abutting the basal cell membranes of the epithelial sheet
- A 50-nm-thick dense, matlike layer, known as the **lamina densa**, which occupies the region between the lamina lucida and the lamina reticularis

Some investigators suggest, however, that the lamina lucida is a fixation artifact, and that the basal lamina is composed only of the lamina densa. In addition to separating epithelium from connective tissue, basal laminae, referred to as **external laminae**, are also noted to surround Schwann cells, skeletal and smooth muscle cells, and fat cells. A thickened basal lamina is present in the glomerulus of the kidney.

BASAL LAMINA AND LAMINA RETICULARIS

The lamina lucida component (whether or not present as a morphological entity) of the **basal lamina** (see Fig. 4.5) houses the extracellular portions of the integral cell membrane proteins, **integrin** and **dystroglycan**, both of which are laminin receptors. Additionally, **laminin** and **entactin**, two structural glycoproteins, form a thin sheath on the surface of the lamina densa, the dense-appearing matlike component of the basal lamina whose main constituent is **type IV collagen** (see Fig. 4.5). The lamina lucida and the lamina reticularis–facing surfaces of the lamina densa are coated with the **heparan sulfate–** rich proteoglycan, **perlacan**. Additionally, the lamina reticularis–facing surface of the lamina densa is rich in fibronectin.

Because laminin binds to integrins and dystroglycans of epithelial cells and to heparan sulfate and type IV collagen of the lamina densa, the epithelium is securely anchored to the basal lamina. The lamina densa is firmly bound to the underlying lamina reticularis by means of fibronectin, type VII collagen (anchoring fibrils), and microfibrils (fibrillin), ensuring the firm attachment of the epithelium not only to the basal lamina, but also to the lamina reticularis.

The basal lamina functions:

- In ensuring epithelial attachment
- As a molecular filter owing to its type IV collagen component and to the negative charge of its heparan sulfate molecules
- In enhancing mitotic activity of cells
- In binding signaling molecules
- In facilitating rearrangement of integral cell membrane proteins
- As an aid in the re-epithelialization of wounds and in the regeneration of myoneural junctions

The **lamina reticularis** (see Fig. 4.5), composed of types I and III collagens, is synthesized by fibroblasts. It is of variable thickness, depending on the abrasive forces acting on the epithelium superficial to it; it is thick deep to the epithelium of the palms of the hand and soles of the foot and thin beneath the epithelium of the lung tissue. The collagens of the lamina reticularis arise from and are continuous with the collagens of the connective tissue, forming a secure bond not only between the basal lamina and the lamina reticularis, but also between the connective tissue and the lamina reticularis, and in that fashion firmly securing the epithelium to the connective tissue.

Integrins and Dystroglycans

Integrins are transmembrane proteins whose extracellular moiety binds, in the presence of divalent cations, with certain ligands present in ECM, and their intracellular carboxyl ends bind to **talins** and **α-actinins** of the cytoskeleton. Integrins are able to transduce extracellular signals into intracellular molecular events that result in cell division or regulation of gene expression or both.

Dystroglycans are also heterodimer transmembrane proteins whose extracellular moiety binds to a particular site on laminin, whereas their intracellular moiety binds with **dystrophin**, an actin-binding protein that forms a bond with the cytoskeleton.

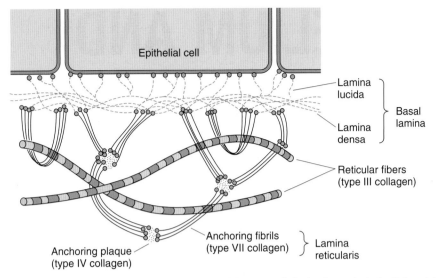

Figure 4.5 The basement membrane has two components, the basal lamina and the lamina reticularis. *(Adapted from Fawcett DW: Bloom and Fawcett's a Textbook of Histology, 12th ed. New York, Chapman & Hall, 1994.)*

CLINICAL CONSIDERATIONS

Goodpasture syndrome is an autoimmune condition that involves the kidneys and the lungs. If only the kidneys are involved, the condition is referred to as **anti–glomerular basement membrane antibody glomerulonephritis**. In either condition, the autoimmune reaction is against the type IV collagen of the basal lamina. The onset of Goodpasture syndrome is usually subsequent to a respiratory tract infection, and the lung involvement is related to smoking. Patients are usually young men, although both sexes and all ages have been affected. The disease can rapidly progress to renal failure and the need for renal transplant. Treatment in the early stages is with corticosteroids, the administration of cytotoxic compounds, and plasmapheresis. Frequently, the disease is fatal, and even with aggressive treatment the survival rate is only 50% within 2 years of the onset of the disease.

Alport syndrome (hereditary nephritis) is a genetic disease caused by a mutation in the *COL4A5* gene responsible for the coding for type IV collagen; these patients do not form normal basal laminae. The glomerular basal lamina of these patients is abnormally thick and appears to split into interweaving layers as if it were composed of blisters. The syndrome is more prevalent and severe in males, although both sexes are affected. The disease progresses to end-stage renal failure by the fifth decade of life in most men and in about 20% of women. Additionally, at least 50% of patients of both sexes experience progressive hearing loss and damage to the lenses of the eyes.

CLINICAL CONSIDERATIONS

Some cases of osteoarthritis are treated by repeated injections of hyaluronic acid, a component of synovial fluid, directly into the joint to lubricate it providing relief for a prolonged period.

5 EPITHELIUM AND GLANDS

The human body consists of more than 200 cell types organized into the four basic tissues: epithelium, connective tissue, muscle, and nervous tissue. Combinations of these tissues form functional entities known as *organs,* which are combined into organ systems.

Epithelial Tissue

Epithelial tissue can exist as sheets of adjoining cells covering or lining the body surface or as glands, secretory organs derived from epithelial cells. Most epithelia originate from ectoderm and endoderm, although mesoderm also gives rise to some epithelia.

- **Ectoderm** gives rise to the epidermis of the skin, lining of the mouth and nasal cavity, cornea, sweat and sebaceous glands, and mammary glands.
- **Endoderm** gives rise to the lining of the gastrointestinal and respiratory systems and to the glands of the gastrointestinal system.
- **Mesoderm** gives rise to the uriniferous tubules of the kidney, the lining of the reproductive and circulatory systems, and the lining of the body cavities.

Epithelium, an avascular tissue organized into sheets, receives its nutrients from the vascular supply of the adjacent connective tissue. It is composed of closely packed cells, held together by junctional complexes, with little intervening extracellular space and a scant amount of extracellular matrix. The two tissues are separated from each other by the epithelially derived basal lamina. Epithelial tissue functions in:

- **Protection** of the tissues that it covers or lines,
- **Transcellular transport** of molecules across epithelial sheets,
- **Secretion** of various substances by glands,
- **Absorption** (e.g., intestinal tract and kidney tubules),
- **Control of movement of ions and molecules** via selective permeability, and
- **Detection of sensations** (e.g., taste, sight, hearing).

> **KEY WORDS**
> - **Epithelium**
> - **Simple epithelium**
> - **Stratified epithelium**
> - **Microvilli**
> - **Junctional complex**
> - **Unicellular exocrine glands**
> - **Multicellular exocrine glands**
> - **Endocrine glands**

CLASSIFICATION OF EPITHELIAL MEMBRANES

The epithelium can be classified based on the number of layers of cells between the basal lamina and the free surface and the morphology of the cells. A single layer of epithelial cells is called **simple epithelium**, whereas two or more layers constitute a **stratified epithelium**. The epithelial cells abutting the free surface may be squamous (flat), cuboidal, or columnar, giving rise to the various types of epithelia (Table 5.1 and Fig. 5.1). Two additional types of epithelia are pseudostratified columnar and transitional.

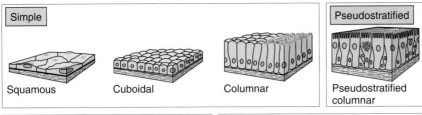

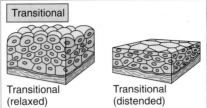

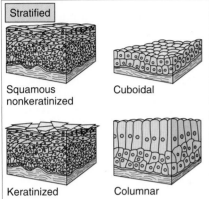

Figure 5.1 Types of epithelia. *(From Gartner LP, Hiatt JL: Color Textbook of Histology, 3rd ed. Philadelphia, Saunders, 2007, p 87.)*

Table 5.1 CLASSIFICATION OF EPITHELIA

Type	Shape of Surface Cells	Sample Locations	Functions
Simple			
Simple squamous	Flattened	*Lining*: pulmonary alveoli, loop of Henle, parietal layer of Bowman's capsule, inner and middle ear, blood and lymphatic vessels, pleural and peritoneal cavities	Limiting membrane, fluid transport, gaseous exchange, lubrication, reducing friction (aiding movement of viscera), lining membrane
Simple cuboidal	Cuboidal	Ducts of many glands, covering of ovary, form kidney tubules	Secretion, absorption, protection
Simple columnar	Columnar	*Lining*: oviducts, ductuli efferentes of testis, uterus, small bronchi, much of digestive tract, gallbladder, and large ducts of some glands	Transportation, absorption, secretion, protection
Pseudostratified	All cells rest on basal lamina, but not all reach epithelial surface; surface cells are columnar	*Lining*: most of trachea, primary bronchi, epididymis and ductus deferens, auditory tube, part of tympanic cavity, nasal cavity, lacrimal sac, male urethra, large excretory ducts	Secretion, absorption, lubrication, protection, transportation
Stratified			
Stratified squamous (nonkeratinized)	Flattened (with nuclei)	*Lining*: mouth, epiglottis, esophagus, vocal folds, vagina	Protection, secretion
Stratified squamous (keratinized)	Flattened (without nuclei)	Epidermis of skin	Protection
Stratified cuboidal	Cuboidal	*Lining*: ducts of sweat glands	Absorption, secretion
Stratified columnar	Columnar	Conjunctiva of eye, some large excretory ducts, portions of male urethra	Secretion, absorption, protection
Transitional	Dome-shaped (relaxed), flattened (distended)	*Lining*: urinary tract from renal calyces to urethra	Protection, distensible

From Gartner LP, Hiatt JL: Color Textbook of Histology, 3rd ed. Philadelphia, Saunders, 2007, p 86.

POLARITY AND CELL SURFACE SPECIALIZATIONS

Epithelial cells generally possess specific regions—**domains**—that impart a distinct polarity to the cell. These domains are defined by their location at the apex or at the basolateral region of the cell. Tight junctions, which are a specialization of the cell membrane, encircle the apex of the cell, separating the two domains from each other and imparting a polarity to the cell. Each domain possesses specific modifications.

Apical Domain

The apical domain, the region of the epithelial cell facing the free surface, has an abundance of ion channels, carrier proteins, H^+-ATPase, aquaporins, glycoproteins, and hydrolytic enzymes. Additionally, it serves as the region where regulated secretory products leave the cell to enter the extracellular space. Surface modifications of the apical domain, such as microvilli and associated glycocalyx, cilia, stereocilia, and flagella, assist in performing many of the cell's functions.

- **Microvilli** (Fig. 5.2) are 1- to 2-μm-long membrane-bound, finger-like projections of the apical cell surfaces of simple cuboidal and simple columnar epithelia. They represent the striated and brush borders of light microscopy and, when closely packed, may increase the surface area as much as 20-fold.
  - The core of each microvillus is composed of 25 to 30 actin filaments that are held to each other by **villin** and **fimbrin**; those at the periphery of the bundle adhere to the plasmalemma via **calmodulin** and **myosin I**.
  - The plus ends of the actin filaments reach the tip of the microvillus, where they are embedded in an amorphous substance.
  - The cytoplasmic ends of the actin bundle are fixed to the terminal web and composed of intermediate filaments, spectrin, actin, and other cytoskeletal components.
  - The extracellular aspect of the microvillar membrane is coated with a glycocalyx whose composition depends on the location and function of the cell.
  - Long, nonmotile, rigid microvilli, present only in the epididymis and on the sensory hair cells of the cochlea (inner ear), are called **stereocilia**. They function in increasing surface to facilitate absorption in the epididymis, whereas in the ear they assist the hair cells in signal generation.
- **Cilia** (Fig. 5.3) are long (7 to 10 μm in length and 0.2 μm in diameter), finger-like structures projecting from the apical domain of the cell. They are highly conserved structures that are present in unicellular organisms, in plants, and in all members of the animal kingdom. Cilia are contractile structures that allow unicellular organisms to move through water; in higher animals, where an epithelial sheet, such as that lining the respiratory tract, can have 2 billion cilia/cm², their coordinated action can propel a fluid along an epithelial sheet.
  - The core of the cilium, known as the **axoneme**, is a highly organized longitudinal arrangement of nine **doublets** surrounding two **singlet** microtubules, dynein, and associated elastic proteins.
  - Each doublet comprises a whole microtubule (**subunit A**), which is composed of 13 protofilaments, and a partial microtubule (**subunit B**), which has 10 protofilaments and shares 3 protofilaments of the whole microtubule.
  - Subunit A of each doublet possesses **dynein arms** located at prescribed intervals of 24 nm along its entire length, resembling the legs of a millipede. The free ends of these arms possess adenosine triphosphate (ATP)–dependent binding sites for subunit B.
  - The elastic proteins associated with the axoneme are arranged in the following manner: the two central singlets are surrounded by a **central sheath**, and a **radial spoke** projects toward the central sheath from each subunit A.
  - Additionally, subunit A of one doublet is connected to subunit B of the adjacent doublets by a **nexin bridge**.
  - Viewed in three dimensions, the central sheet is a cylinder around the singlets; each nexin bridge and each radial arm is a quadrilateral sheet of elastic material.

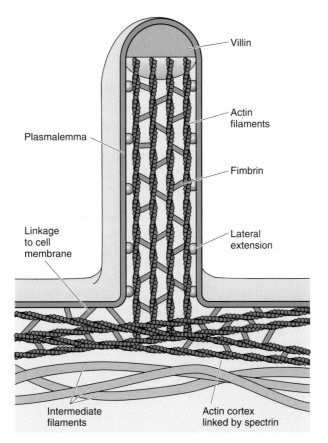

Figure 5.2 Structure of a microvillus. *(From Gartner LP, Hiatt JL: Color Textbook of Histology, 3rd ed. Philadelphia, Saunders, 2007, p 94.)*

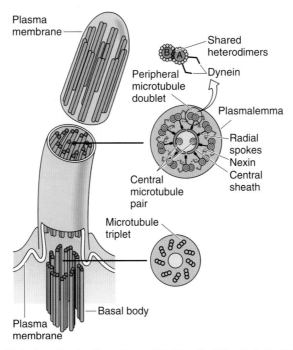

Figure 5.3 Structure of a cilium with its basal body. *(From Gartner LP, Hiatt JL: Color Textbook of Histology, 3rd ed. Philadelphia, Saunders, 2007, p 95.)*

Ciliary Movement, Basal Body, and Flagella

During ciliary movement in the presence of ATP, the dynein arms fleetingly attach to and detach from subunit B of the adjacent doublet climbing up toward the cilium tip. Nexin and the radial spokes tend to restrain the climbing action, however, and the cilium bends instead.

- The bending of the cilium (a process that requires ATP) stretches the elastic proteins; however, when the dynein arms cease their climbing action, the elastic proteins return to their normal length, and the cilium resumes its straight position (an ATP-independent process).
- Alternating these two processes in rapid progression permits the cilia to propel substances along the epithelial surface.

The axoneme arrangement ceases at the base of the cilium where it is attached to the **basal body** (Fig. 5.4), a structure composed of nine **triplet microtubules** (subunits A, B, and C) with no central singlets. The basal body resembles a centriole and develops from **procentriole organizers**.

- **Subunits A and B** of the cilium are continuous with subunits A and B of the basal body.
- **Subunit C** of the basal body does not continue into the cilium.

Certain cells, including fibroblasts, neurons, and certain epithelial cells such as those of kidney tubules, may possess a single nonmotile cilium whose axoneme has no dynein arms. These are known as **primary cilia**, and they are believed to function as sensory organs or signal receptors.

Flagella, present only on spermatozoa in humans, are modified cilia that possess an axoneme and a robust elastic protein complex that is designed to propel the spermatozoa along the female reproductive tract. Flagella are described in Chapter 21.

Basolateral Domain

Two regions constitute the basolateral domain of epithelia, the lateral and basal plasma membranes. Specialized junctional complexes and signal receptors, ion channels, and Na$^+$,K$^+$-ATPase abound in these regions, which also function as sites for constitutive secretion.

Lateral Membrane Specializations

Terminal bars, as viewed by light microscopy, are sites of apparent attachment of epithelial cells that have been shown to be structures that are continuous around the circumference of the entire cell. Terminal bars occupy restricted regions of the cell located in the vicinity of its apex. When examined with the electron microscope, the terminal bars were resolved to be **junctional complexes** that facilitate the adherence of contiguous cells to each other (Fig. 5.5). Three types of cell junctions constitute the terminal bar: the apicalmost **zonula occludens** and just basal to it, the **zonula adherens**, both of which are continuous, beltlike junctions around the circumference of the cell, and the **maculae adherentes (desmosomes)**, which are spot junctions rather than continuous around the cell's perimeter. Additional types of cell junctions are located in regions of the cell other than at terminal bars and do not belong to the junctional complex. These are **gap junctions**, **desmosomes**, **hemidesmosomes**, and **actin-linked cell-matrix adhesions**. From a functional perspective, there are three types of epithelial cell junctions:

- **Occluding junctions (zonulae occludentes)** provide an impermeable, or selectively permeable, barrier that prevents material from traversing an epithelial membrane between adjoining cells (paracellular route).
- **Anchoring junctions (zonulae adherentes, maculae adherentes, hemidesmosomes, actin-linked cell-matrix adhesions)** permit epithelial cells to adhere to each other or to the basal lamina or both.
- **Communicating junctions (gap junctions)** permit the transcytoplasmic movement of ions and small molecules between adjacent cells, coupling them electrically and metabolically.

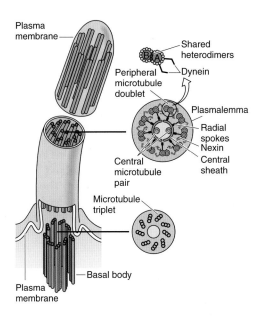

Figure 5.4 Structure of a cilium with its basal body. *(From Gartner LP, Hiatt JL: Color Textbook of Histology, 3rd ed. Philadelphia, Saunders, 2007, p 95.)*

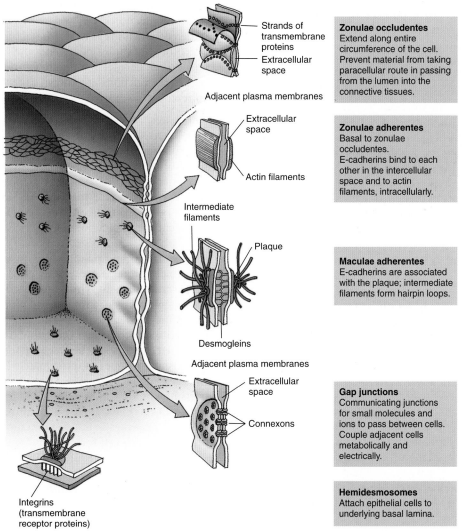

Zonulae occludentes
Extend along entire circumference of the cell. Prevent material from taking paracellular route in passing from the lumen into the connective tissues.

Zonulae adherentes
Basal to zonulae occludentes.
E-cadherins bind to each other in the intercellular space and to actin filaments, intracellularly.

Maculae adherentes
E-cadherins are associated with the plaque; intermediate filaments form hairpin loops.

Gap junctions
Communicating junctions for small molecules and ions to pass between cells. Couple adjacent cells metabolically and electrically.

Hemidesmosomes
Attach epithelial cells to underlying basal lamina.

Figure 5.5 Junctional complexes. *(From Gartner LP, Hiatt JL: Color Textbook of Histology, 3rd ed. Philadelphia, Saunders, 2007, p 97.)*

Zonulae occludentes (tight junctions), the most apical component of the junctional complex, are formed by the fusion of the outer leaflets of adjacent cell membranes (Fig. 5.6). The fusion extends along the entire circumference of epithelial cells and, when viewed with freeze fracture electron microscopy, **fusion strands**, linear arrangements of transmembrane proteins, are evident on the P-face, and concomitant linear grooves are noted on the E-face.

- Depending on the integrity of the tight junction, several instances of fusion may be present, resembling a diverging system of fusion strands, so that some zonulae occludentes are more leaky, having fewer fusion strands, or less leaky, possessing more fusion strands.
- These transmembrane proteins are present in the membranes of both cells, and they contact each other, in a calcium-independent manner, in the extracellular space, obliterating that space. There are three types of transmembrane proteins present in tight junctions:
  - **Claudins** are the most important of the three components; this protein blocks the extracellular space when two cells contact one another.
  - **Tricellulin**, instead of claudin, is present in regions where *three* cells contact each other.
  - **Occludins** are the third type of protein; their function is not understood.
- Tight junctions are reinforced by the other two components of the junctional complex, zonulae adherentes and maculae adherentes.
  - Three cytoplasmic scaffolding proteins—tight junction proteins (zonula occludens) ZO1, ZO2, and ZO3—ensure the proper alignment of the claudins, occludins, and tricellulins of cells facing each other, but the mechanism of their actions is not understood.
  - Attached to the ZO1 protein is another complex of molecules, **afadin-nectin complex**, which is believed to meet its counterpart from the adjoining cell and reinforce the adherence of the claudins to each other.

Tight junctions limit or prevent paracellular movement of material across the epithelial sheet, and prevent the migration of integral proteins between the apical and basolateral domains of the cell membrane.

Zonulae adherentes, similar to zonulae occludentes, are *beltlike* junctions that encircle the cell (see Fig. 5.6). These adhesion junctions rely on calcium-dependent **transmembrane linker proteins**, **cadherins**, to hold adjacent cells to one another. The calcium-sensitive moiety of cadherins is extracellularly located and is a flexible, hingelike structure.

- In the presence of Ca^{++}, the hinge region is unable to flex, and as it extends, it contacts and binds to the extended moiety of the cadherin of the adjacent cell, but the two membranes cannot be more than 15 to 20 nm apart. The intracellular moieties of cadherins are affixed to actin filament bundles that course parallel to the cell membrane.
- The links to the actin filaments occur via catenins, vinculin, and α-actinin. In this fashion, the transmembrane linker cadherins attach the cytoskeleton of one cell to the cytoskeleton of its neighboring cell. As in the zonulae occludentes, an **afadin-nectin complex** reinforces this adhesion junction.
- Adherens junctions may also be *ribbonlike* attachments, as in capillary endothelia, where they do not encircle the perimeter of the cell; here these junctions are known as **fasciae adherentes**.

Other *weldlike* cell junctions, known as **desmosomes** (approximately $400 \times 250 \times 10$ nm), appear to be haphazardly located on the basolateral plasmalemmae of cells of simple epithelia and on the adjacent cell membranes of stratified squamous epithelia, such as that of the epidermis (see Fig. 5.6). Each half of a desmosome pairs up on the intracellular surfaces of the membranes of adjoining epithelial cells.

- **Desmoplakins** and **pakoglobins** function as attachment proteins composing each plaque.
- Cytokeratin filaments (**intermediate filaments**) are thought to reduce the shearing forces on the cell as they penetrate the plaque and turn back on themselves to reenter the cytoplasm.
- The intercellular space between opposing desmosome plaques (approximately 30 nm in width) contains filamentous Ca^{++}-dependent **transmembrane linker proteins** of the cadherin family, **desmoglein** and **desmocollin**.
- If Ca^{++} is present, the transmembrane linker proteins of each cell form a bond with each other. When calcium is unavailable, the bond is broken, and the two halves of the desmosome are unable to maintain their firm contact, and the cells become detached from each other.

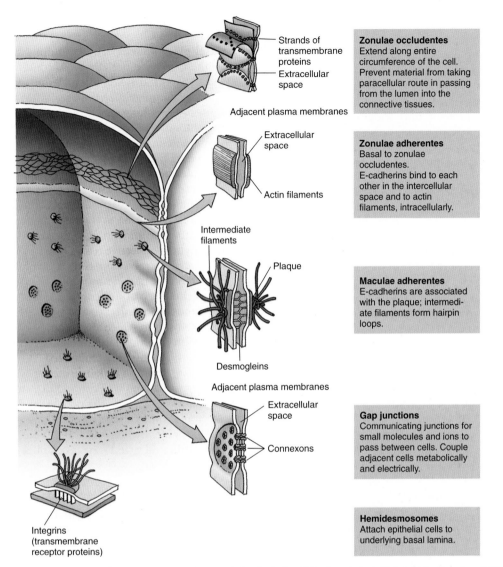

Zonulae occludentes
Extend along entire circumference of the cell. Prevent material from taking paracellular route in passing from the lumen into the connective tissues.

Zonulae adherentes
Basal to zonulae occludentes.
E-cadherins bind to each other in the intercellular space and to actin filaments, intracellularly.

Maculae adherentes
E-cadherins are associated with the plaque; intermediate filaments form hairpin loops.

Gap junctions
Communicating junctions for small molecules and ions to pass between cells. Couple adjacent cells metabolically and electrically.

Hemidesmosomes
Attach epithelial cells to underlying basal lamina.

Figure 5.6 Junctional complexes. *(From Gartner LP, Hiatt JL: Color Textbook of Histology, 3rd ed. Philadelphia, Saunders, 2007, p 97.)*

CLINICAL CONSIDERATIONS

Pemphigus vulgaris is an autoimmune disease of the skin in which antibodies are produced against desmosomal proteins. Antibodies bind to the desmosomal proteins disturbing cell adhesion. This disturbance leads to blistering of the epidermis causing loss of tissue fluids. If this condition is left untreated, death occurs. Systemic steroids and immunosuppressants are used to control this disease.

The most abundant of the junctional complexes, gap junctions, are present in most epithelial tissues and neurons and in cardiac and smooth muscle cells. Gap junctions are sites of intercellular communication because they permit small molecules to pass through the narrow (2 to 4 nm) wide intercellular space. These gap junctions couple cells chemically and electrically to each other, facilitating intercellular communications in adult and embryonic tissues.

- Six **connexins**, transmembrane channel–forming proteins, gather to form aqueous channels, known as **connexons**, in the cell membrane (Fig. 5.7).
- The number of connexons that are present in a gap junction varies from a few to several thousands.
- Connexons of one side of the gap junction that are in register with connexons on the opposing side of the gap junction bind to each other forming a hydrophilic communication channel, 1.5 to 2 nm in diameter, through which molecules less than 1 kDa in size can pass between adjoining cells.
- Although the manner in which passage of material through gap junctions is not understood, it is known that an increase in cytosolic Ca^{++} concentrations or a decrease in cytosolic pH closes gap junctions, whereas gap junctions open if the cytoplasmic pH is high, or Ca^{++} concentration is low.

Basal Surface Specializations

Basal lamina, cell membrane plications, and hemidesmosomes are the three principal specializations of the basal surfaces of epithelial cells (see Fig. 5.7). Hemidesmosomes, located on the basal surface of the cell, contribute to anchoring the basal plasma membrane to the underlying basal lamina.

- The **basal lamina**, a product of the epithelium located at the interface between the epithelium and the underlying connective tissue, was discussed in Chapter 4.
- **Basal plasma membrane enfoldings** of epithelial cells, especially those concerned with ion transport, increase plasmalemma surface area and compartmentalize the basal cytoplasm into mitochondria-housing segments. The presence of mitochondria coupled with the plicated plasma membrane makes the cell appear striated when viewed by light microscopy.
- **Hemidesmosomes** appear to be half of a desmosome and are located on the basal plasma membrane. They assist in the attachment of the basal plasmalemma to the basal lamina, facilitating the anchoring of the cell to the underlying connective tissue.
  - Located on the cytoplasmic side of the plasma membrane, hemidesmosomes display **attachment plaques** composed of desmoplakins, plectin, and other minor proteins, into which the terminal ends of **keratin intermediate filaments (tonofilaments)** are embedded.
  - **Transmembrane linker proteins**, which are integrins, a family of extracellular matrix receptors, penetrate the plaque on the cytoplasmic side and pass through the cell membrane; their extracellular moiety binds to **laminin** and **type IV collagen** present in the basal lamina.

Renewal of Epithelial Cells

There is a high replacement rate for cells of an epithelium, but this rate is faster in some organs, as in the lining of the gastrointestinal tract, and slower in other regions, as in the epidermis of skin. The renewal rate for a particular organ is generally constant, however. In the event that numerous cells are lost because of infection or injury, mitotic activity is increased to restore the cell population to normal levels.

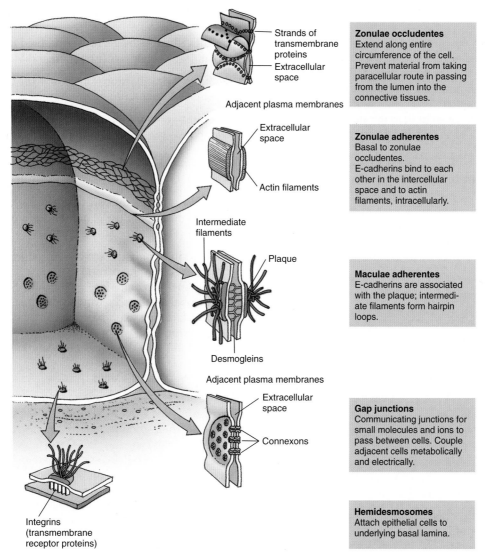

Zonulae occludentes
Extend along entire circumference of the cell. Prevent material from taking paracellular route in passing from the lumen into the connective tissues.

Zonulae adherentes
Basal to zonulae occludentes. E-cadherins bind to each other in the intercellular space and to actin filaments, intracellularly.

Maculae adherentes
E-cadherins are associated with the plaque; intermediate filaments form hairpin loops.

Gap junctions
Communicating junctions for small molecules and ions to pass between cells. Couple adjacent cells metabolically and electrically.

Hemidesmosomes
Attach epithelial cells to underlying basal lamina.

Figure 5.7 Junctional complexes. *(From Gartner LP, Hiatt JL: Color Textbook of Histology, 3rd ed. Philadelphia, Saunders, 2007, p 97.)*

CLINICAL CONSIDERATIONS

Nonsyndromic deafness and the skin disease **erythrokeratodermia variabilis** are the result of connexin gene mutations. Mutations of connexin genes are also associated with aberrant migration of neural crest cells leading to developmental defects in the pulmonary vessels of the heart.

Diverse populations of epithelial cells display their own distinctive characteristics that are based on many factors, including location and environment, but all are related to function. Under certain pathological conditions, epithelial cells may be transformed into another epithelial type via a process called **metaplasia**. The respiratory epithelium (pseudostratified ciliated columnar epithelium) of a heavy smoker may undergo **squamous metaplasia** resulting in an epithelial transformation to a stratified squamous epithelium, restricting function. This transformation may be reversed after the environmental insult is removed.

Epithelial cell tumors may be benign or malignant. The malignant tumors that arise from epithelia are known as **carcinomas**. Malignant tumors of glands are called **adenocarcinomas**. Cancers in children younger than 10 years are least likely to be derived from epithelia, whereas adenocarcinomas are most prominent in adults. About 90% of all cancers in adults older than 45 years originate in epithelia.

Glands

During the development of certain regions of the body, epithelial cells invade the underlying connective tissue, form the **parenchyma** (secretory units and ducts) of glands, and surround themselves with a basal lamina that they secrete. The surrounding connective tissue, referred to as the **stroma**, supports the parenchyma of the gland by providing vascular and neural supplies, and its structural elements such as capsules, which envelop the entire gland, and septa, which subdivide the gland into lobes and lobules. The individual cells of the gland's secretory units synthesize secretory products and store them in intracellular compartments known as **secretory granules** until the secretion is released. Depending on the gland, these secretory products may be as varied as:

- A hormone, such as insulin from the islets of Langerhans;
- An enzyme, such as salivary amylase from the parotid gland, or a bicarbonate-rich fluid from Brunner's glands of the duodenum; or
- A tear, a watery secretion from the lacrimal gland.

Two principal categories of glands exist based on the manner of delivery of their secretory products:

- **Exocrine glands** possess ducts through which their secretory products are delivered onto an epithelial surface.
- **Endocrine glands** are **ductless**; consequently, their secretory product is delivered directly into the bloodstream or lymphatic vessels.

Frequently, cells communicate with each other by releasing **cytokines**, which are signaling molecules designed to act on specific cells known as **target cells**. Cells secreting cytokines are known as **signaling cells**, and their signaling molecules bind to receptors inducing these target cells to perform a specific function (see Chapter 2). The effects of cytokines may be classified into three categories, based on the distance between the signaling cell and the target cell:

- **Autocrine**: The signaling cell and the target cell are the same—the cell stimulates itself.
- **Paracrine**: The target cell and signaling cell are near each other, so the cytokine can diffuse to the target cell.
- **Endocrine**: A great enough distance separates the signaling cell from the target cell so that the cytokine has to enter the blood or lymphatic system to reach its destination.

EXOCRINE GLANDS

Exocrine glands may be classified by the number of cells that compose the gland:

- **Unicellular**—a single cell is the entire gland (e.g., goblet cell)
- **Multicellular**—the gland is composed of more than just a single cell (e.g., submandibular gland).

Additional classifications are based on the type of secretion the gland produces:

- **Serous**—watery (e.g., parotid gland)
- **Mucous**—viscous (e.g., minor salivary glands of the palate)
- **Mixed**—serous and mucous (e.g., sublingual gland)

Still other classifications are based on the mechanism whereby the cells of the gland release their secretory products (Fig. 5.8):

- **Merocrine**—only the secretory product is released (as in the parotid gland)
- **Apocrine**—a small piece of the cell's cytoplasm accompanies the secretory product (as, perhaps, in the lactating mammary gland)
- **Holocrine**—the entire cell dies and becomes the secretion (as in the sebaceous gland)

Unicellular Exocrine Glands

The **goblet cell**, located in the epithelial lining of the small and large intestines and of the conducting portion of the respiratory tract, is the principal example of a unicellular exocrine gland (Fig. 5.9). The narrow base of the goblet cell, known as the **stem**, contacts the basal lamina. The **theca**, the apical portion of the cell, expanded by the numerous **mucinogen**-containing secretory granules, abuts the lumen of the intestine or that of the conducting portion of the respiratory system. Mucinogen, released as a result of noxious chemical stimulation or by neurotransmitter substances derived from the parasympathetic nervous system, is hydrated to form the viscous slippery substance known as **mucin**, which, when mixed with other components located in the lumen, is known as **mucus**.

CLINICAL CONSIDERATIONS

Sjögren syndrome is a chronic inflammatory autoimmune disease of the salivary and lacrimal glands in which the secretory units of these exocrine glands are rendered unable to release their secretions, resulting in dry mouth and dry eyes. This condition may occur in isolation, or it may be associated with underlying disorders, such as rheumatoid arthritis, lupus, and scleroderma; it is also associated with the development of lymphoma. Sjögren syndrome affects women nine times more frequently than men. Currently, this disease is incurable.

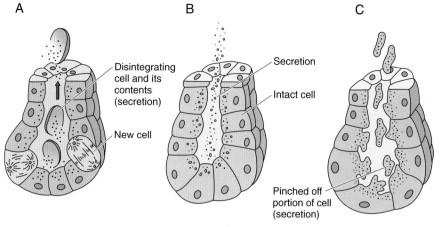

A, Holocrine — Disintegrating cell and its contents (secretion); New cell

B, Merocrine — Secretion; Intact cell

C, Apocrine — Pinched off portion of cell (secretion)

Figure 5.8 Modes of glandular secretion. **A,** Holocrine. **B,** Merocrine. **C,** Apocrine. *(From Gartner LP, Hiatt JL: Color Textbook of Histology, 3rd ed. Philadelphia, Saunders, 2007, p 105.)*

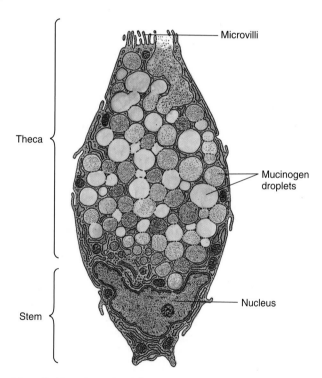

Theca — Microvilli; Mucinogen droplets

Stem — Nucleus

Figure 5.9 Ultrastructure of a goblet cell. *(From Lentz TL: Cell Fine Structure: An Atlas of Drawings of Whole-Cell Structure. Philadelphia, Saunders, 1971.)*

Multicellular Exocrine Glands

Secretory cells that are grouped together and organized to act as secretory organs are **multicellular exocrine glands**. Some multicellular glands display a simple structure (e.g., gastric mucosa and in the uterus), or they may be complex structures that exhibit assorted types of secretory units along with compound branching (e.g., submandibular gland). Multicellular glands are classified according to the shape and organization of their secretory units and their duct components. They may be classified as:

• **Simple**, where the ducts do not branch, or
• **Compound**, where the ducts branch.

The morphology of the secretory units on the compound ducts is classified as **acinar (alveolar)**, **tubular**, or **tubuloalveolar** (Fig. 5.10).

Collagenous connective tissue forms capsules that encase large multicellular glands and form strands called **septa** that add structural support to the gland by subdividing the gland into **lobes** and **lobules** (Fig. 5.11). Nerves, blood vessels, and ducts access and exit the glands via the passageways of the septa.

Myoepithelial cells—cells of epithelial origin that possess the ability to contract—are present in major salivary glands and sweat glands, where they share the same basal lamina as the glandular acini. Glandular acini and small ducts are wrapped by fibrillar strands of cytoplasm that extend from these myoepithelial cells. Contractions of these cells squeeze the acini and small ducts, assisting them in delivering their secretory product.

ENDOCRINE GLANDS

The endocrine glands include the suprarenal (adrenal), thyroid, pituitary, parathyroid, ovaries, testes, placenta, and pineal glands. Because these glands are ductless, they must release their secretions (hormones) into the blood or into the lymphatic vessels so that they can be distributed to the target organs. Certain of these endocrine glands (e.g., the islets of Langerhans of the pancreas and the interstitial cells of Leydig in the testes) are simply composed of clusters of cells embedded within the connective tissue stroma of those organs.

Hormones secreted by endocrine glands include proteins, peptides, steroids, modified amino acids, and glycoproteins (see Chapter 13). Endocrine secretory cells are arranged as cords or as follicles. Cords, the most common, frequently anastomose around capillaries or blood sinusoids. Their hormone, stored within the cell, is released on receiving a neural stimulation or a signaling molecule. Endocrine glands of the cord arrangement include the parathyroid and suprarenal glands and the anterior lobe of the pituitary gland. Endocrine glands of the **follicle** arrangement possess follicular cells (secretory cells) that surround a depression or a cavity, and because they do not store the secretory product, they release it into the cavity where it is stored. On receiving the proper signal, the stored hormone is resorbed from the cavity by the follicular cells and then released into blood capillaries located within the associated connective tissue (e.g., the thyroid gland).

Other glands of the body are mixed—that is, they contain exocrine and endocrine secretory units. The pancreas, ovaries, and testes each possess both kinds of glands. The exocrine portion empties its secretion into a duct, and the endocrine portion empties its secretion into the bloodstream.

Diffuse Neuroendocrine System

Endocrine cells are also scattered among the epithelial cells lining the digestive tract and the respiratory system. These particular endocrine cells represent the **diffuse neuroendocrine system (DNES)**. Certain paracrine and endocrine hormones are products of these DNES cells. The DNES designation has replaced the terms **argentaffin cells**, **argyrophil cells**, and **APUD cells** (see Chapter 17).

CLINICAL CONSIDERATIONS

Carcinoid tumors originate from DNES cells mostly in the digestive system. Before 2000, this name was applied to benign and malignant forms of DNES growths. Since that year, benign DNES growths are known as **neuroendocrine tumors**, but if they migrate to other parts of the body, they are called **carcinoids**. The following terms apply to cancers: *neuroendocrine cancers* (carcinomas), *well differentiated* (less aggressive), and *poorly differentiated* (more aggressive). Many physicians still prefer to use the term *carcinoid* for benign and well-differentiated cancers. These DNES tumors and cancers release hormone-like substances as they grow and spread causing face flushing, wheezing, diarrhea, and rapid heartbeat; these symptoms are called **carcinoid syndrome**. Additionally, these tumors and cancers can cause symptoms throughout the body.

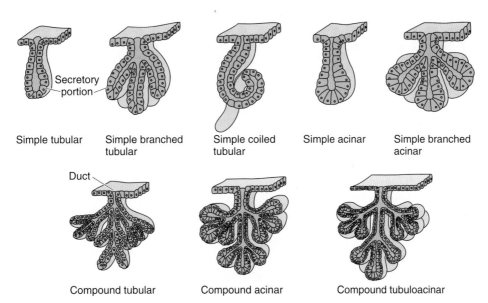

Simple tubular   Simple branched tubular   Simple coiled tubular   Simple acinar   Simple branched acinar

Duct

Compound tubular   Compound acinar   Compound tubuloacinar

Secretory portion

Figure 5.10 Classification of multicellular exocrine glands. *(From Gartner LP, Hiatt JL: Color Textbook of Histology, 3rd ed. Philadelphia, Saunders, 2007, p 107.)*

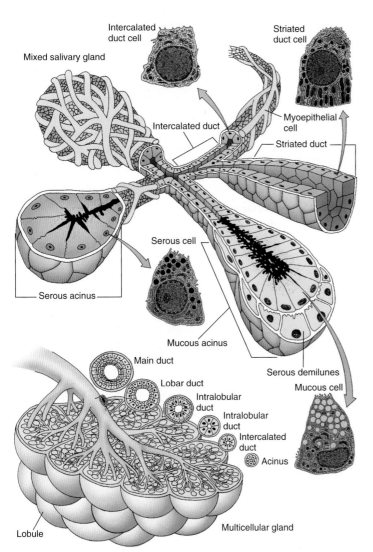

Intercalated duct cell

Striated duct cell

Mixed salivary gland

Intercalated duct

Myoepithelial cell

Striated duct

Serous cell

Serous acinus

Mucous acinus

Serous demilunes

Mucous cell

Main duct

Lobar duct

Intralobular duct

Intralobular duct

Intercalated duct

Acinus

Lobule

Multicellular gland

Figure 5.11 Salivary gland: its organization, secretory units, and system of ducts. *(From Gartner LP, Hiatt JL: Color Textbook of Histology, 3rd ed. Philadelphia, Saunders, 2007, p 108.)*

6 CONNECTIVE TISSUE

Connective tissue, one of the four basic tissues of the body, is derived mostly from **mesoderm**, and serves to connect those tissues and different types of connective tissues to each other. During embryonic development, multipotential **mesenchymal cells** of the primitive embryonic connective tissue known as **mesenchyme** migrate throughout the body to differentiate into mature cells of specialized connective tissue, such as tissues of cartilage, bone, and blood. Mesenchymal cells also give rise to cells of connective tissues that are not specialized—**connective tissue proper**, including fibroblasts, adipocytes, and mast cells.

The various types of connective tissues have diverse and far-ranging functions:

- Cartilage, bone, tendons, ligaments, and capsules of organs provide structural **support**.
- Blood, lymph, and connective tissue proper act as a **medium for exchange** by delivering nutrients, waste products, and signaling molecules to and from cells of the body.
- Certain cells that travel in the bloodstream leave the blood and enter connective tissue proper to **defend** and **protect** the body from potentially deleterious agents.
- Adipose cells store lipids and congregate to form adipose tissue serving as local storage depots of fat.

Connective tissue proper is composed of **extracellular matrix** and **cells**, some of which function in manufacturing the matrix in which they and other cells are embedded. Depending on the function of a particular connective tissue, cells or the extracellular matrix predominates and forms the essential component. Fibers are more important than their cells, the fibroblasts, for the function of tendons and ligaments, whereas in loose connective tissue, fibroblasts serve a more important function than do the fibers. In other instances, such as during immunological responses, the function of the ground substance supersedes the functions of cells and fibers because the defense of the body depends on the characteristics of the ground substance.

Extracellular matrix, the nonliving component of connective tissue, composed of ground substance and fibers, is described in Chapter 4, but its salient features are reviewed here. Ground substance is composed of:

- **Glycosaminoglycans**, either sulfated (e.g., keratan sulfate, heparin, chondroitin sulfates, dermatan sulfate, and heparan sulfate) or nonsulfated (e.g., hyaluronic acid).
- **Proteoglycans**, which, by being covalently bound to hyaluronic acid, form macromolecules of aggrecan aggregates, producing the gel state of the extracellular matrix.
- Some **adhesive glycoproteins**, such as **fibronectin**, which is dispersed throughout the extracellular matrices, and **laminin**, which is also widespread as it is localized in the basal lamina. Others, such as **chondronectin**, are located in cartilage, and **osteonectin** is located in bone.

Fibers, also nonliving substances, are of two types:

- **Collagen fibers** are of 25 different types depending on the amino acid sequence of their three alpha chains, but only 6 are of major importance for the purpose of this textbook (Table 6.1). Most collagen fibers have great tensile strength. Glycine, proline, hydroxyproline, and hydroxylysine are the most common amino acids of collagen.
- Elastin and microfibrils compose **elastic fibers**. The amorphous protein **elastin**, composed mostly of **glycine** and **proline**, is responsible for their elasticity (e.g., elastic fibers may be stretched 150% of their length), whereas microfibrils are responsible for their stability. Elastin also contains a high concentration of lysine, responsible for the formation of desmosine bonds that are elastic and deformable.

> **KEY WORDS**
> - **Extracellular matrix**
> - **Cells of connective tissue**
> - **Lipid storage by fat cells**
> - **Inflammatory response**
> - **Connective tissue types**

Table 6.1 MAJOR TYPES AND CHARACTERISTICS OF COLLAGEN

Molecular Type	Molecular Formula	Synthesizing Cells	Function	Location in Body
I (fibril-forming); most common of all collagens	$[\alpha(I)]_2\alpha2(I)$	Fibroblasts, osteoblasts, odontoblasts, cementoblasts	Resists tension	Dermis, tendon, ligaments, capsules of organs, bone, dentin, cementum
II (fibril-forming)	$[\alpha1(II)]_3$	Chondroblasts	Resists pressure	Hyaline cartilage, elastic cartilage
III (fibril-forming); also known as reticular fibers; highly glycosylated	$[\alpha1(III)]_3$	Fibroblasts, reticular cells, smooth muscle cells, hepatocytes	Forms structural framework of spleen, liver, lymph nodes, smooth muscle, adipose tissue	Lymphatic system, spleen, liver, cardiovascular system, lung, skin
IV (network-forming); do not display 67-nm periodicity, and alpha chains retain propeptides	$[\alpha1(IV)]_2\alpha2(IV)$	Epithelial cells, muscle cells, Schwann cells	Forms meshwork of lamina densa of basal lamina to provide support and filtration	Basal lamina
V (fibril-forming)	$[\alpha1(V)]_2\alpha2(V)$	Fibroblasts, mesenchymal cells	Associated with type I collagen, also with placental ground substance	Dermis, tendon, ligaments, capsules of organs, bone, cementum, placenta
VII (network-forming); form dimers that assemble into anchoring fibrils	$[\alpha1(VII)]_3$	Epidermal cells	Forms anchoring fibrils that fasten lamina densa to underlying lamina reticularis	Junction of epidermis and dermis

From Gartner LP, Hiatt JL: Color Textbook of Histology, 3rd ed. Philadelphia, Saunders, 2007, p 76.

CLINICAL CONSIDERATIONS

Ehlers-Danlos syndrome is a group of rare *genetic disorders* affecting humans caused by defective *collagen* synthesis. Symptoms vary widely based on the type of Ehlers-Danlos syndrome the patient has. In each case, the symptoms are ultimately due to faulty or reduced amounts of collagen, the most common of which include unstable joints that are easily dislocated and hypermobile because of overstretchable ligaments that are composed of defective collagen. Some forms affect the skin, and others affect the walls of blood vessels. The severity of the syndromes of this incurable disease can vary from mild to life-threatening.

Marfan syndrome is an autosomal dominant disorder in which the elastic tissue is weakened because of a mutation in the fibrillin gene. This disorder affects the elastic fibers of the cardiovascular, ocular, and skeletal systems. Individuals with Marfan syndrome are unusually tall, with very long arms, fingers, legs, feet, and toes. Cardiovascular problems are life-threatening and include valvular problems and dilation of the ascending aorta. Ocular disorders include myopia and detached lens. Skeletal disorders include abnormally weak periosteum because of defects in the elastic fibers being unable to provide an appositional force in bone development.

Connective Tissue Cells

The **cells of connective tissue** proper are classified into two categories: **fixed** (resident), referring to cells that do not migrate, and **transient**, referring to cells that use the blood and lymph vascular system(s) to relocate to regions of connective tissue proper where they have a particular function to perform, and then they either die there or leave to go to a different location (Table 6.2).

FIXED CELLS OF CONNECTIVE TISSUE

Fibroblasts

Fibroblasts (Figs. 6.1 and 6.2), the most abundant cells of connective tissue, are derived from mesenchymal cells and are responsible for synthesizing the extracellular matrix. Fibroblasts are either active or quiescent; myofibroblasts are a subcategory of fibroblasts:

- **Active fibroblasts** lie parallel to the long axis of collagen bundles as elongated, fusiform cells with pale-staining cytoplasm and a dark, large ovoid nucleus. During matrix production, the Golgi apparatus and rough endoplasmic reticulum (RER) are well developed. Myosin is located throughout the cytoplasm, and actin and α-actinin are localized at the cell periphery.
- **Inactive fibroblasts** are smaller, display acidophilic cytoplasm, and have a denser, deeply stained nucleus. RER and the Golgi apparatus are reduced in these cells, but ribosomes are abundant.
- Fibroblasts may be modified to become **myofibroblasts** in regions of wound healing. They possess characteristics of fibroblasts and smooth muscle cells, but in contrast to smooth muscle, they do not have an external lamina. Myofibroblasts function in wound contraction, and as resident cells of the periodontal ligament they may assist in tooth eruption.

Table 6.2 FIXED AND TRANSIENT CELLS

Fixed Cells	Transient Cells
Fibroblasts	Plasma cells
Adipose cells	Lymphocytes
Pericytes	Neutrophils
Mast cells	Eosinophils
Macrophages	Basophils
	Monocytes
	Macrophages

Pericytes

Pericytes, derived from mesenchymal cells, partially surround endothelial cells of capillaries and small venules (see Fig. 6.2). They possess their own basal lamina, which may fuse with that of adjacent endothelial cells. Pericytes share some of the characteristics of smooth muscle and endothelial cells, and they may give rise to fibroblasts, endothelial cells, or vascular smooth muscle cells in response to injury.

Adipose Cells

Fat cells (**adipocytes**) are amitotic and function in the synthesis and storage of triglycerides (see Fig. 6.2). There are two types of adipose cells—**unilocular** and **multilocular**.

- **Unilocular fat cells**, large round cells (≤120 μm in diameter) filled with a single drop of lipid, constitute the principal population of white adipose tissue. Electron microscopy shows a thin peripheral cytoplasm rich in ribosomes with a small Golgi complex, few mitochondria, RER, and numerous pinocytotic vesicles along the cytoplasmic aspect of the cell membrane.
- **Multilocular fat cells** are polygonal in shape, are smaller than white fat cells, and store fat in small droplets throughout the cytoplasm. Electron micrographs show abundant mitochondria, which are responsible for the cell's darker coloration—hence their being called *brown fat cells*, the principal component of brown adipose tissue.

CLINICAL CONSIDERATIONS

Although fibroblasts are considered to be fixed cells, they are able to display some limited movement. These cells may undergo cell division under special conditions, such as in wound healing. Additionally, when tendons are stressed because of overuse, fibroblasts may be stimulated to become chondrocytes and form cartilage matrix around themselves and transform the tendon into fibrocartilage. Additionally, fibroblasts may differentiate into adipose cells; under pathological conditions, fibroblasts may even differentiate into osteoblasts.

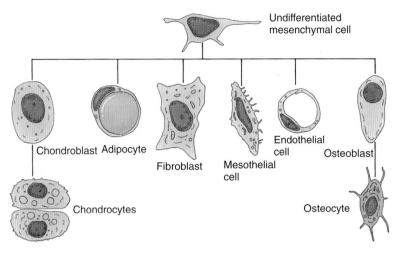

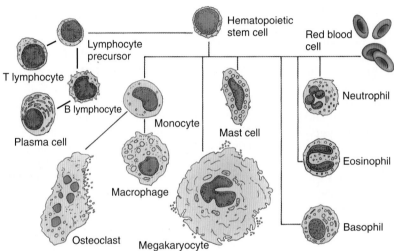

Figure 6.1 Origins of connective tissue cells. *(From Gartner LP, Hiatt JL: Color Textbook of Histology, 3rd ed. Philadelphia, Saunders, 2007, p 112.)*

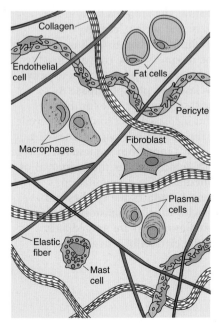

Figure 6.2 Cell types and fiber types in loose connective tissue. *(From Gartner LP, Hiatt JL: Color Textbook of Histology, 3rd ed. Philadelphia, Saunders, 2007, p 113.)*

Storage and Release of Fat by Adipose Cells

During digestion, fats in the lumen of the small intestine are catabolized by **pancreatic lipase** into **fatty acids** and **glycerol**, substances that are absorbed by surface absorptive cells of the epithelial lining. When in the cytoplasm of these cells, the fatty acids and glycerol enter the smooth endoplasmic reticulum, where they are re-esterified and conveyed to the Golgi apparatus, where they are invested with a protein coat. These proteinated triglycerides, called **chylomicrons**, are released into the lamina propria of the small intestine to enter lymph channels, known as **lacteals**, and eventually are released into the bloodstream.

Capillaries that vascularize adipose tissue have an enzyme, **lipoprotein lipase**, manufactured by adipocytes, on the luminal surface of their endothelial cells (Fig. 6.3). This enzyme catabolizes chylomicrons and other blood-borne lipids, such as very-low-density lipoproteins (VLDL), into glycerol and fatty acids. The fatty acids leave the capillaries; penetrate the adipocyte plasmalemma; and within the cytoplasm of fat cells are formed into triglycerides, which are stored in the pool of lipid droplets, an efficient and low weight method of energy storage. When **norepinephrine** and **epinephrine** bind to their respective receptor sites on the fat cell membrane, the adipocyte's **adenylate cyclase system** is activated to form **cyclic adenosine monophosphate (AMP)**, which induces the cytoplasmic enzyme **hormone-sensitive lipase** to degrade triglycerides of the lipid droplet. The fatty acids and glycerol leave the adipocyte to enter the surrounding capillaries (see Fig. 6.3).

Mast Cells

Mast cells (20 to 30 μm in diameter) are derived from precursors in the bone marrow and enter the connective tissue compartment where they mature, live for a few months, and only seldom enter the cell cycle. These ovoid cells with a centrally placed nucleus have membrane bound granules (Fig. 6.4 and Table 6.3) that are responsible for their **metachromasia**. Mast cells store some pharmacologic agents, known as **primary or preformed mediators**, in granules and synthesize others, known as **secondary mediators**, as they are required.

- **Primary mediators** are **histamine** and **heparin** (in connective tissue mast cells) or histamine and **chondroitin sulfate** (in mucosal mast cells of the mucosa of the respiratory tract and alimentary canal), **neutral proteases** (tryptase, chymase, and carboxypeptidases), **aryl sulfatase**, β-glucuronidase, kininogenase, peroxidase, superoxide dismutase, **eosinophil chemotactic factor**, and **neutrophil chemotactic factor**.
- **Secondary mediators**, synthesized from membrane arachidonic acid precursors, include leukotrienes (C_4, D_4, and E_4), thromboxanes (thromboxane A_2 and thromboxane B_2), and prostaglandins (prostaglandin D_2).
- **Secondary mediators** that are not derived from arachidonic acid precursors include platelet-activating factor, bradykinins, interleukins (IL-4, IL-5, and IL-6), and tumor necrosis factor-α. (See Table 6.3 for a list of the major primary and secondary mediators released by mast cells.)

Mast Cell Activation and Degranulation

The plasma membranes of mast cells possess high-affinity cell surface Fc receptors (FcεRI) for IgE molecules that project into the extracellular space. These cells have the ability to release pharmacologic agents that set off a localized response known as **immediate hypersensitivity reaction** or, in extreme cases, a widespread, possibly fatal response known as an **anaphylactic reaction**. Certain drugs, venoms of some insects, various pollens, and other antigens may elicit these responses in the following manner (see Fig. 6.4):

1. Mast cells become **sensitized** when they bind IgE antibodies against a particular antigen to their FcεRI receptors, but the mast cells do not respond to the first exposure to the antigen.
2. If the same antigens enter the connective tissue for a second time, the antigens bind to the IgE on the mast cell surface, causing the immunoglobulin molecules to be linked to each other and the receptors to be crowded together, stimulating **receptor coupling factors** to activate **adenylate cyclase** and **phospholipase A_2**.
3. **Adenylate cyclase** is responsible for the formation and increased concentration of **cyclic AMP** within the plasma cell cytosol, inducing the release of **Ca^{++} ions** from sequestered storage compartments, which induces the exocytosis of **preformed mediators** by degranulation.
4. **Phospholipase A_2** induces the synthesis of **arachidonic acid**, which is transformed into **secondary mediators** that are immediately released into the extracellular space.

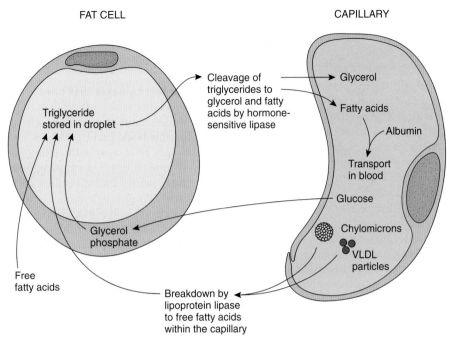

FAT CELL

CAPILLARY

Figure 6.3 Transport of lipid between a capillary and an adipocyte. *(From Gartner LP, Hiatt JL: Color Textbook of Histology, 3rd ed. Philadelphia, Saunders, 2007, p 119.)*

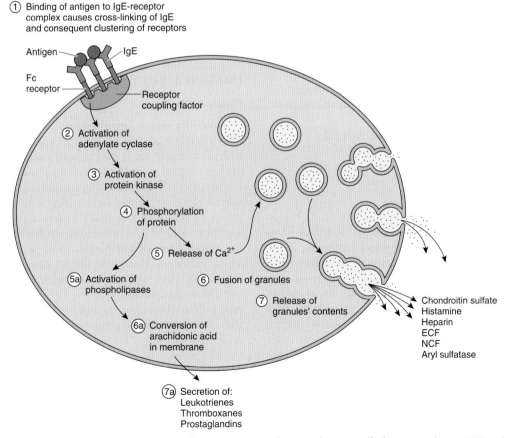

① Binding of antigen to IgE-receptor complex causes cross-linking of IgE and consequent clustering of receptors

Antigen   IgE

Fc receptor

Receptor coupling factor

② Activation of adenylate cyclase

③ Activation of protein kinase

④ Phosphorylation of protein

⑤ Release of Ca²⁺

⑤ₐ Activation of phospholipases

⑥ Fusion of granules

⑥ₐ Conversion of arachidonic acid in membrane

⑦ Release of granules' contents

Chondroitin sulfate
Histamine
Heparin
ECF
NCF
Aryl sulfatase

⑦ₐ Secretion of:
Leukotrienes
Thromboxanes
Prostaglandins

Figure 6.4 Binding of antigens and cross-linking of IgE receptor complexes on the mast cell plasma membrane. ECF, eosinophil chemotactic factor; NCF, neutrophil chemotactic factor. *(From Gartner LP, Hiatt JL: Color Textbook of Histology, 3rd ed. Philadelphia, Saunders, 2007, p 120.)*

Mast Cells and the Inflammatory Response

The release of mediators (both primary and secondary) by mast cells (see Table 6.3) in response to the binding of antigens to their surface IgE results in the following sequence of events:

1. **Histamine** is a vasodilator, and its effects are to increase vascular permeability; it also is a bronchoconstrictor, and it not only reduces the luminal diameter of bronchioles, but also causes an increase in mucus production.
2. The leakage of plasma from the blood vessels brings **complement** into the connective tissue spaces, which is catabolized by **neutral proteases** into macromolecules that contribute to the inflammatory process.
3. **Neutrophil** and **eosinophil chemotactic factors** recruit **neutrophils** and **eosinophils** to the site of inflammation; neutrophils kill microorganisms, and eosinophils phagocytose antigen-antibody complexes and kill parasites.
4. **Bradykinins** also increase vascular permeability and elicit pain in the area of inflammation.
5. **Leukotrienes** C_4, D_4, and E_4 have similar functions as histamine, but are much more potent in their action; they do not affect mucus production, however.
6. **Prostaglandin** D_2 causes contraction of bronchiolar smooth muscles and increases mucus production.
7. **Platelet-activating factor** attracts neutrophils and eosinophils to the site of inflammation, increases the permeability of blood vessels, and is a bronchoconstrictor.
8. **Thromboxane** A_2, although it is rapidly inactivated by being converted into thromboxane B_2, is a vasoconstrictor and induces aggregation of platelets.

Macrophages

Macrophages, irregularly shaped cells about 10 to 30 μm in diameter, are phagocytes, belonging to the **mononuclear phagocyte system**, all of whose members are derived from common bone marrow precursor cells. They travel in the bloodstream as **monocytes**, but when they enter connective tissue, they mature and become macrophages. Some macrophages remain in the area of the body that they enter and are known as **resident (fixed) macrophages** (e.g., Kupffer cells, Langerhans cells, dust cells, microglia), whereas others are **transient (free, elicited) macrophages** that perform their function and then either die or migrate from the area of their activity.

Some macrophages that have to eliminate larger substances fuse with each other to be able to perform their duties; examples of such cells are **osteoclasts** and **foreign body giant cells**. The macrophage cell membranes have a smooth outline, unless they are actively moving or phagocytosing foreign substances or cellular debris, and then they develop folds and pleats on their plasmalemma. To be able to perform their functions, some macrophages have to be activated by signaling molecules released by lymphocytes that are participating in an immune response (see Chapter 12). As macrophages mature, their cytoplasm possesses numerous vacuoles, a prominent Golgi apparatus, a copious amount of lysosomes, many microtubules, and numerous profiles of RER. Their nuclei are dense and characteristically kidney shaped. The principal functions of macrophages, other than phagocytosis of invading microorganisms and cellular and extracellular debris, are to synthesize and release signaling molecules, such as **tumor necrosis factor-α** and **IL-1**, and to act as **antigen presenting cells** that display antigenic fragments on their membrane bound receptors to lymphocytes inducing them to initiate an immune response.

TRANSIENT CONNECTIVE TISSUE CELLS

Plasma Cells

Plasma cells, derived from a subcategory of lymphocytes (B cells) that have been activated by contact with an antigen, are large (approximately 20 μm in diameter), oval cells, the heterochromatin of whose acentric, dense nucleus displays a characteristic *clockface* or *cartwheel* configuration (Fig. 6.5). The cytoplasm of these cells is richly endowed with Golgi apparatus and RER because they are responsible for the manufacture of **antibodies** in response to antigenic challenges. These cells live for approximately 2 to 3 weeks. They are present throughout the connective tissue compartment of the body, but they are especially numerous in regions of chronic inflammation and areas that are susceptible to antigenic or microbial invasions, such as the lamina propria of the alimentary canal and respiratory tract.

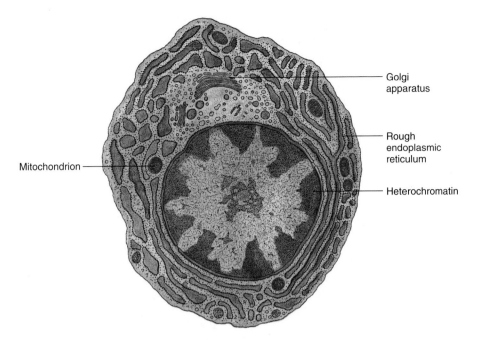

Mitochondrion

Golgi apparatus

Rough endoplasmic reticulum

Heterochromatin

Figure 6.5 Drawing of a plasma cell as observed on an electron micrograph. *(From Lentz TL: Cell Fine Structure: An Atlas of Drawings of Whole-Cell Structure. Philadelphia, Saunders, 1971.)*

Table 6.3 PRINCIPAL PRIMARY AND SECONDARY MEDIATORS RELEASED BY MAST CELLS

Substance	Type of Mediator	Source	Action
Histamine	Primary	Granule	Increases vascular permeability, vasodilation, smooth muscle contraction of bronchi, mucus production
Heparin	Primary	Granule	Anticoagulant binds and inactivates histamine
Chondroitin sulfate	Primary	Granule	Binds to and inactivates histamine
Aryl sulfatase	Primary	Granule	Inactivates leukotriene C_4, limiting inflammatory response
Neutral proteases	Primary	Granule	Protein cleavage to activate complement (especially C3a); increases inflammatory response
Eosinophil chemotactic factor	Primary	Granule	Attracts eosinophils to site of inflammation
Neutrophil chemotactic factor	Primary	Granule	Attracts neutrophils to site of inflammation
Leukotrienes C_4, D_4, and E_4	Secondary	Membrane lipid	Vasodilator; increases vascular permeability; causes contraction of bronchial smooth muscle
Prostaglandin D_2	Secondary	Membrane lipid	Causes contraction of bronchial smooth muscle; increases mucus secretion; vasoconstriction
Thromboxane A_2	Secondary	Membrane lipid	Causes platelet aggregation, vasoconstriction
Bradykinins	Secondary	Formed by activity of enzymes located in granules	Causes vascular permeability and is responsible for pain sensation
Platelet-activating factor	Secondary	Activated by phospholipase A_2	Attracts neutrophils and eosinophils; causes vascular permeability and contraction of bronchial smooth muscle

From Gartner LP, Hiatt JL: Color Textbook of Histology, 3rd ed. Philadelphia, Saunders, 2007, p 121.

Leukocytes

Leukocytes, or white blood cells, circulate in the blood and enter the connective tissue compartments to which they are recruited by cytokines or that they recognize by their own homing receptors (see Fig. 6.4). These cells are discussed in detail in Chapters 10 and 12.

- **Monocytes** are discussed in the previous section on Macrophages.
- **Neutrophils** respond to neutrophil chemotactic factor released by mast cells to act in acute inflammation, where they phagocytose and digest bacteria. After they degranulate and destroy the bacteria, they die and become a component of pus.
- **Eosinophils** are recruited to the site by eosinophil chemotactic factor released by mast cells to act in acute inflammation. They kill parasites and phagocytose antibody-antigen complexes.
- **Basophils** are similar to mast cells and perform the same function as mast cells.
- **Lymphocytes** are most numerous at sites of chronic inflammation.

Classification of Connective Tissue

There are three categories of connective tissue. **Embryonic connective tissue** exists only during the embryonic and fetal stages of development, although some authors consider it to belong to the category of **connective tissue proper**, which is distributed throughout the body. **Specialized connective tissue** consists of cartilage, bone, and blood. Table 6.4 summarizes the various categories and subcategories of the connective tissues.

EMBRYONIC CONNECTIVE TISSUE

There are two types of embryonic connective tissues:

- **Mesenchymal connective tissue** is widespread throughout the embryo and fetus and is composed of a gelatinous **ground substance** rich in **hyaluronic acid** in which **reticular fibers (type III collagen fibers)** and **mesenchymal cells** are embedded. Mesenchymal cells are multipotential cells whose relatively long processes extend in various directions away from the cell body. Each mesenchymal cell has a single, pale, ovoid nucleus displaying a well-defined nucleolus surrounded by a slender array of fine chromatin threads. With the exception of a few regions of the body, mesenchymal cells are not present in the adult.
- **Mucoid connective tissue**, located only deep to the embryonic skin and in the umbilical cord, is composed of a hyaluronic acid–rich ground substance in which fibroblasts and slender type I and type III collagen fibers are embedded. Within the umbilical cord, the mucoid connective tissue is known as **Wharton's jelly**.

CLINICAL CONSIDERATIONS

Hay fever victims experience localized edema and swelling of the nasal mucosa, which hinders breathing and results in the *stuffed up* feeling. These symptoms result from histamine being released by the mast cells of the nasal mucosa, increasing permeability of the small blood vessels and localized edema. Difficulty in breathing also accompanies patients with **asthma** resulting from **leukotrienes** being released in the lungs that brings about **bronchospasm**.

Mast cell degranulation is normally a localized condition bringing on a typical mild inflammatory response. **Hyperallergic** individuals are at risk, however, because they may experience **systemic anaphylaxis** after a second exposure to the allergen (e.g., bee sting). This exposure, characterized by systemic and severe immediate hypersensitivity reaction, is called **anaphylactic shock**. The symptoms occur almost immediately to within a few minutes, and if they are left untreated, death may occur within a few hours. Symptoms include sudden decrease in blood pressure and shortness of breath. Wearing a medical emergency bracelet is suggested for hyperallergic individuals because it informs an emergency health provider of the need for immediate medical attention.

Normally, the extracellular fluid within the tissues is returned to capillaries directly or to lymph vessels and then to the bloodstream. During an inflammatory response, there is an accumulation of extracellular fluid within loose connective tissue that prevents the return of extracellular fluid to the bloodstream. This condition results in **edema** (gross swelling), which may be due to the excessive release of histamine and leukotrienes C_4 and D_4, products of mast cells that increase capillary permeability. Edema can also be caused by venous or lymphatic vessel obstructions.

Adult obesity develops in two forms:

- **Hypertrophic obesity** develops from an imbalance between energy intake and energy expenditure resulting in accumulation and storage of fat in unilocular fat cells, quadrupling their size.
- **Hypercellular (hyperplastic) obesity** develops as a result of an excessive number of adipocytes. Mature adipocytes do not undergo cell division. Their precursors do undergo cell division for a short time postnatally, however. Significant evidence exists that overfeeding newborns even for a few weeks increases the adipocyte precursor population, resulting in abnormally increasing the adipocyte population and leading to hyperplastic obesity that may begin in childhood. Infants who are overweight are three or more times likely to develop obesity as adults compared with infants of average weight.

Adipose tissue tumors may be either benign or malignant. **Lipomas** are benign tumors of adipocytes, whereas **liposarcomas** are malignant tumors of adipocytes or their precursors Liposarcoma is common with approximately 2000 cases per year in the United States. There are three types of liposarcoma:

- **Well-differentiated or dedifferentiated liposarcoma** (approximately 50%; the most frequent type) develops in the abdominal cavity or in an extremity, as a large painless mass. Primary therapy is surgical, with a 70% to 80% recurrence risk in the abdomen. The "dedifferentiated" version is the more aggressive form, but still not a high-grade sarcoma.
- **Myxoid or round cell liposarcoma** (approximately 40%).
- **Pleomorphic liposarcoma** (10%; the least common) affects an extremity and is aggressive and may spread to other sites, including the lung and soft tissue.

Fat accumulation is regulated by two different sets of hormones—those responsible for **short-term weight control**, ghrelin and peptide YY, and those for **long-term weight control**, leptin and insulin.

- **Ghrelin** is manufactured by **P/D1 cells** of the gastric epithelium and of the pancreas and induces a feeling of hunger, whereas **peptide YY**, manufactured by **L cells** of the epithelial lining of the ileum and colon, induces a feeling of satiation. It is interesting to note that sleep deprivation increases ghrelin levels and induces a feeling of hunger.
- **Leptin**, manufactured by white adipocytes and by the ovary and muscle cells, binds to receptors of cells in the "**appetite center**" of the **hypothalamus** and induces a feeling of satiety. Some individuals are resistant to leptin and, even though they have high serum leptin levels, may be morbidly obese. Recombinant human leptin has been very effective in treating these patients. **Insulin** increases the amount of fat stored in unilocular white blood cells by inducing the conversion of glucose to triglycerides in these cells.

Table 6.4 CLASSIFICATION OF
CONNECTIVE TISSUE

A. Embryonic Connective Tissues
   1. Mesenchymal connective tissue
   2. Mucous connective tissue
B. Connective Tissue Proper
   1. Loose (areolar) connective tissue
   2. Dense connective tissue
      a. Dense irregular connective tissue
      b. Dense regular connective tissue
         (1) Collagenous
         (2) Elastic
   3. Reticular tissue
   4. Adipose tissue
C. Specialized Connective Tissue
   1. Cartilage
   2. Bone
   3. Blood

From Gartner LP, Hiatt JL: Color Textbook of Histology, 3rd ed. Philadelphia, Saunders, 2007, p 126.

CONNECTIVE TISSUE PROPER

Connective tissue proper may be divided into four major categories: loose connective tissue, dense connective tissue, reticular tissue, and adipose tissue. Each of these different types possesses specific characteristics and functions.

Loose (Areolar) Connective Tissue

The extracellular matrix of **loose (areolar) connective tissue** is composed of a loose, apparently haphazard arrangement of **types I and III collagen fibers** interspersed with long, slender **elastic fibers** embedded in a gelatinous **ground substance**. Cells of connective tissue proper are also present in healthy loose connective tissue, and they are nourished by the **extracellular fluid** that percolates through the ground substance as it leaves the abundance of arterioles and the arterial side of capillary beds to return to the venous side of capillary beds and to the profusion of venules and lymph vessels. Loose connective tissue is present deep to the skin and envelopes neurovascular bundles.

Reticular Tissue

Reticular tissue, composed mostly of type III collagen fibers, constitutes the netlike framework of some organs such as liver, spleen, bone marrow, smooth muscle, adipose tissue, and lymph nodes. Usually, reticular fibers are manufactured by fibroblasts, although the smooth muscle cells manufacture type III collagen fibers in smooth muscle.

Dense Connective Tissue

Dense connective tissue is much richer in fibers and much poorer in cells than loose connective tissue. Depending on the precision in the orientation of the fibers, dense connective tissue may be classified as irregular or regular:

- The type I collagen fiber bundles of **dense irregular collagenous connective tissue** are arranged in an apparently random orientation that provides this tissue a great deal of flexibility and elasticity, but at the same time imparts to it the ability to resist tensile forces. Dense irregular collagenous connective tissue forms the dermis of skin, the capsules of many organs, and the connective tissue sheaths that surround nerves and larger blood vessels.
- **Dense regular connective tissue** is of two types—collagenous and elastic—depending on the majority of the fiber type composing it.
  - **Dense regular collagenous connective tissue** forms tendons, aponeuroses, and ligaments. It is composed mostly of thick, coarse, parallel bundles of type I collagen fibers packed so closely that only a scant amount of ground substance and compressed fibroblasts are present among the fiber bundles.
  - **Dense regular elastic connective tissue** is composed of densely packed elastic fiber bundles disposed parallel to each other with fibroblasts among the bundles. Dense regular elastic connective tissue is arranged in perforated sheets, as in the fenestrated membrane of the aorta, or as thick, short bundles, as in the ligamentum nuchae of the spinal column.

Adipose Tissue

There are two categories of **adipose tissue** depending on the type of fat cells that compose it—the unilocular fat cells of white adipose tissue or the multilocular adipocytes of brown fat. Brown fat develops prenatally, whereas white fat develops postnatally.

- **Brown (multilocular) adipose tissue** is even more lobular than white adipose tissue, and in contrast to in white fat, the nerve fibers serve blood vessels and the multilocular adipocytes. In appearance, brown fat is present only in embryos and neonates in humans; after birth the fat droplets coalesce to appear as if they were unilocular. In some older individuals with wasting diseases, multilocular adipocytes may reappear.
- **White (unilocular) adipose tissue** consists of unilocular adipocytes (Fig. 6.6) arranged in lobules that are incompletely separated from each other by connective tissue septa that convey nerve fibers and blood vessels to the tissue. The rich vascular supply forms extensive capillary beds within the lobules so that each adipocyte is closely associated with nearby capillaries. In addition to its location in the subcutaneous connective tissue, omentum, mesenteries, and buttocks, there is also a gender-specific accumulation of white adipose tissue. In women, it is prominent in the breasts, hips, and thighs, whereas in men it is prominent in the neck, shoulder, and hips.

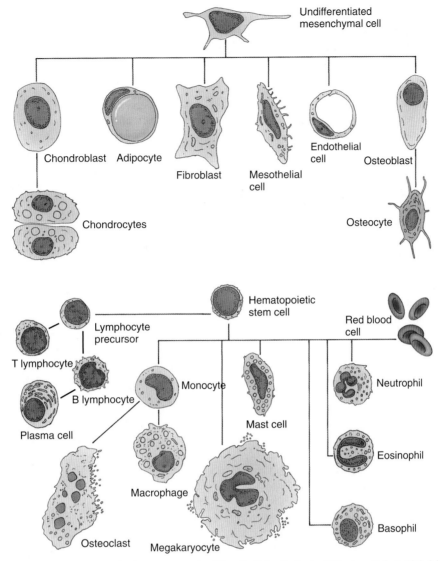

Figure 6.6 Origins of connective tissue cells. *(From Gartner LP, Hiatt JL: Color Textbook of Histology, 3rd ed. Philadelphia, Saunders, 2007, p 112.)*

CLINICAL CONSIDERATIONS

Multilocular adipocytes are prominent in animals that hibernate. These cells, on the proper signal—the release of norepinephrine from nerve fibers synapsing with multilocular fat cells—begin to generate heat and bring the animal out of hibernation. Brown adipocytes are able to generate heat because the inner membranes of their mitochondria possess a transmembrane protein, known as **uncoupling protein-1 (UPC-1)**, also known as **thermogenin**, that is specific only to these cells. UPC-1, instead of permitting the flow of protons through the enzyme complex adenosine triphosphate (ATP) synthase, directs a reverse flow of the protons, uncoupling oxidation from phosphorylation. The proton flow, instead of generating ATP, is dissipated and generates heat. The blood in the rich vascular supply of brown adipose tissue is dispersed throughout the animal's body, and the increasing body temperature brings the animal out of its hibernating state.

7 CARTILAGE AND BONE

Cartilage and bone are the two specialized connective tissues discussed in this chapter. Cartilage is a smooth, firm structure containing a flexible matrix, whereas the matrix of bone is calcified, making it inflexible. As the cells of cartilage and bone secrete their respective matrices, they become entrapped in that matrix. Cartilage and bone are intimately related through their function in resisting stresses and in supporting various elements of the body; also, during embryonic development, hyaline cartilage is elaborated first to form the template on which long bone develops. As bone is being elaborated, the cartilage is resorbed in a process called **endochondral bone formation**. Most of the remaining bones of the skeleton are formed by another method called **intramembranous bone formation**, in which bone is formed within a membranous sheath in the absence of a cartilage template.

> **KEY WORDS**
> - **Hyaline cartilage**
> - **Elastic cartilage**
> - **Bone matrix**
> - **Cells of bone**
> - **Lamellar systems**
> - **Bone formation**
> - **Bone remodeling**
> - **Bone repair**

Cartilage

Cells of cartilage known as **chondroblasts** and **chondrocytes** secrete an **extracellular matrix** composed of **glycosaminoglycans** and **proteoglycans** reinforced by collagen and elastic fibers. During their secretory process, the chondroblasts become entrapped within the matrix they secreted and become known as chondrocytes, occupying small cavities called **lacunae**. Because cartilage does not possess a vascular supply, nourishment must reach these cells by diffusion through the matrix from the vascular supply located in the connective tissue, **perichondrium**, surrounding the cartilage. The flexible nature of cartilage and its resistance to compression enable it to:

- Absorb shock
- Cover the surfaces of most bony joints; its smooth surface eliminates frictional forces during articulation

There are three types of cartilage, and they are defined by the fibers present in their matrix (Fig. 7.1 and Table 7.1):

- **Elastic cartilage** resembles hyaline cartilage except for the presence of coarse elastic fibers in its matrix that impart an opaque yellowish tinge to it and a greater degree of flexibility. There are additional subtle differences between them: the

chondrocytes of elastic cartilage are more numerous and larger than the chondrocytes of its hyaline counterpart, and the matrix of elastic cartilage is less abundant than the matrix of hyaline cartilage. Elastic cartilage is present in the pinna of the ear, larynx, epiglottis, and external and internal auditory tubes.

- **Fibrocartilage** has no perichondrium and resembles tendon because it is composed of thick parallel bundles of type I collagen fibers with very little matrix. Fibrocartilage matrix, composed mostly of dermatan sulfate and chondroitin sulfates, surrounds small chondrocytes lodged between these coarse collagen fiber bundles. Frequently, fibrocartilage is formed when the tensile forces placed on tendons become excessive; fibroblasts differentiate into chondrocytes that form matrix, transforming the tendon into fibrocartilage because it is better able to resist the powerful tensile forces placed on the tendon. Fibrocartilage is present in articular disks, intervertebral disks, pubic symphysis, and at sites where tendons and ligaments attach to bone.

- **Hyaline cartilage** is located throughout the body, including the rib/sternum joints, the skeleton of the air passageways in the respiratory system, and the skeleton of the larynx and much of the nose. It also covers the articular surfaces of bony joints. Epiphyseal plates located at the ends of developing long bones are composed of hyaline cartilage. Hyaline cartilage formed during embryonic development becomes the template on which bone is elaborated during endochondral bone formation.

> **CLINICAL CONSIDERATIONS**
>
> Although fibrocartilage is very strong, sometimes the forces on the vertebral column may be excessive causing the intervertebral disk to herniate or to rupture. These conditions may often be very painful because the slipped disk may impinge on spinal nerves in its vicinity. Slipped and ruptured disks occur most often on the posterior aspects of the lumbar region.

HYALINE CARTILAGE

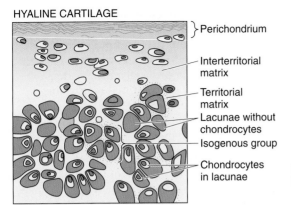

} Perichondrium

— Interterritorial matrix

— Territorial matrix

— Lacunae without chondrocytes

— Isogenous group

— Chondrocytes in lacunae

Figure 7.1 Types of cartilage. *(From Gartner LP, Hiatt JL: Color Textbook of Histology, 3rd ed. Philadelphia, Saunders, 2007, p 132.)*

ELASTIC CARTILAGE

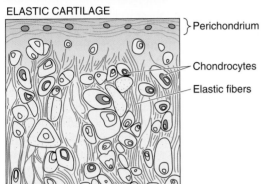

} Perichondrium

— Chondrocytes

— Elastic fibers

FIBROCARTILAGE

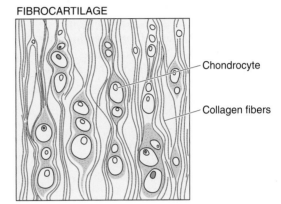

— Chondrocyte

— Collagen fibers

Table 7.1 TYPES OF CARTILAGE

Type	Characteristics	Perichondrium	Location
Hyaline	Type II collagen, basophilic matrix, chondrocytes usually arranged in groups	Perichondrium present in most places	Articular ends of long bones, nose, larynx, trachea, bronchi, ventral ends of ribs
Elastic	Type II collagen, elastic fibers	Perichondrium present	Pinna of ear, walls of auditory canal, auditory tube, epiglottis, cuneiform cartilage of larynx
Fibrocartilage	Type I collagen, acidophilic matrix, chondrocytes arranged in parallel rows between bundles of collagen fibers	Perichondrium absent	Intervertebral disks, articular disks, pubic symphysis, insertion of some tendons

From Gartner LP, Hiatt JL: Color Textbook of Histology, 3rd ed. Philadelphia, Saunders, 2007, p 133.

HISTOGENESIS AND GROWTH OF HYALINE CARTILAGE

Mesenchymal cells located in the vicinity where cartilage is to form assemble into **chondrification centers**, express the gene *Sox9*, and differentiate into **chondroblasts**. These newly formed cells secrete cartilage matrix, which surrounds chondroblasts, trapping each in a small space known as a **lacuna** (Fig. 7.2). These cells still possess the ability to divide; they are now known as **chondrocytes**.

- During **interstitial growth** of cartilage, a chondrocyte divides to form a collection of two or four cells, called **isogenous groups**, within the lacuna. As each cell of the isogenous group secretes matrix, the lacuna is separated into two or four compartments, the chondrocytes move farther away from each other, and the cartilage increases in size.
- Other mesenchymal cells surrounding the forming cartilage differentiate into fibroblasts that form a dense, vascular connective tissue—the two-layered **perichondrium**.
  - The **outer fibrous layer**, composed of fibrous tissue, houses fibroblasts and a rich vascular supply.
  - The **inner cellular layer** possesses mitotically active **chondrogenic cells** that become chondroblasts.
- **Chondroblasts** of the inner layer of the perichondrium form cartilage matrix on the periphery of the cartilage, a process known as **appositional growth**. Appositional growth is the major method of growth of cartilage except in locations where a perichondrium is absent (e.g., at articular joints and epiphyseal plates of long bones).

Chondrogenic cells differentiate into not only chondroblasts, but also, under high oxygen tension, into bone precursors known as *osteoprogenitor cells*. The growth and development of hyaline cartilage are affected by various hormones and vitamins (Table 7.2).

MATRIX OF HYALINE CARTILAGE

Type II collagen is the major component of the matrix (40% of dry weight and slight amounts of types IX, X, and XI collagens), whereas the remainder is composed of glycoproteins (chondroitin 4-sulfate, chondroitin 6-sulfate, and heparan sulfate), proteoglycans (chondronectin), and extracellular fluid. Two specialized regions of the matrix exist:

- **Territorial matrix**, immediately surrounding each lacuna.
- **Interterritorial matrix**, constituting the matrix between territorial matrices. The territorial matrix is collagen-poor, but rich in chondroitin sulfates, whereas interterritorial matrix is rich in collagen, but possesses fewer proteoglycans.
- A narrow band of the territorial matrix, the **pericellular capsule**, resembles a basal lamina and is in direct contact with the chondrocytes, perhaps protecting them from physical insults.

Cartilage matrix possesses abundant **aggrecans**, large proteoglycan molecules of protein cores to which glycosaminoglycans are covalently linked. Many of these aggrecan molecules bind to **hyaluronic acid**, forming giant, negatively charged **aggrecan composites** that are 3 to 4 μm in length and, due to their negative charge, attract Na^+ ions. Water molecules are attracted to this sheath of positively charged elements, forming a sheath of hydration around the aggrecan composites responsible for the high water content of hyaline cartilage (approximately 80%), and permitting hyaline cartilage to resist compression. **Type II collagen fibers** embedded in this matrix not only form electrostatic bonds with the matrix, but also resist tensile forces. The adhesive glycoprotein **chondronectin** has binding sites to the cells of cartilage, type II collagen, and components of the aggrecans composite, and in this manner facilitates the adhesion among the various cellular and extracellular elements of hyaline cartilage. The smoothness of this cartilage surface and its ability to resist forces of compression and tension make hyaline cartilage an ideal substance to cover the articular surfaces of long bones.

CLINICAL CONSIDERATIONS

Chondrocytes of hyaline cartilage that undergo hypertrophy and die leave behind a calcified matrix that results in degeneration of the cartilage. This sequence of hyaline cartilage deterioration represents the normal course of events during endochondral bone formation; however, these same events accompany the normal pattern in aging with the consequence of acute and chronic joint pain and limited mobility. Regeneration of cartilage is mostly confined to children with only limited restoration in older adults, and when it does occur, chondrogenic cells migrate from the perichondrium to the lesion. If the defect is not too large, new cartilage fills the lesion; otherwise, dense collagenous tissue is formed to fill it.

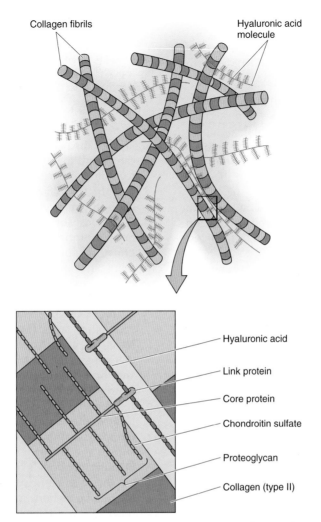

Figure 7.2 Diagrammatic representation of the extracellular matrix. *Top,* Lower magnification showing the banded collagen fibers with the adherent proteoglycans. *Bottom,* Glycosaminoglycans attached to their protein core and the link proteins that attach them to hyaluronic acid, forming huge macromolecules that may be hundreds of millions of daltons in size. *(From Gartner LP, Hiatt JL: Color Textbook of Histology, 3rd ed. Philadelphia, Saunders, 2007, p 72.)*

Table 7.2 EFFECTS OF HORMONES AND VITAMINS ON HYALINE CARTILAGE

Substance	Effects
Hormones	
Thyroxine, testosterone, and somatotropin (via insulin-like growth factors)	Stimulate cartilage growth and matrix formation
Cortisone, hydrocortisone, and estradiol	Inhibit cartilage growth and matrix formation
Vitamins	
Hypovitaminosis A	Reduces width of epiphyseal plates
Hypervitaminosis A	Accelerates ossification of epiphyseal plates
Hypovitaminosis C	Inhibits matrix synthesis and deforms architecture of epiphyseal plate; leads to scurvy
Absence of vitamin D, resulting in deficiency in absorption of calcium and phosphorus	Proliferation of chondrocytes is normal, but matrix does not become calcified properly; results in rickets

From Gartner LP, Hiatt JL: Color Textbook of Histology, 3rd ed. Philadelphia, Saunders, 2007, p 135.

Bone

Bone, the third hardest tissue, is always being remodeled by responding to pressure by undergoing resorption and to tension by adding more bone.

- The bony skeleton not only supports the body, but also forms a defensive armor to protect vital organs, such as the brain and spinal cord.
- Skeletal muscles attach to bones across joints permitting movement of parts of the body against each other and locomotion of the entire body.
- Almost all of the body's calcium is stored in the bony skeleton; acting as a reservoir, the calcium can be liberated from the skeleton to maintain the proper blood calcium level.
- Bone also houses **bone marrow** in its **marrow cavity**, which is responsible for **hematopoiesis**.

The outer surface of bone is covered by a soft connective tissue, the two-layered **periosteum**:

- The **outer fibrous layer** is composed of dense irregular collagenous connective tissue.
- The **inner cellular layer** is osteogenic, housing **osteoprogenitor cells** (osteogenic cells), some **osteoblasts**, and, occasionally, **osteoclasts**.

The marrow cavities are lined by **endosteum**, a thin cellular layer composed of osteoprogenitor cells, osteoblasts, occasionally osteoclasts, and slender connective tissue elements.

Bone matrix is composed of inorganic and organic components:

- Calcium and phosphorus constitute most of the inorganic components (about 65% of the dry weight). Most of the calcium and the phosphorus are present as **hydroxyapatite crystals** $[Ca_{10}(PO_4)_6(OH)_2]$ that are inserted into the gap regions of and are aligned along the length of type I collagen fibers. The crystals attract water, forming a **hydration shell** that facilitates ion exchange with the extracellular fluid.
- Type I collagen, the principal constituent of the organic component, forms approximately 80% to 90% of the organic portion of bone. The bulk of the remaining organic component is in the form of **aggrecan composites**, whereas **osteocalcin**, **osteopontin**, **bone sialoproteins**, and **adhesive glycoproteins** complete the organic component of bone matrix. Glycoproteins facilitate the adherence of bone matrix proteins to hydroxyapatite crystals and to integrins present in the plasma membranes of bone cells.

CELLS OF BONE

Bone possesses four classes of cells, the first three of which—osteoprogenitor cells, osteoblasts, and osteocytes—belong to the same cell lineage, whereas the fourth class, osteoclasts, are derived from monocyte precursors (Fig. 7.3).

- **Osteoprogenitor cells** populate the inner cellular layer of the periosteum; they line haversian canals and the marrow cavities. They proliferate, forming more osteoprogenitor cells and **osteoblasts** when oxygen tension is high, or **chondrogenic cells** when oxygen tension is low.
- **Osteoblast formation** requires the presence of **bone morphogenetic proteins** and **transforming growth factor-β**. Osteoblasts form a layer of cells that secrete the organic components of bone matrix, as well as the signaling molecules, receptor for activation of nuclear factor kappa β ligand (**RANKL**) and macrophage colony-stimulating factor (**M-CSF**). As the osteoblasts secrete their matrix, they form slender processes that contact the processes of adjacent osteoblasts and form **gap junctions** with them. As the bone matrix accumulates around the osteoblasts, these cells become incarcerated in the matrix that they formed; they become known as **osteocytes**, and the space that they occupy in their matrix is known as a **lacuna**. Osteoblasts not only manufacture bone matrix and become osteocytes, but they also participate in the calcification of the matrix. As bone formation is completed, its outer surface retains a layer of inactive osteoblasts that no longer manufacture bone matrix, but become flattened, and are known as **bone-lining cells**. These cells and osteocytes are separated from the calcified bone matrix by a thin layer of noncalcified matrix, known as **osteoid**. If the need arises, bone-lining cells can be activated to form bone matrix. The cell membranes of osteoblasts possess **integrins** and **parathyroid hormone (PTH) receptors**; the former permit osteoblasts to adhere to bone matrix components, and the latter, when they bind PTH, prompt the secretion of RANKL and **osteoclast-stimulating factor** by osteoblasts. RANKL facilitates the transformation of **preosteoclasts** to **osteoclasts**, and osteoclast-stimulating factor induces osteoclasts to resorb bone. Before they can do that, however, osteoblasts have to remove the osteoid from the bone surface, permitting the osteoclasts to gain access to the calcified bone.

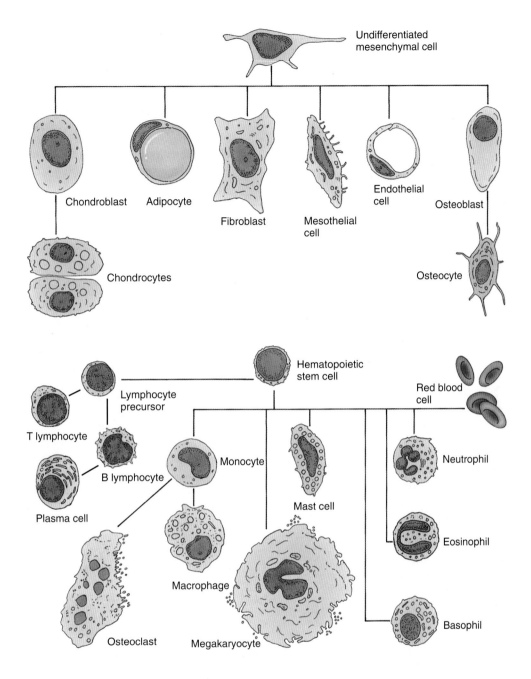

Figure 7.3 Origins of connective tissue cells (see osteoblasts, osteocytes, and osteoclasts). *(From Gartner LP, Hiatt JL: Color Textbook of Histology, 3rd ed. Philadelphia, Saunders, 2007, p 112.)*

CLINICAL CONSIDERATIONS

Alkaline phosphatase is richly represented in the cell membranes of osteoblasts. When bone is being elaborated, these cells secrete high levels of alkaline phosphatase, elevating the blood level of this enzyme. By evaluating alkaline phosphatase blood levels, it is possible to monitor bone formation.

CELLS OF BONE (cont.)

- **Osteocytes** occupy lacunae in bone, and their slender **osteocytic processes** extend through **canaliculi**, narrow channels in the calcified bone matrix, to contact the osteocytic processes of adjacent osteocytes, where they form **gap junctions** with one another and with the processes of osteoblasts, thus facilitating communications among the cells of bone. Extracellular fluid infiltrates the **periosteocytic spaces** and the canaliculi, providing nutrients and signaling molecules for these cells, and removing waste products and signaling molecules released by these cells. These spaces house more than 1 L of extracellular fluid into which osteocytes can release as much as 20 g of calcium in a short time.
- **Osteoclasts**, derived from the **mononuclear-phagocyte system**, are large (150 μm in diameter), multinucleated cells (≤50 nuclei) that resorb bone and possess numerous cell surface receptors, which include **osteoclast-stimulating factor-1 receptor**, **calcitonin receptor**, and **RANK**. Osteoclasts are *activated* to resorb bone by osteoblasts that have been stimulated by **PTH**, and are *inhibited* by **calcitonin** that binds to **calcitonin receptors** on their plasmalemma. **M-CSF**, secreted by osteoblasts, bind to **M-CSF receptors** on osteoclast precursor cells, stimulating them to proliferate and to express cell membrane **RANK** receptors. Simultaneously, osteoblasts express receptors for RANK, **RANKL**, allowing osteoclast precursors to bind to osteoblasts.
  - The RANK-RANKL interaction induces the **trimerization** of RANK on the surface of the osteoclast precursor cell, activating its adaptor molecules to trigger nuclear transcription.
  - The nuclear factors that are produced convert the *mononuclear* osteoclast precursor into an inactive *multinuclear* **osteoclast**, which detaches from the osteoblast.
  - Osteoblasts also manufacture **osteoprotegerin (OPG)**, a ligand that possesses a strong affinity for RANKL, blocking its availability for RANK and preventing the binding of osteoclast precursor to an osteoblast, preventing osteoclast formation.
  - In the presence of **PTH**, osteoblasts manufacture more RANKL than OPG, and in this manner they facilitate **osteoclastogenesis** (development of osteoclasts).

- Inactive osteoclasts express $\alpha_v\beta_3$ **integrins** allowing these cells to adhere to the bone surface.
- After osteoblasts remove osteoid from the bone surface, they leave, and their previous location becomes populated by inactive osteoclasts that, by adhering to the bone surface, become active osteoclasts. Shallow depressions located on the bone surface, called **Howship's lacunae**, house these active osteoclasts.

Osteoclasts have four recognizable regions when resorbing bone (Fig. 7.4):

- The **basal zone** contains most of the organelles of the osteoclast except for the mitochondria, which preferentially concentrate at the ruffled border.
- The **ruffled border** is located at the osteoclast-bone interface where resorption occurs. The osteoclast exhibits motile finger-like cytoplasmic extensions whose plasma membrane is thickened to protect the cell as it is resorbing bone forming a **subosteoclastic compartment**.
- The **clear zone**, the organelle-free region at the periphery of the ruffled border, expresses $\alpha_v\beta_3$ **integrins** whose extracellular aspect binds with osteopontin on the bone surface to form a **sealing zone**, isolating the microenvironment of the subosteoclastic compartment. Intracellularly, the integrin molecules contact actin filaments that form an **actin ring**.
- The **vesicular zone**, the region of the osteoclast located between the basal zone and the ruffled border, is rich in exocytotic and endocytotic vesicles. The former transport **cathepsin K**, which degrades collagens and other proteins of the bone matrix, into the subosteoclastic compartment, whereas the latter transport degraded bone products into the osteoclast.

MECHANISM OF BONE RESORPTION

The acidic environment leaches the inorganic components from the bone matrix, and the dissolved minerals enter the osteoclast cytoplasm, where they are exocytosed for delivery into the local capillaries in the vicinity of the basal zone. Osteoclasts secrete cathepsin K into the subosteoclastic compartment to degrade the organic components of the bone matrix. The resultant partially degraded materials are endocytosed by the osteoclasts, where they undergo further degradation before their release at the basal region (see Fig 7.4).

OSTEOCLAST

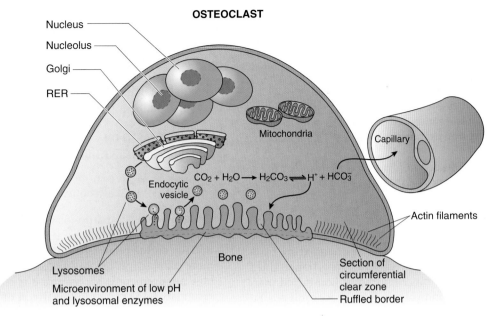

Figure 7.4 Osteoclastic function. RER, rough endoplasmic reticulum. *(From Gartner LP, Hiatt JL, Strum JM: Cell Biology and Histology [Board Review Series]. Philadelphia, Lippincott Williams & Wilkins, 1998, p. 100.)*

CLINICAL CONSIDERATIONS

Osteopetrosis results from a genetic defect in which osteoclasts are formed that are unable to resorb bone because they cannot form a ruffled border. Patients with osteopetrosis present with very dense bones and possibly anemia because of a reduced volume of marrow cavity. These individuals are also susceptible to blindness, deafness, and cranial nerve anomalies as a consequence of narrowing of the foramina through which cranial nerves exit the skull.

GROSS OBSERVATION OF BONE

Based on their external morphology, bones are categorized as:

- **Long bones**—composed of a slender shaft, **diaphysis**, and two heads, **epiphyses**
- **Short bones**—length and width are similar
- **Flat bones**—composed of two flat plates of compact bone sandwiching a layer of spongy bone
- **Irregular bones**—no definitive morphology
- **Sesamoid bones**—formed within the substance of tendons

Based on density, bone may be dense, as in **compact bone**, or spongelike, as in **cancellous (spongy) bone**. Spongy bone is always surrounded by compact bone. The **marrow cavity** of long bones, lined by a thin layer of cancellous bone, houses **red marrow** in young individuals, but it accumulates fat deposits as one ages and becomes known as **yellow marrow** in adults. Red marrow produces blood cells, whereas yellow marrow does not produce blood cells, but does retain its hematopoietic potential. Cancellous bone has resting osteoblast-lined marrow spaces that contain red marrow, and the bone tissue that forms the perimeter of the marrow spaces has smaller and larger irregular lamellae of bone—**spicules** and **trabeculae**.

The articulating surfaces of the epiphyses are composed of a thin layer of compact bone that overlies spongy bone and is covered by hyaline cartilage. In individuals still growing, an **epiphyseal plate** of hyaline cartilage is interposed between the epiphysis and the diaphysis. The **metaphysis** is a flared zone of the shaft, located between the diaphysis and the epiphyseal plate.

The external surface of the diaphysis and the nonarticulating surfaces of the epiphyses are covered by a two-layered **periosteum** that is inserted into the bone via collagen fibers, **Sharpey's fibers** (Fig. 7.5).

- The **outer fibrous layer** of the periosteum is composed of dense irregular fibrous connective tissue whose neurovascular elements serve the outer region of compact bone.
- The **inner cellular layer** possesses osteoprogenitor cells and osteoblasts.

Bones of the calvaria (**skull cap**) are composed of the **outer** and **inner tables** of compact bone with a layer of spongy bone known as the **diploë** interposed between them. The periosteum covering the outer table of the bones of the cranium is known as the **pericranium**, but the periosteum covering the inner table of the bones of the calvaria is the **dura mater**, the outermost layer of the meninges covering and protecting the brain. The dura also serves as the periosteum of the inner table.

BONE TYPES BASED ON MICROSCOPIC OBSERVATIONS

Two types of bone may be observed from microscopic studies—primary bone and secondary bone.

- **Primary bone** (**immature** or **woven bone**) is the first bone to be formed and it is the bone formed initially during bone repair. Primary bone is more cellular, it is less calcified, and its collagen fiber arrangement is haphazard. It is replaced by secondary bone except in the alveoli of teeth and tendon insertions.
- **Secondary bone** (**mature** or **lamellar bone**) is highly organized into concentric bony lamellae (3 to 7 μm thick), and because it is more calcified and has a precise arrangement of collagen fiber bundles, it is stronger than primary bone. **Osteocytes** housed in **lacunae** are distributed at regular intervals between, or infrequently within, lamellae (see Fig. 7.5). These cells communicate with one another via their **osteocytic processes** that form gap junctions with each other in narrow channels known as **canaliculi**.

Lamellar Systems of Compact Bone

Compact bone consists of very thin bony layers called **lamellae**, arranged in four lamellar systems—outer and inner circumferential lamellae, interstitial lamellae, and osteons (haversian canal systems)—that are readily observable in long bones (see Fig. 7.5).

- The outermost calcified layer of the diaphysis, located just deep to the periosteum, is the **outer circumferential lamellar system**, into which Sharpey's fibers insert.
- Lamellae of bone that encircle the marrow cavity are known as the **inner circumferential lamellar system**. Spongy bone lining this lamellar system extends trabeculae and spicules into the marrow cavity.

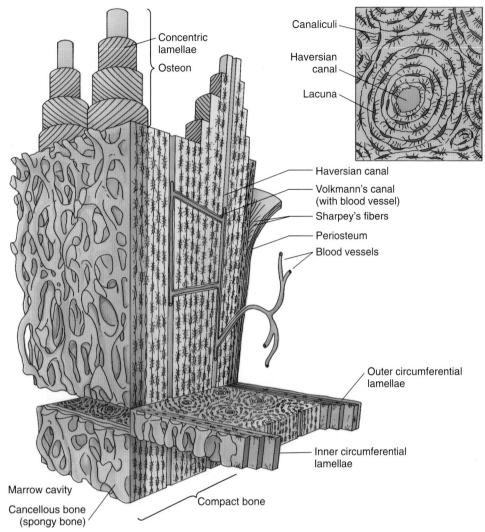

Concentric lamellae
Osteon
Canaliculi
Haversian canal
Lacuna
Haversian canal
Volkmann's canal (with blood vessel)
Sharpey's fibers
Periosteum
Blood vessels
Outer circumferential lamellae
Inner circumferential lamellae
Marrow cavity
Cancellous bone (spongy bone)
Compact bone

Figure 7.5 Diagram of bone illustrating compact cortical bone, osteons, lamellae, Volkmann's canals, haversian canals, lacunae, canaliculi, and spongy bone. *(From Gartner LP, Hiatt JL: Color Textbook of Histology, 3rd ed. Philadelphia, Saunders, 2007, p 144.)*

Lamellar Systems of Compact Bone (cont.)

- **Haversian canal systems (osteons)**, about 20 to 100 µm in diameter, constitute the predominant lamellar system in compact bone. Osteons are composed of wafer-thin lamellae of calcified bone that form concentric cylinders whose central, **haversian canal** contains a neurovascular supply and are lined by osteoprogenitor cells and osteoblasts (Fig. 7.6). As the vascular supply branches and bifurcates, osteons mirror this organization. Osteons are delimited by a boundary, known as a **cementing line**, composed of calcified ground substance containing only few collagen fibers.
  - The **helical arrangement** of collagen fibers is strictly organized, so that, when viewed in cross section, the fibers parallel each other within a particular lamella, but are perpendicular to collagen fibers of adjacent lamellae. This pattern is created by varying the pitch of the helix, lessening the chances of bone fracture.
  - Haversian canals are connected to the canals of their neighboring osteon via oblique channels, **Volkmann's canals**, which allow blood vessels access to other haversian canals (see Fig. 7.6).
  - Osteons are formed as follows: the outermost lamella, the one bordering the cementing line, is formed first; succeeding lamellae line the last one that was formed; and the innermost lamella, bordering the haversian canal, is the last one to be formed. Because osteocytes depend on the inefficient canaliculi for their sustenance, the thickness of each osteon is limited to approximately 20 lamellae.
- Bone is being continually remodeled as osteons are resorbed by osteoclasts and are replaced by osteoblasts. This process leaves remnants of the old osteons, which appear as arc-shaped fragments of lamellae, known as **interstitial lamellae**, trapped among unresorbed osteons.

HISTOGENESIS OF BONE

Bone develops in the embryo either by **intramembranous bone formation** or by **endochondral bone formation**. Although these two methods are grossly different, *histologically*, the final products are indistinguishable from each other. Regardless of the mode of development, primary bone is the first to form; this is resorbed and replaced by secondary bone, which is mature bone that continues to be resorbed and remodeled as it responds to environmental forces placed on it throughout life (Fig. 7.7).

- **Intramembranous bone formation** is the method by which most of the flat bones develop.
  - Formation begins in a highly vascular environment of mesenchymal tissue in which mesenchymal cells maintain contact with each other.
  - These mesenchymal cells express the osteogenic master regulators, **transcription factors Cbfa1/Runx2** and the zinc finger transcription factor **osterix**, and differentiate into **osteoblasts**, which secrete **bone matrix**.
  - In the absence of osterix, the mesenchymal cells differentiate into preosteoblasts, but cannot make the transition into fully competent, matrix-secreting osteoblasts.
  - Osteogenesis begins as the initial matrix forms trabecular complexes whose surfaces are occupied by osteoblasts. This area now represents a **primary ossification center** forming primary bone.
  - When osteoid is secreted, calcification begins trapping osteoblasts in **lacunae**. These cells, surrounded by their matrix, are now known as **osteocytes**. The matrix calcifies, and **canaliculi** are formed around processes of osteocytes.
  - **Trabeculae** enlarge and increase in number forming networks around the vascular elements, which become transformed into **bone marrow**.
  - Additional **ossification centers** are necessary in the larger flat bones, such as those of the skull. As bone formation continues, these ossification centers fuse forming a single bone. An exception is in the **fontanelles** of the newborn skull, where the ossification centers of the frontal and parietal bones do not fuse until after birth when the membranous *soft spots* are replaced by bone.
  - Regions of the mesenchymal connective tissue that do not participate in bone formation become transformed into the **periosteum** and **endosteum**.

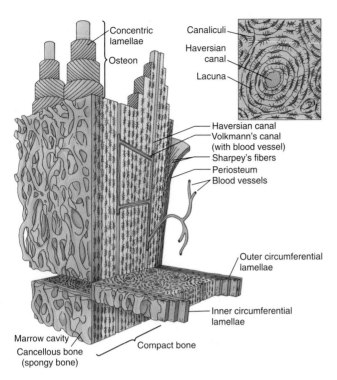

Figure 7.6 Diagram of bone illustrating compact cortical bone, osteons, lamellae, Volkmann's canals, haversian canals, lacunae, canaliculi, and spongy bone. *(From Gartner LP, Hiatt JL: Color Textbook of Histology, 3rd ed. Philadelphia, Saunders, 2007, p 144.)*

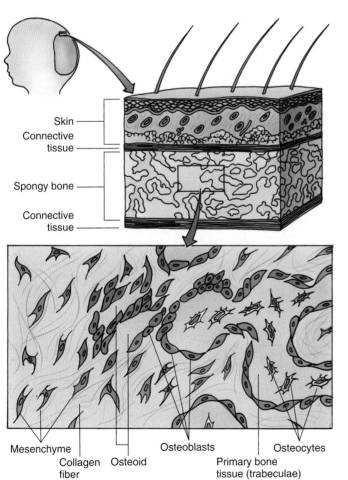

Figure 7.7 Intramembranous bone formation. *(From Gartner LP, Hiatt JL: Color Textbook of Histology, 3rd ed. Philadelphia, Saunders, 2007, p 146.)*

Endochondral Bone Formation

With the exception of the flat bones, most of the bones of the body are developed via **endochondral bone formation**, a method employing several phases. These processes are presented graphically in Figure 7.8 and summarized in Table 7.3.

- A **hyaline cartilage model** becomes a scaffold for development of bone.
- As the bone being formed becomes stable enough to support the body, the cartilage model is **resorbed** and replaced by the forming **bone**.

- The first area of the cartilage model to be replaced is the diaphysis, the **primary center of ossification**, to be followed by bone formation in the epiphyses, the **secondary centers of ossification**.

The process of endochondral bone formation is represented by a dynamic series of interrelated events that begin in fetal life and continue into adulthood and beyond as bone may need repair. Even in adulthood, these processes are in action as bone is in a dynamic state and must be remodeled constantly to accommodate environmental forces.

Table 7.3 EVENTS IN ENDOCHONDRAL BONE FORMATION

Event	Description
Hyaline cartilage model formed	Miniature hyaline cartilage model formed in region of embryo where bone is to develop. Some chondrocytes mature, hypertrophy, and die. Cartilage matrix becomes calcified
Primary Center of Ossification	
Perichondrium at midriff of diaphysis becomes vascularized	Vascularization of perichondrium changes it to periosteum. Chondrogenic cells become osteoprogenitor cells
Osteoblasts secrete matrix, forming subperiosteal bone collar	Subperiosteal bone collar is formed of primary bone (intramembranous bone formation)
Chondrocytes within diaphysis core hypertrophy, die, and degenerate	Presence of periosteum and bone prevents diffusion of nutrients to chondrocytes. Their degeneration leaves lacunae, opening large spaces in septa of cartilage
Osteoclasts etch holes in subperiosteal bone collar, permitting entrance of osteogenic bud	Holes permit osteoprogenitor cells and capillaries to invade cartilage model, now calcified, and begin elaborating bone matrix
Formation of calcified cartilage/calcified bone complex	Bone matrix laid down on septa of calcified cartilage forms this complex. Histologically, calcified cartilage stains blue, calcified bone stains red
Osteoclasts resorbing calcified cartilage/calcified bone complex	Destruction of calcified cartilage/calcified bone complex enlarges marrow cavity
Subperiosteal bone collar thickens, begins growing toward epiphyses	This event, over time, completely replaces diaphyseal cartilage with bone
Secondary Center of Ossification	
Ossification begins at epiphysis	Begins in same way as primary center except there is no bone collar. Osteoblasts lay down bone matrix on calcified cartilage scaffold
Growth of bone at epiphyseal plate	Cartilaginous articular surface of bone remains. Epiphyseal plate persists—growth added at epiphyseal end of plate. Bone added at diaphyseal end of plate
Epiphysis and diaphysis become continuous	At end of bone growth, cartilage of epiphyseal plate ceases proliferation. Bone development continues to unite diaphysis and epiphysis

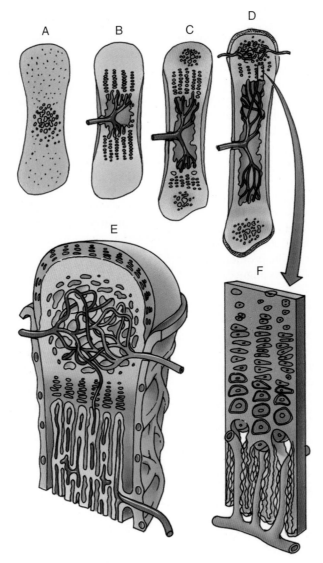

Figure 7.8 Endochondral bone formation. *Blue* represents the cartilage model on which bone is formed. Bone then replaces cartilage. **A,** Hyaline cartilage model. **B,** Cartilage at the midriff (diaphysis) is invaded by vascular elements. **C,** Subperiosteal bone collar is formed. **D,** Bone collar prevents nutrients from reaching cartilage cells, so they die leaving confluent lacunae. **E,** Calcified bone/calcified cartilage complex at the epiphyseal ends of the growing bone. **F,** Enlargement of the epiphyseal plate at the end of the bone where bone replaces cartilage. *(From Gartner LP, Hiatt JL: Color Textbook of Histology, 3rd ed. Philadelphia, Saunders, 2007, p 147.)*

Bone Growth in Length

The proliferation of chondrocytes located in the epiphyseal plate is responsible for bone elongation. The epiphyseal side of the plate is cartilaginous, whereas at the diaphyseal side of the plate, bone is replacing cartilage. The epiphyseal plate presents five distinct zones beginning at the epiphyseal side of the epiphyseal plate as follows (Fig. 7.9):

- **Zone of reserve cartilage**: Mitotically active chondrocytes are haphazardly arranged.
- **Zone of proliferation**: Chondrocytes secrete the protein **Indian hedgehog**, which hinders hypertrophy of chondrocytes and induces the release of **PTH-related protein (PTH-RP)**, which promotes cell division among the chondrocytes of the zone of proliferation. The proliferating chondrocytes form parallel rows aligned in the direction of bone growth.
- **Zone of maturation and hypertrophy**: Maturing chondrocytes amass glycogen and express the transcription factors **Cbfa1/Runx2**, which permits them to hypertrophy. These chondrocytes also release type X collagen and **vascular endothelial growth factor**, which promotes vascular incursion.
- **Zone of calcification**: Hypertrophied cells attract **macrophages** to destroy the calcified walls between their adjacent, enlarged lacunae; chondrocytes undergo apoptosis and die.
- **Zone of ossification**: Osteoprogenitor cells enter the zone of ossification and form osteoblasts, which deposit bone matrix that becomes calcified on the surface of the calcified cartilage. The calcified cartilage/calcified bone complex becomes resorbed and is replaced by bone.

Bone continues to grow in length as long as there is a balance between the zone of proliferation and the rate of resorption in the zone of ossification. By the time the individual reaches 20 or so years of age, the mitotic rate in the proliferation zone is surpassed by the resorption rate in the zone of ossification depleting the zone of reserve cartilage. When the last calcified cartilage/calcified bone complex is resorbed, the epiphyseal plate no longer separates the epiphysis from the diaphysis, the marrow cavities of the two regions become continuous, and the bone is unable to continue growing in length.

Bone Growth in Width

Bone growth in length occurs by interstitial growth of the cartilage of the epiphyseal plate, whereas bone growth in width is accomplished by appositional growth occurring deep to the periosteum. Osteoblasts derived from **osteoprogenitor cells** of the periosteum secrete bone matrix on the bone surface, a process known as **subperiosteal intramembranous bone formation**, which continues during bone development and growth.

Throughout life, the processes of bone resorption and bone deposition must be in balance. Bone formation on the external surface of the diaphysis must be balanced with osteoclastic activity resorbing the internal aspect to enlarge the marrow cavity.

CALCIFICATION OF BONE

Although the process of calcification is not fully understood, it is known that **proteoglycans**, **osteonectin**, and **bone sialoprotein** stimulate calcification. The calcification theory currently accepted involves release of membrane-bound **matrix vesicles** (100 to 200 nm in diameter) by osteoblasts.

- **Matrix vesicles** contain high concentrations of Ca^{++} and PO_4^{3-} ions, adenosine triphosphate (ATP), alkaline phosphatase, cyclic adenosine monophosphate, ATPase, pyrophosphatase, calcium-binding proteins, and phosphoserine.
- Matrix vesicle membranes have **calcium pumps** that transport Ca^{++} ions into the vesicle; increased concentrations of Ca^{++} ions cause the formation of calcium hydroxyapatite crystals that grow in size and eventually puncture the vesicle membrane causing it to disperse its contents.
- Freed calcium hydroxyapatite crystals serve as **nidi of crystallization** within the matrix.
- **Enzymes** released from matrix vesicles liberate phosphate ions that combine with calcium ions and calcify the matrix around the nidi of crystallization.
- **Water is resorbed** from the matrix, and hydroxyapatite crystals are deposited within the gap regions of the collagen molecules.
- The various nidi of mineralization enlarge and fuse with each other, and the entire matrix becomes calcified.

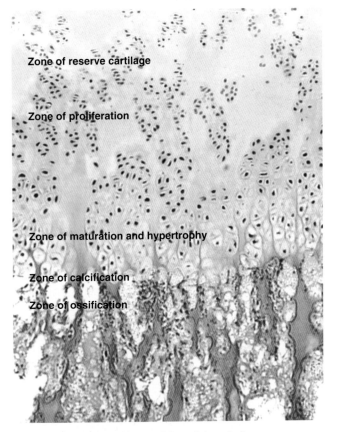

Zone of reserve cartilage

Zone of proliferation

Zone of maturation and hypertrophy

Zone of calcification

Zone of ossification

Figure 7.9 Zones of the epiphyseal plate.

CLINICAL CONSIDERATIONS

Children who are deficient in somatotropin exhibit **dwarfism**, whereas individuals possessing an excess of somatotropin during their years of growth exhibit **pituitary gigantism**. Adults who produce excess somatotropin display increased bone deposition without normal bone resorption. This condition, called **acromegaly**, causes thickening of the bones particularly in the face, causing disfigurement of the overlying soft tissues.

BONE REMODELING

Adult bone is remodeled constantly, and haversian systems are continuously being replaced to counter the changing environmental stresses placed on it as some bone is resorbed from one area, and some bone is added to another area.

- The generalized shape of bones continues to mirror the form of the embryonic cartilage templates even though they are many times larger than their embryonic counterparts. This ability is a product of **surface remodeling** because bone deposition and bone resorption act in concert on the periosteal and on the endosteal surfaces of bone.
- Cells of compact bone respond to the systemic factors **calcitonin** and **PTH**, whereas cancellous bone is remodeled in response to local bone marrow–derived factors, such as **colony-stimulating factor-1**, **tumor necrosis factor**, **interleukin-1**, osteoprotegerin (**OPG**, a RANK homolog), **osteoprotegerin ligand** (**OPGL**, a RANK L homolog), and **transforming growth factor-β**.
- When haversian systems are replaced, the osteocytes die, and some portions of the old haversian systems are resorbed by osteoclasts, whose activities create **resorption cavities**.
- As osteoclastic activity is continued, the resorption cavities enlarge and become invaded by blood vessels.
- Bone formation begins as osteoblasts manufacture successive lamellae surrounding the blood vessels, forming a new haversian system. This resorption followed by bone replacement is known as **coupling**; the remnants of resorbed osteons remain as the interstitial lamellar system.

BONE REPAIR

When bone injury is severe, the ends of a broken bone may be displaced or bone fragments may be detached from the injured bone or both. Additionally, blood vessels are severed near the break, causing localized hemorrhaging, forming a blood clot that fills the injury site (Fig. 7.10).

- Blood supply to the region ceases retrograde from the injury site back to where anastomosing vessels may later develop collateral circulation to the region.
- Many haversian systems lose their vascular supply, which causes their osteocytes to die,

resulting in empty lacunae and enlarging the zone of injury.

- The periosteum and the bone marrow are less affected by this loss of a vascular supply because their tissues are exceptionally well vascularized from many areas.
- Within 2 days of injury, small capillaries and fibroblasts invade the blood clot that fills the injury site and form **granulation tissue**.
- The osteogenic layer of the periosteum, endosteum, and undifferentiated cells of the bone marrow proliferate, forming osteoprogenitor cells, which differentiate into osteoblasts.
- The newly formed osteoblasts secrete bone matrix cementing dead bone in the injury site to the healthy bone, beginning the formation of a collar of bone—the **external callus**.
- Concurrently, the clot within the marrow cavity is invaded by multipotential cells of the bone marrow and by osteoprogenitor cells originating from the endosteum to form, within less than 1 week after injury, the **internal callus** composed of bony trabeculae.

Proliferation of osteoprogenitor cells in the region of the external callus outpaces the growth of capillaries; some of the **osteoprogenitor cells** located farther away from the capillary bed are exposed to a reduced oxygen tension. These cells become **chondrogenic cells** that differentiate into chondroblasts and secrete cartilage matrix on the surface of the bone collar. Osteoprogenitor cells that are still in the presence of capillaries continue to proliferate forming more osteoprogenitor cells. The **external callus** is composed of three layers:

- Layer of bone collar cemented to bone
- Layer of cartilage forming an intermediate layer
- Surface layer containing osteogenic cells

Cartilage matrix adjacent to the woven bone of the collar becomes calcified and is ultimately replaced with primary bone via **endochondral bone formation**. Eventually, all of the bone fragments become united by cancellous bone. Finally, the injury site is remodeled by replacing the primary bone with secondary bone and resorbing the callus. The injury zone ultimately is restored to its original shape and strength. Intramembranous and endochondral bone formation are necessary for successful repair of bone fractures.

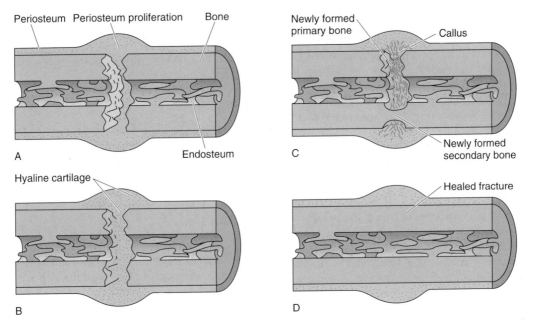

Figure 7.10 Events in bone fracture repair. *(From Gartner LP, Hiatt JL: Color Textbook of Histology, 3rd ed. Philadelphia, Saunders, 2007, p 153.)*

CLINICAL CONSIDERATIONS

When bone is damaged so severely that it may be necessary to remove some of its fragments, the distance between the remaining bone segments may be too great to form a callus bridge and form a **bony union**. In this instance, viable bone for grafting is secured from a bone bank where bone is harvested and frozen to maintain its osteogenic potential. Three different kinds of bone for grafting are available. **Autographs** are grafts of bone from the recipient and are the most successful. **Homografts** are grafts of bone from another individual of the same species. These pose risks of immunological rejection. **Heterografts** are grafts of bone from a different species and are the least successful.

Androgens and **estrogens** produced by the male and female gonads influence skeletal maturation by affecting the closure of the epiphyseal plates. Skeletal development is stunted when sexual maturation occurs early because this stimulates the epiphyseal plates to close prematurely. The opposite is true in individuals whose sexual maturity is retarded. Skeletal growth in these individuals continues for a longer time because their epiphyseal plates remain functional beyond the normal time frame.

Osteoporosis is related to decreasing bone mass and affects about 10 million Americans, especially postmenopausal women and women older than 40 years. The decreased estrogen production by these women reduces the number of osteoblasts recruited to secrete bone matrix. Additionally, osteoclastic activity is increased beyond that of bone deposition, resulting in a decreased bone mass. The severity of the reduction may be great enough that the affected individual's bones become fragile. To ameliorate the disease process, estrogen replacement therapy was initiated in these women. It was discovered, however, that estrogen replacement therapy increased the risk for heart disease, breast cancer, stroke, and blood clots. Consequently, instead of estrogen replacement therapy, a new group of drugs (bisphosphonates) are employed to reduce the incidence of osteoporosis-induced fractures.

MAINTENANCE OF BLOOD CALCIUM LEVELS

Calcium levels in the blood are carefully controlled and maintained at a blood plasma concentration of 9 to 11 mg/dL. The body's reservoir for calcium is in bone, where about 99% of the body's calcium is stored in hydroxyapatite crystals; the remaining (1%) is available for rapid recruitment from newly formed osteons whose labile calcium ions are more readily available. A constant exchange occurs between calcium ions present in bone and those in blood.

HORMONAL EFFECTS

When blood calcium levels decrease, the parathyroid glands secrete PTH, activating osteoblasts to secrete **osteoclast-stimulating factor** and **OPGL** and to cease bone formation. As a result, dormant osteoclasts are activated, and the formation of new osteoclasts is induced, initiating bone resorption and ultimately leading to calcium ions being released from the bone and transferred to the bloodstream.

Plasma calcium ion levels are monitored by parafollicular cells (C cells) of the thyroid gland. Increased levels of calcium ions in the plasma prompt these cells to secrete **calcitonin**, a hormone that sensitizes receptors on the osteoclasts, restraining them from resorbing bone. At the same time, osteoblasts are signaled to increase osteoid synthesis, and calcium is recruited and deposited in newly forming bone. The anterior lobe of the pituitary gland secretes **somatotropin** that controls bone development by encouraging **insulin-like growth factors**, formerly called **somatomedins**, which stimulate epiphyseal plate growth. Additional factors affecting bone metabolism are:

- **Interleukin-1**, derived from osteoblasts, activates proliferation of osteoclast precursors and indirectly stimulates osteoclasts.
- **Interleukin-6**, derived from bone cells, induces the formation of new osteoclasts.
- **OPG** restrains osteoclast differentiation.
- **Tumor necrosis factor**, formed by activated macrophages, resembles interleukin-1 in function.
- **Interferon-γ**, formed by T lymphocytes, prevents the formation of osteoclasts.
- **Colony-stimulating factor-1**, formed by stromal cells, stimulates osteoclast formation.
- **Transforming growth factor-β**, released from bone matrix during bone degradation, induces osteogenesis and inhibits osteoclast formation.

In addition to hormones, vitamins also affect skeletal development (Table 7.4).

JOINTS

A bone may articulate with another bone at a movable joint, or two bones may closely approximate each other in a nonmovable joint. Classification of joints is based on whether there is a lack of movement (**synarthrosis joints**) or there is freedom of movement (**diarthrosis joints**) between the two bones of the joint (Fig. 7.11).

Synarthrosis joints are of three types:

- **Synostosis**: Minimal or no movement; bone is joint-uniting tissue (e.g., right and left parietal bones of the adult skull).
- **Synchondrosis**: Only a limited amount of movement; hyaline cartilage is joint-uniting tissue (e.g., sternocostal joint).
- **Syndesmosis**: Little movement; dense connective tissue is the joint-uniting tissue (e.g., inferior tibiofibular articulation joined by the interosseous ligament.

Diarthrosis joints are the most common joints of the extremities (see Fig. 7.10). The articulating surfaces of the bones of these joints are permanently covered by **hyaline cartilage** (**articular cartilage**). Contact between the bony members of the joint is usually maintained by ligaments that are attached to both bones of the joint. A **joint capsule** encloses and seals the joint. The outer **fibrous layer** of the capsule is composed of dense connective tissue, which becomes continuous with the periosteum of both bones of the joint. The inner layer of the capsule, the cellular **synovial layer** (**synovial membrane**), covers all of the joint surfaces except the articulating surfaces. The synovial layer is composed of two cell types:

- **Type A cells** are macrophages that phagocytose debris present in the joint cavity.
- **Type B cells** secrete **synovial fluid**.

Synovial fluid supplies nutrients and oxygen to the chondrocytes of the articular cartilage. It possesses leukocytes, a high concentration of **hyaluronic acid**, and **lubricin**, a glycoprotein that is combined with plasma filtrate to lubricate the joint.

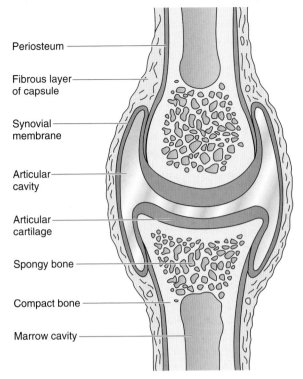

Periosteum

Fibrous layer of capsule

Synovial membrane

Articular cavity

Articular cartilage

Spongy bone

Compact bone

Marrow cavity

Figure 7.11 Anatomy of a diarthrodial joint. *(From Gartner LP, Hiatt JL: Color Textbook of Histology, 3rd ed. Philadelphia, Saunders, 2007, p 156.)*

Table 7.4 VITAMINS AND THEIR EFFECTS ON SKELETAL DEVELOPMENT

Vitamin	Effects on Skeletal Development
Vitamin A deficiency	Inhibits proper bone formation as coordination of osteoblast and osteoclast activities fails. Failure of resorption and remodeling of cranial vault to accommodate the brain with serious damage to central nervous system
Hypervitaminosis A	Erosion of cartilage columns without increases of cells in proliferation zone. Epiphyseal plates may become obliterated, ceasing growth prematurely
Vitamin C deficiency	Mesenchymal tissue affected as connective tissue is unable to produce and maintain extracellular matrix. Deficient production of collagen and bone matrix results in retarded growth and delayed healing. Scurvy
Vitamin D deficiency	Ossification of epiphyseal cartilages disturbed. Cells become disordered at metaphysis, leading to poorly calcified bones, which become deformed by weight bearing. In children—rickets. In adults—osteomalacia

CLINICAL CONSIDERATIONS

Osteoarthritis is a degenerative disease of the synovial joints related to wear and tear on the articular cartilage of the condyles of one or both bony members of the joint. The hyaline cartilage begins to degenerate and eventually erodes, and the cortical bones of the condyles contact each other during articulation, causing pain severe enough to restrict movement at the joint and debilitate the individual.

Rheumatoid arthritis is a disease of synovial joints related to destruction of the synovial membrane. The synovial membrane becomes thickened and infiltrated with plasma cells and lymphocytes. The articular cartilage is eventually destroyed and replaced with fibrovascular connective tissue resulting in severe pain during movement at the joint.

Rickets is a disease of infants and children caused by vitamin D deficiency. When vitamin D is absent, the mucosa of the intestines cannot absorb calcium even when the diet is adequate. Without calcium, there are bone ossification

disorders in the epiphyseal cartilages and confused orientation of metaphysis cells resulting in insufficiently calcified bone matrix. Rickets causes a child's bones, especially those of the legs, to be deformed and weakened because the bones can no longer bear the body weight.

Osteomalacia is a prolonged vitamin D deficiency disease in adults (adult rickets). When vitamin D has been absent for an extended time, newly formed bone in the remodeling process does not calcify in a proper fashion. During pregnancy, this condition may become severe for the woman because the fetus requires calcium, and the only source for the fetus is from the mother.

Scurvy is a vitamin C deficiency disease. When intake of vitamin C is inadequate, there is deficient collagen production resulting in inadequate formation of bone matrix and bone development. This condition is also problematic because healing is delayed in the absence of proper levels of collagen.

8 MUSCLE

Animals are able to move and have the capacity of moving blood and other material along the lumina of tubular structures because of elongated muscle cells that specialize in the ability to contract. These muscle cells are of two types—**striated**, which display alternating light and dark bands, and **smooth**, which lack such striations. There are two types of striated muscle:

- **Skeletal**, for voluntary movements, and
- **Cardiac**, for pumping blood (Fig. 8.1).

These specialized cells have their own nomenclature. Their cell membranes are known as *sarcolemma,* their smooth endoplasmic reticulum is referred to as *sarcoplasmic reticulum,* and their mitochondria are sometimes referred to as *sarcosomes.* Because their length far exceeds their girth, they are frequently referred to as *muscle fibers.* All three are mesodermal derivatives.

> **KEY WORDS**
> - **Skeletal muscle**
> - **Myofibrils**
> - **Sarcomere**
> - **Myofilaments**
> - **Muscle contraction**
> - **Neuromuscular junction**
> - **Cardiac muscle**
> - **Smooth muscle**

Skeletal Muscle

Skeletal muscle cells are formed by hundreds of **myoblasts** that line up end to end and coalesce into a **myotube.** Each myotube manufactures its own contractile elements, **myofilaments,** which are distinctively arranged to form **myofibrils,** and cytoskeletal components and organelles. Skeletal muscle cells:

- May be several centimeters long and 10 to 100 μm in diameter, and
- Are arranged so that they not only are parallel to each other, but also the dark and light bands of adjacent cells are aligned with each other.

The extracellular spaces between neighboring cells are occupied by **continuous capillaries.**

Skeletal muscle strength is a function of the number and diameter of the muscle fibers composing a particular muscle.

- **White fibers** (e.g., chicken breast) are designed for fast contractility but are easily fatigued.
- **Red fibers** (e.g., dark meat) contract slower but are not fatigued easily.
- Fibers that are in between red and white are **intermediate fibers.**

White fibers have a poorer vascular supply, fewer mitochondria, fewer oxidative enzymes, and less of the oxygen-transporting protein **myoglobin** than red fibers, but their diameters are larger, and their sarcoplasmic reticulum is more extensive. The nerve supply determines whether a muscle fiber is red or white, and switching the fiber of one muscle cell type to that of the other switches the characteristic of the muscle cell to the modality of its new innervation.

The connective tissue elements of skeletal muscle not only harness the contraction-derived energy of the muscle but also conduct neurovascular elements to each muscle cell and subdivide the muscle mass into smaller units, known as **fascicles.** Each fascicle, enveloped by its **perimysium** (see Fig. 8.1), is composed of numerous skeletal muscle fibers, each with its own, slender connective tissue investment—the **endomysium,** whose reticular fibers interweave with those of adjacent cells. The connective tissue surrounding the entire muscle, the **epimysium** (see Fig. 8.1), is continuous with the **tendons** and **aponeuroses** of the whole muscle and is intimately related to the reticular fibers of the endomysium that interdigitate with the fluted ends of the muscle cell; this relationship is the **myotendinous junction.**

LIGHT MICROSCOPY OF SKELETAL MUSCLE

Along the length of the skeletal muscle fiber, small regenerative cells, known as **satellite cells** and possessing a single nucleus, are present, sharing the external lamina of the muscle fiber. Occasional **fibroblasts** are also noted in the endomysium. The cytoplasm of skeletal muscle cells is packed with cylindrical **myofibrils.**

- Myofibrils are precisely arranged so that their dark and light bands are aligned with those of their neighbors; these bands are aligned along the length of the muscle fiber.
- **I bands** are transected by a thin **Z disk (line).**
- Dark bands, **A bands,** are bisected by a light area, the **H band,** which is transected by a thin **M line.**
- The contractile unit of skeletal muscle, the **sarcomere,** extends from Z disk to Z disk.
- During muscle contraction, the sarcomere shortens; the Z disks are closer to each other, the H band disappears, and the I bands become narrower, but the A band does not change.

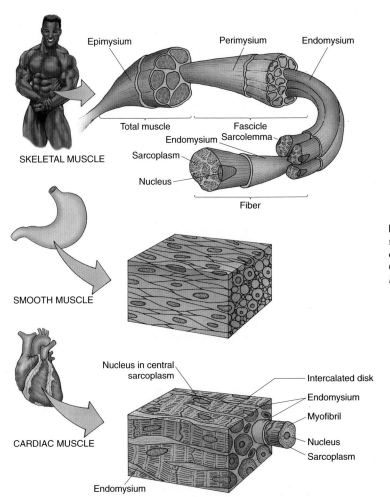

Epimysium
Perimysium
Endomysium
Total muscle
Fascicle
Sarcolemma
Endomysium
Sarcoplasm
Nucleus
Fiber

SKELETAL MUSCLE

SMOOTH MUSCLE

CARDIAC MUSCLE

Nucleus in central sarcoplasm
Intercalated disk
Endomysium
Myofibril
Nucleus
Sarcoplasm
Endomysium

Figure 8.1 Diagram of the three types of muscle: skeletal (*top*), smooth (*middle*), and cardiac (*bottom*). *(From Gartner LP, Hiatt JL: Color Textbook of Histology, 3rd ed. Philadelphia, Saunders, 2007, p 159.)*

CLINICAL CONSIDERATION

Temporary myositis is a mild to severe inflammation of skeletal muscles that results from accidental injury, infection, strenuous exercise, viral infection, or certain prescription drugs. Symptoms include muscle pain, muscle weakness, tenderness of the area over the region of the muscle, warmth, and reduced or impaired function. As its name suggests, the condition is not serious; it is temporary, and the problem resolves itself when the offending condition is removed.

Myositis can be a very serious condition that includes numerous **inflammatory myopathies**—dermatomyositis, inclusion body myositis, the juvenile form of myositis, and polymyositis. All of these diseases are idiopathic, although they may be autoimmune diseases. The general symptoms for all of these myopathies are painful, weak muscles; general malaise; reduced mobility (especially in climbing stairs and standing up after falling down); and frequently difficulties in deglutition (dysphagia).

ELECTRON MICROSCOPY OF SKELETAL MUSCLE

The sarcolemma is similar in most respects to other cell membranes except that in skeletal muscle it forms numerous deep, tubular invaginations.

- **T tubules** (Fig. 8.2) extend into the cytoplasm and interweave, always at the junction of the I and A bands, throughout the interior of the muscle fiber. Two T tubules for each sarcomere spread waves of depolarization into the interior of the muscle fiber.
- Two **terminal cisternae**, expanded regions of the sarcoplasmic reticulum that store calcium, flank each T tubule at the I–A junctions (known as a **triad**) around every myofibril.
- Voltage-gated **calcium release channels** (**ryanodine receptors**) of the terminal cisternae are in close association with the **voltage-sensitive dihydropyridine-sensitive receptors (DHSR)** of the T tubules (this complex is known as **junctional feet**). As the wave of depolarization is conducted into the interior of the muscle cell, the DHSR causes calcium release channels to open, and calcium leaves the terminal cisternae to enter the sarcoplasm (Fig. 8.3; see Fig. 8.2).

The A and I bands of adjacent myofilaments are closely aligned with each other.

- This relationship is maintained by **desmin**, which wraps around the Z disks of adjacent myofibrils, fastening them to each other and to Z disks via the assistance of **plectin**.
- The heat shock protein **αB-crystallin** protects desmin from stresses placed on it.
- Actin-binding protein **dystrophin** fixes desmin to the **costamere** regions of the sarcolemma.
- Long, tubular mitochondria occupy spaces among myofilament bundles and the periphery of the sarcoplasm deep to the cell membrane. The sarcoplasm is rich in **myoglobin**.

STRUCTURAL ORGANIZATION OF MYOFIBRILS

The dark and light bands seen in light microscopy are due to the presence of parallel, interdigitating:

- **Thin myofilaments** (1 μm in length, 7 nm in diameter, and composed mainly of **actin**) and
- **Thick myofilaments** (1.5 μm long, 15 nm in diameter, and composed principally of **myosin II**).

Thin filaments extend from each side of the Z disk in opposite directions toward the middle of successive sarcomeres. The two Z disks of a single sarcomere have thin filaments pointing toward the center of that sarcomere and pointing toward the center of the sarcomeres to its right and left sides.

If the skeletal muscle cell is not contracted, neither the thin nor the thick filaments extend the entire length of the sarcomere, and the area on either side of a particular Z disk, composed only of thin filaments, is the I band of light microscopy.

- An **I band** is composed of two halves, each belonging to adjacent sarcomeres.
- The area of a particular relaxed sarcomere that is composed of the entire length of the thick filament is the **A band**. The center of the A band of a relaxed sarcomere is void of thin filaments, and this represents the **H band**, an area rich in **creatine kinase**, the enzyme that catalyzes the transfer of high-energy phosphate from **creatine phosphate** to form **adenosine triphosphate (ATP)**.
- In the center of the H band is the **M line**, composed mainly of **C protein** and **myomesin**, macromolecules that interconnect the thick filaments to each other and assist in maintaining their proper position to permit the interdigitation of the thick filaments with the thin filaments.

When a muscle cell contracts, the thin filaments slide past the thick filaments and drag the Z disks closer to each other, shortening the sarcomere by approximately 0.4 μm. Because a single skeletal muscle cell may have 100,000 sarcomeres in sequence, a change in length of 0.4 μm per sarcomere means that the contracted muscle becomes 4 cm shorter. For the thin filaments to be able to interact with the thick filaments as they slide past them, the morphologic arrangements must be very precise.

In mammalian skeletal muscle, each thick filament is surrounded by six thin filaments at 60-degree intervals so that in cross section the thin filaments form a hexagon with a thick filament in the center (Fig. 8.4). Five proteins are responsible for maintaining the correct relationships among the sarcomere components:

- Two **titin** molecules, large, elastic proteins extend from each Z disk of the same sarcomere to the M line, ensure that the thick filaments remain in the correct position.
- **α-Actinins** anchor thin filaments to the Z disk.
- Two **nebulin** molecules extend from the Z disk to the end of each thin filament, ensuring that the thin filaments are in their proper positions, and that they are exactly the correct length.
- The length of the thin filament is also controlled by **Cap Z** and **tropomodulin**, molecules that prevent the addition to or deletion of G actin to or from the thin filament. Cap Z acts at the barbed **plus end** (at the Z disk), whereas tropomodulin acts at the pointed **minus end** of the thin filament (see Fig. 8.4).

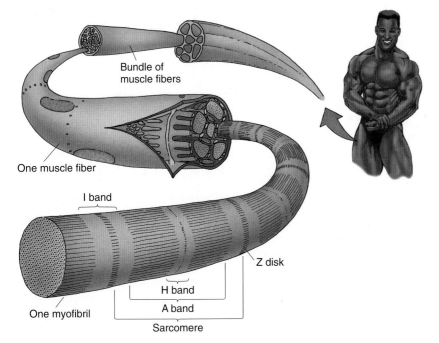

Figure 8.2 Organization of sarcomeres and myofibrils of a skeletal muscle cell. *(From Gartner LP, Hiatt JL: Color Textbook of Histology, 3rd ed. Philadelphia, Saunders, 2007, p 161.)*

Bundle of muscle fibers

One muscle fiber

I band

Z disk

H band

A band

One myofibril

Sarcomere

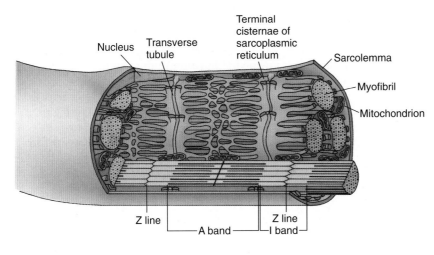

Nucleus

Transverse tubule

Terminal cisternae of sarcoplasmic reticulum

Sarcolemma

Myofibril

Mitochondrion

Z line

A band

Z line

I band

Figure 8.3 Organization of triads and sarcomeres of skeletal muscle fibers. *(From Gartner LP, Hiatt JL: Color Textbook of Histology, 3rd ed. Philadelphia, Saunders, 2007, p 162.)*

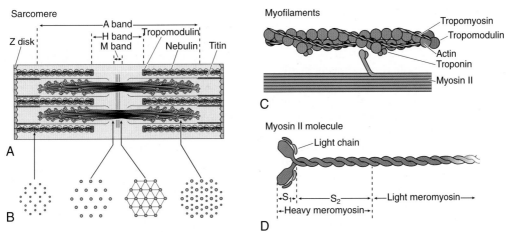

Sarcomere

A band

H band

M band

Tropomodulin

Nebulin

Titin

Z disk

A

B

Myofilaments

Tropomyosin

Tropomodulin

Actin

Troponin

Myosin II

C

Myosin II molecule

Light chain

S_1

S_2

Light meromyosin

Heavy meromyosin

D

Figure 8.4 A–D, Myofilaments of a sarcomere. *(From Gartner LP, Hiatt JL: Color Textbook of Histology, 3rd ed. Philadelphia, Saunders, 2007, p 164.)*

Thick Filaments

Approximately 300 **myosin II** molecules, each 2 to 3 nm in diameter and 150 nm long, are present in a thick filament. Myosin II molecules are composed of:

- Two heavy chains
- Two pairs of light chains; each pair consists of an essential light chain and a regulatory light chain (Fig. 8.5), and the regulatory light chain can be phosphorylated by myosin light chain kinase (MLCK)

Each of the two identical heavy chains resembles a golf club, and the polypeptide chains (handles) of the two form an α-helix as they wrap around each other. Each heavy chain can be enzymatically cleaved by trypsin into:

- Rodlike light meromyosin
- Heavy meromyosin, two globular heads with a short stalk, composed of two polypeptide chains wrapped around each other; papain cleaves heavy meromyosin into two globular regions (S_1) and the short stalk (S_2)

Each S_1 subfragment has three binding sites— ATP, light-chain myosin, and F actin binding sites. Myosin molecules are arranged head to tail in a thick filament so that the center of the thick filament is smooth, and the two ends appear barbed because of the projection of the S_1 subfragments. Myosin molecules possess two pliant regions—one at the junction of the S_1 and S_2 moieties, and one at the junction of the heavy and light meromyosins—that allow myosin II to contact and drag the thin filament toward the center of the sarcomere.

Thin Filaments

Thin filaments, composed of F actin, tropomyosin, and troponin, have a barbed plus end attached to the Z disk and a pointed minus end capped by tropomodulin (Fig. 8.6).

- **F actin** consists of two chains of **G actin** polymers, which resemble two strands of pearls twisted around each other. The two shallow grooves formed in this fashion are each occupied by 40-nm-long linear **tropomyosin molecules** arranged head to toe.
- The tropomyosin molecules mask the **active site** of each G actin molecule so that it is unavailable for contact by the S_1 subunit of the myosin II molecule.
- A tripartite **troponin** molecule is bound to each tropomyosin. The three components are

troponin C (TnC), which binds free calcium; **troponin T (TnT)**, which binds the troponin molecule to tropomyosin; and **troponin I (TnI)**, which inhibits the interaction of the S_1 subunit with G actin.

- If free calcium ions are available, they bind to TnC causing a conformational change in the troponin molecule that pushes the tropomyosin molecule deeper into the groove of the F actin filament and, by unmasking the active site, allows temporary binding with the S_1 subunit.

MUSCLE CONTRACTION

Muscle contraction usually occurs after a nervous impulse, and for each individual muscle cell, it follows the **all-or-none law**, which is that either the cell contracts or it does not. The amount of shortening is a function of the number of sarcomeres in a particular myofibril, and the strength of contraction of an entire muscle depends on the number of muscle cells that are contracting. Myofilaments do not contract; instead, according to the **Huxley sliding filament theory**, the thin filaments slide past the thick filaments as follows:

- T tubules convey the impulse generated at the myoneural junction to the terminal cisternae. Voltage-gated calcium release channels of the terminal cisternae open, and Ca^{++} ions, released into the sarcoplasm, bind to TnC, altering its conformation and pushing the tropomyosin deeper into the groove, unmasking the myosin binding site of G actin molecules.
- Hydrolysis of ATP on the S_1 moiety of myosin II results in the formation of adenosine diphosphate (ADP) and inorganic phosphate (P_i), both of which remain attached to the S_1 moiety. The myosin head swivels, and the entire complex becomes bound to the myosin binding site of G actin (see Fig. 8.6).
- P_i leaves the complex; this not only results in a stronger bond between the myosin and the actin, but also the S_1 moiety alters its conformation and releases ADP, and the conformation of the myosin head alters and pulls the thin filament toward the center of the sarcomere. This movement is referred to as the **power stroke** of muscle contraction.
- The S_1 moiety accepts a new ATP, releasing the bond between actin and myosin (see Fig. 8.6).
- For muscle contraction to be complete, the attachment and release cycles must be repeated approximately 200 to 300 times, and each cycle necessitates the hydrolysis of an ATP.

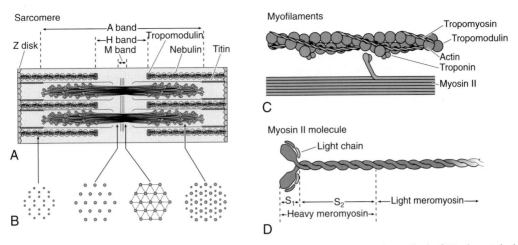

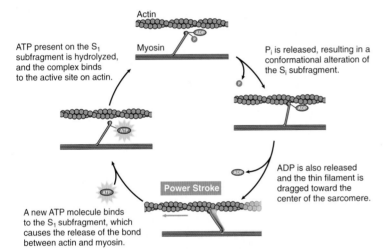

Figure 8.5 A–D, Thick and thin filaments within a sarcomere. *(From Gartner LP, Hiatt JL: Color Textbook of Histology, 3rd ed. Philadelphia, Saunders, 2007, p 164.)*

Figure 8.6 Role of ATP in muscle contraction. *(Modified from Alberts B, Bray D, Lewis J, et al: Molecular Biology of the Cell. New York, Garland Publishing, 1994.)*

CLINICAL CONSIDERATION

Mutations in some of the structural proteins that are responsible for the integrity of the myofibrillar organization of skeletal muscle can be devastating. If the primary structure of the intermediate filament desmin or of the heat shock protein αB-crystallin is altered, the myofibrils cannot be fixed in their proper position in three-dimensional space, and the myofibrils become destroyed under conditions of stressful contractile forces.

Rigor mortis is a condition that occurs after death. During muscle contraction in a living individual, ATP on the S_1 moiety (myosin head) of myosin II is hydrolyzed into ADP and P_i, but neither ADP nor P_i leaves the myosin head. A change in conformation of myosin II allows the head to contact the myosin binding site of G actin of the thin filament. This contact is followed by the release of P_i and a stronger bond between myosin and actin, and then ADP is released from the myosin head resulting in the power stroke. New ATP binds to the myosin head releasing the bond between the S_1 moiety of myosin II and the G actin of the thin filament. In a dead individual, ATP is not regenerated, and after a while the muscle's ATP supply becomes exhausted; the sarcoplasmic reticulum can no longer sequester calcium, and muscle contraction continues until ATP is no longer available to detach the S_1 moiety of myosin II from the thin filament, and a sustained muscle contraction (i.e., muscle rigidity) ensues. This rigidity is known as rigor mortis. Depending on the ambient temperature, a little while later, lysosomal enzymes escape from the lysosomes and break down the actin and myosin, resolving rigor mortis. During late spring in temperate zones, rigor mortis begins 3 to 8 hours after death, and the stiffness lasts 16 to 24 hours; by 36 hours after death, the muscles are no longer rigid.

MUSCLE RELAXATION

The process of muscle contraction requires the presence of free calcium ions in the sarcoplasm. When the neural stimulus ceases, and the T tubules no longer convey the wave of depolarization into the interior of the muscle cell, the voltage-gated calcium release channels of the terminal cisternae close.

- The sarcoplasmic calcium is driven back into the sarcoplasmic reticulum by the action of calcium pumps to be sequestered by calsequestrin.
- Because calcium is no longer abundant, TnC releases its calcium ions and regains its relaxed conformation; the tropomyosin molecule occupies its previous position, hiding the active site of the G actin molecule, and myosin and actin are unable to bind to each other.

INNERVATION OF SKELETAL MUSCLE

Skeletal muscle cells receive motor nerve fibers, which induce muscle contraction; sensory nerve fibers, which supply muscle spindles and Golgi tendon organs that protect the muscle from injury; and autonomic fibers, which control the vascular supply of the muscle. Depending on the degree of fine coordination of a particular muscle, it may have a:

- **Rich nerve supply**, as in the muscles of the eyes, in which a single motoneuron may control only five muscle cells, or
- **Crude nerve supply**, as in the muscles of the back, in which a single motoneuron may control several hundred muscle cells.

The motoneuron and all of the muscle cells that it controls are known as a **motor unit**. All the muscle fibers of a particular motor unit either contract simultaneously or do not contract at all.

Impulse Transmission at the Neuromuscular Junction

Skeletal muscle cells are innervated by the **myelinated** axons of **α-motoneurons**. These axons use the connective tissue elements of the muscle as they arborize to reach each skeletal muscle cell of their motor unit. As an axon branch reaches its muscle cell, it loses its myelin sheath, but retains its **Schwann cell** cover, and forms an expanded **axon terminal (presynaptic membrane)** over the **motor end plate (postsynaptic membrane)**, a modified region of the sarcolemma. The combination of the motor end plate, **(primary) synaptic cleft** (the space between the presynaptic and postsynaptic membranes), and

axon terminal is known as a **neuromuscular junction** (Fig. 8.7).

The postsynaptic membrane has numerous folds, and the spaces between these folds are referred to as **secondary synaptic clefts (junctional folds)**. The folds and secondary synaptic clefts are lined by an **external lamina**. The axon terminal is covered by Schwann cells, and it houses mitochondria, sarcoplasmic reticulum, and several hundred thousand **synaptic vesicles** that contain the neurotransmitter **acetylcholine**, **proteoglycans**, ATP, and various other substances. The presynaptic membrane displays **dense bars** in the vicinity of which the membrane houses **voltage-gated calcium channels**. The transmission of a stimulus occurs in the following manner:

- A stimulus, traveling along the axon, reaches and depolarizes the presynaptic membrane, causing an opening of the voltage-gated calcium channels and the influx of calcium into the axon terminal.
- With each impulse, approximately 120 synaptic vesicles fuse with the **active sites** of the presynaptic membrane along the dense bars, releasing a **quantum** of acetylcholine (approximately 20,000 molecules), proteoglycans, and ATP into the primary synaptic cleft (Fig. 8.8).
- Acetylcholine receptors of the postsynaptic (muscle) membrane bind the released acetylcholine, opening **ligand-gated sodium channels** of the postsynaptic membrane, and the influx of sodium causes depolarization of the sarcolemma and T tubule. The wave of depolarization reaches the terminal cisternae, and calcium is released at the I–A junction to initiate muscle contraction.
- In less than 500 msec, the enzyme **acetylcholinesterase**, located in the external lamina of the primary and secondary synaptic clefts, degrades acetylcholine into choline and acetate; the resting membrane potential of the postsynaptic membrane is re-established, preventing a single release of acetylcholine from precipitating multiple contractions.
- The sodium concentration gradient powers a sodium-choline symport to ferry the choline back into the axon terminal where activated acetate, derived from mitochondria, combines with the choline facilitated by the action of the enzyme **choline O-acetyltransferase**. The acetylcholine is conveyed into synaptic vesicles by a proton gradient powered by antiport carrier proteins.
- The surface area of the presynaptic membrane remains constant because of the membrane-trafficking mechanism.

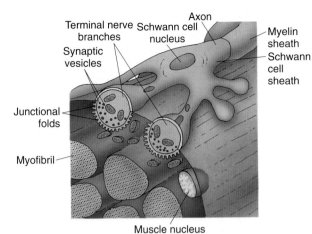

Figure 8.7 Neuromuscular junction. *(From Gartner LP, Hiatt JL: Color Textbook of Histology, 3rd ed. Philadelphia, Saunders, 2007, p 171.)*

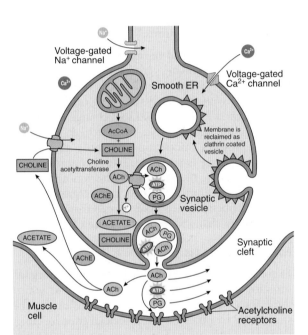

Figure 8.8 Events occurring at a synapse of a motoneuron with a skeletal muscle cell. AcCoA, acetyl coenzyme A; ACh, acetylcholine; AChE, acetylcholinesterase; ER, endoplasmic reticulum; PG, prostaglandin. *(Modified from Katzung BG: Basic and Clinical Pharmacology, 4th ed. East Norwalk, CT, Appleton & Lange, 1989.)*

CLINICAL CONSIDERATION

Clostridium tetani is a common, spore-forming bacterium that lives in the soil and, under anaerobic conditions, forms a toxin that blocks glycine, an inhibitory neurotransmitter produced by certain neurons of the central nervous system. Usually, the infection occurs when the bacterium is introduced by soil or contaminant into a penetrating wound. The proliferating bacteria release the toxin, which enters the spinal cord and inhibits the release of glycine, resulting in spasmodic muscle contraction, known as **tetanus**. The initial symptoms, stiffness of the muscles of mastication, may be noted 2 to 50 days after the infection. The initial stiffness may develop into a lack of ability to open the mouth, commonly referred to as **lockjaw**. Additional symptoms include stiffness of other muscles; in severe conditions, the muscles of the neck, abdomen, and back can go into violent spasms causing the forward arching of the thorax and abdomen and the posteriorward stretching of the head and lower extremities, a typical position in late tetanus referred to as *opisthotonos*. The global death toll is approximately 50,000 people per year. The best prevention is the administration of tetanus vaccination followed by a booster shot every 10 years. Treatment involves an antibiotic regimen with accompanying tetanus immunoglobulin to inactivate the toxin. Analgesics, sedation, muscle relaxants, and ventilation may be required to assist the patient in breathing.

SENSORY SYSTEM OF SKELETAL MUSCLE

The activity of a muscle has to be monitored to ensure that the muscle or its tendons are not injured.

- **Muscle spindles** monitor the alteration and its rate in the length of a muscle.
- The **Golgi tendon organ** monitors the tensile forces and the rate at which the tensile forces develop in a tendon as the muscle shortens.

Information gathered by these two sensory organs reaches the spinal cord for processing. The information is also transmitted to the cerebellum for subconscious processing and to the cerebral cortex where the information may reach conscious levels so that the individual can become aware of the position of his or her muscles.

Muscle Spindles

Muscle spindles (Fig. 8.9) are encapsulated sensory receptors interspersed among skeletal muscle fibers that cause stretched muscles to contract automatically, a proprioceptive response known as the **stretch reflex**. These encapsulated muscle spindles are composed of a few modified skeletal muscle cells, known as **intrafusal fibers**, located within the fluid containing **periaxial space**; they are arranged parallel to the longitudinal axis of the muscle. Although the skeletal muscle cells that surround the muscle spindle are ordinary muscle cells, they are referred to as **extrafusal muscle fibers**.

There are two types of intrafusal fibers: **nuclear bag fibers** and **nuclear chain fibers**. The nuclear bag fibers are wider and fewer in number than the nuclear chain fibers. Both fiber types have their nuclei located in the center of the cell, and their contractile regions are limited to their polar regions.

- Nuclei of the nuclear bag fibers form a clump in the expanded region in the middle of the cell.
- Nuclei of the nuclear chain fibers, aligned in a row, do not form a clump in the middle of these cells.

Nuclear bag fibers are of two types, **dynamic** and **static**. Although the nerve supply of the intrafusal fibers seems to be complex, it is really very straightforward because they receive two types of sensory fibers, which innervate the nuclear regions, and two types of motor fibers, which innervate the contractile regions.

- The nuclear regions of nuclear chain and both types of nuclear bag fibers of a muscle spindle are innervated by branches of a single, large, myelinated **group Ia** (also referred to as **Ia** or **dynamic sensory ending**) nerve fiber that wraps around this region in a spiral fashion.
- The nuclear areas of all nuclear chain fibers and *only* static nuclear bag fibers of a muscle spindle are innervated by branches of a single, sensory **group II** nerve fiber (also referred to as **static** or **II sensory nerve endings**) that wrap around this area of the cells (see Fig. 8.9).
- Motor innervation to the polar (contractile) regions of all nuclear chain fibers and *only* static nuclear bag fibers is by axons of **static γ-motoneurons**, whereas the polar regions of dynamic nuclear bag fibers receive their motor innervation from axons of **dynamic γ-motoneurons**.
- All extrafusal fibers are innervated by myelinated axons of **γ-motoneurons** (see Fig. 8.5A and B).

Stretching of a skeletal muscle stretches the muscle spindle and stimulates group Ia (dynamic) and group II (static) sensory nerve fibers. These fibers fire more often with increased stretching of the muscle. Also, group Ia fibers respond to a change in the rate at which the muscle fiber is stretched; a muscle spindle provides information not only about how rapidly a muscle is stretched, but also about unexpected stretching of the muscle. The γ-motoneurons induce contraction of the two polar regions of the intrafusal fibers, stretching and sensitizing them to even minute changes in the stretching of a muscle.

Golgi Tendon Organs

In contrast to muscle spindles, **Golgi tendon organs** monitor the tensile forces (and the rate at which these forces develop) placed on tendons due to the shortening (contraction) of a skeletal muscle. Golgi tendon organs, situated at the muscle-tendon interface, are about 1 mm long and 0.1 mm in diameter and are parallel to the longitudinal axis of the muscle. They are composed of wavy collagen fibers whose interstices house nonmyelinated branches of **type Ib axons**. As the muscle contracts and places tensile forces on the tendon, the wavy collagen fibers straighten out and compress the free nerve endings. The rate of impulse generation in these nerve fibers is a function of the tensile forces that the tendon is experiencing. If the force approaches critical values so that the tendon, muscle, and bone can be damaged, the Golgi tendon organ acts to inhibit further contraction of the muscle. Muscle spindles monitor the stretching and Golgi tendon organs monitor the contraction of the same muscle to coordinate spinal control over skeletal muscle reflexes.

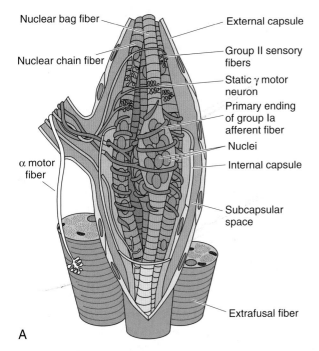

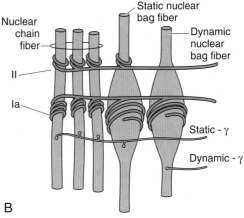

Figure 8.9 A, Schematic diagram showing components of a muscle spindle. **B,** Various fiber types of a muscle spindle and their innervation are presented in a spread-out fashion. (**A,** *Modified from Krstic RV: Die Gewebe des Menschen und der Saugertiere. Berlin, Springer-Verlag, 1978.* **B,** *Modified from Hulliger M: The mammalian muscle spindle and its central control. Rev Physiol Biochem Pharmacol 101:1–110, 1984.)*

CLINICAL CONSIDERATION

MYASTHENIA GRAVIS

Myasthenia gravis is an autoimmune disease that has highest prevalence among women 20 to 40 years old, but can affect individuals of both genders and all ages. Approximately 10% of these patients have tumors of the thymus; the antibodies can cross the placental barrier, and in 10% to 12% of pregnant women, infants are born with a temporary myasthenia gravis that spontaneously resolves before 2 months of age. Patients with myasthenia gravis form antibodies against their acetylcholine receptors, reducing the ability of the muscle to contract properly. Although the blocked receptors are internalized and replaced by the muscle cell, the disease overpowers the ability of the system to repair itself. The disease affects especially the muscles of the face, particularly the extrinsic muscles of the eyes. Additionally, muscles of the throat and the rest of the body become affected resulting in difficulties in speech and swallowing and generalized muscle weakness involving most of the muscles of the body. The degree of weakness fluctuates from mild to severe. The severe condition is known as **myasthenia crisis**, and it may involve the muscles of respiration with fatal consequences. Immunosuppressants and drugs that increase the production of acetylcholine can frequently control the condition.

SIMPLE REFLEX ARC

Muscle spindles, such as the **patellar reflex**, are designed as two neuron reflexes, which react to stretching of their parent muscle by initiating the contraction of that muscle. An example of the importance of such a reflex is shown by the following scenario: As a person is standing at ease, someone approaches the person from the back and kicks him or her in the right popliteal fossa (behind the right knee). That action causes the right leg to bend; the right knee moves forward, and the right leg begins to buckle. As the knee moves forward, the large quadriceps muscle (four muscles in the front of the thigh) of the right leg is stretched; the sensory nerve fibers of the muscle spindles fire, and the wave of depolarization enters the spinal cord. Neurotransmitters are released at the synapse to stimulate the α-motoneurons of the ventral horn of the spinal cord that serve the extrafusal muscle fibers of the right quadriceps muscle and cause them to contract. As the quadriceps muscle of the right leg contracts, the right leg straightens and prevents the person from falling down. This system was designed to be activated when an individual trips and the reflex arc protects the individual from falling down.

Cardiac Muscle

Cardiac muscle is also a striated muscle, but it differs from skeletal muscle in many respects. It is not under voluntary control; it is located in the heart and the beginnings of the great vessels of the heart. The myocardium, the bulk of the heart, is composed of **laminae**, or overlapping sheaths, of cardiac muscle cells. Slender connective tissue elements, carrying blood vessels and neural components, separate laminae from each other. A rich capillary network supplies individual cardiac muscle cells.

- **Cardiac muscle cells** are short cylindrical, branching cells about 80 μm in length and 15 μm in diameter with a single, centrally placed nucleus (or occasionally two nuclei). At either end of the nucleus, the cell possesses glycogen deposits and triglycerides.
- Approximately 50% of the sarcoplasm is occupied by mitochondria that are arranged parallel to the longitudinal axis of the cell interspersed among the myofibrils of the cardiac muscle cell. There is also a copious amount of the oxygen-bearing protein **myoglobin**.

In contrast to skeletal muscle fiber, cardiac muscle cells are able to **contract spontaneously** and possess an **inherent rhythmicity**. Modified heart muscle cells (sinoauricular node, atrioventricular node, bundle of His, and Purkinje fibers), discussed in Chapter 11, function as the neural elements of the heart that regulate and coordinate its pumping action.

- Ventricular muscle cells are larger than atrial muscle cells.
- Atrial muscle cells possess **atrial granules** that contain **atrial natriuretic factor** and **brain natriuretic factor**, diuretic substances that inhibit the release of **aldosterone** by the adrenal cortex and inhibit the release of **renin** by the juxtaglomerular cells of the kidney, decreasing the ability of the kidney to conserve sodium and water, and decreasing blood pressure.

The muscle cells of the heart display fluted ends that interdigitate with each other as they line up end to end and form specialized interdigitating junctions, known as **intercalated disks** (Fig. 8.10). Each **intercalated disk** has:

- A **lateral portion** that is well endowed with gap junctions
- A **transverse portion** that has abundant desmosomes and fasciae adherentes

- **Thin myofilaments** are attached via **α-actinin** and **vinculin** to the fasciae adherentes, which acts as if it were a Z disk.
- Gap junctions facilitate the passage of information between cardiac muscle cells, coordinating the process of contraction in such a fashion that the ventricles twist on themselves so that the blood is pumped efficiently out of the ventricles and into the aorta and pulmonary trunk.

Similar to skeletal muscle fibers, cardiac muscle cells exhibit alternating A and I banding, and the sarcomere arrangements of the two types of striated muscle are identical to each other. The Huxley sliding filament theory applies to cardiac muscle as well. There are differences, however:

- The **T tubules** have a wider diameter (a little more than twice that of skeletal muscle), and they are lined by a negatively charged external lamina that stores calcium ions by loosely binding them. Instead of being positioned at the junction of the I and A bands, in cardiac muscle the T tubules are located at the Z disk of the sarcomere.
- The **sarcoplasmic reticulum** of cardiac muscle cells is less abundant and consequently is unable to sequester enough Ca^{++} ions to initiate contraction.
- Additionally, instead of having dilated cisternae that are placed on either side of a T tubule to form triads, only one sarcoplasmic reticulum profile adjoins a T tubule located at each Z disk, forming **diads**.
- The sarcolemma of cardiac muscle cells possesses **fast sodium channels** (sodium channels of skeletal muscle cells) and **slow sodium channels** (**calcium-sodium channels**) that remain open for several tenths of a second. During depolarization, the slow sodium channels of the T tubules open, and calcium and sodium ions enter the sarcoplasm in the vicinity of the sarcoplasmic reticulum.
- Ca^{++} ions open the **calcium release channels** of the sarcoplasmic reticulum, and even more calcium enters the sarcoplasm. Muscle contraction is initiated in a fashion that is similar to contraction in skeletal muscle. The contraction lasts longer than in a skeletal muscle cell because K^+ cannot readily leave the cardiac muscle cell, retarding the repolarization of the sarcolemma.

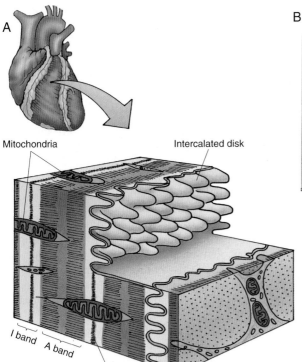

Mitochondria   Intercalated disk

I band   A band

Z disk

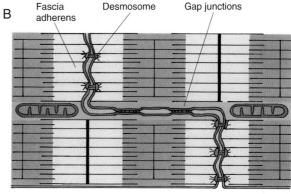

Fascia adherens   Desmosome   Gap junctions

Figure 8.10 **A,** Three-dimensional representation of cardiac muscle at the level of its intercalated disk. **B,** Two-dimensional representation of an intercalated disk showing its transverse and lateral portions. *(From Gartner LP, Hiatt JL: Color Textbook of Histology, 3rd ed. Philadelphia, Saunders, 2007, p 178.)*

CLINICAL CONSIDERATION

MYOCARDIAL INFARCTION

Myocardial infarction refers to damage to the cardiac muscle caused by the lack of blood flow to the affected area. The stoppage of blood flow may be due to an atherosclerotic coronary artery that was completely occluded or a dislodged thrombus that lodged in a vessel whose lumen was small enough to be blocked by the clot. The damage is reversible if blood flow resumes within 20 minutes; after that time, the injury is irreversible and the cardiac muscle cells that are not being perfused die. Dead cardiac muscle cells release **cardiocyte-specific troponin I (cardiocyte-specific TnI)**, a marker that is characteristic of myocardial infarction, within 3 to 10 hours after the injury, and the TnI remains in circulation for approximately 2 to 3 weeks. A less specific marker that is indicative of dead cardiac muscle cells is the presence of **creatine kinase** and **creatine kinase-MB isozyme** in the patient's bloodstream.

ARTIFICIAL PACEMAKERS

When an individual's slow arrhythmia cannot be controlled by medications, an **artificial pacemaker** is implanted. Pacemakers are electronic devices that are placed just under the skin below the clavicle and are connected to a wire that is threaded via the venous system into the right atrium and right ventricle. Depending on the type of pacemaker used, it may continuously control the rate of heartbeat, or it may act on demand and control the heart rate when the biologic pacemakers are not functioning properly. Still other pacemakers can adjust the heart rate depending on the activity of the individual. The batteries of pacemakers last for about 15 years, and battery replacement is a simple process. Implanting a pacemaker may be done on an outpatient basis; the entire procedure lasts 1 to 2 hours or less.

Smooth Muscle

Smooth muscle has neither striations nor T tubules. It is located in the walls of viscera; it is not under voluntary control; it is regulated by local factors, hormones, and the autonomic nervous system; and it may be:

- **Multiunit smooth muscle**, in which each cell is innervated individually, or
- **Unitary (single-unit, or vascular) smooth muscle**, in which only some of the cells have their own nerve supply, and the information is transmitted to other smooth muscle cells via gap junctions.

Smooth muscle cells not only function in contraction, but they also synthesize extracellular matrix macromolecules.

LIGHT MICROSCOPY OF SMOOTH MUSCLE FIBERS

Smooth muscle fibers are short, elongated, fusiform cells that are generally 200 μm or less in length with an average diameter of 5 to 6 μm. The single, oval nucleus is located in the center of the cell from a longitudinal perspective, but is acentric from the perspective of the cell's diameter. During contraction, the entire cell twists on itself, and the nucleus resembles a corkscrew (Fig. 8.11). Smooth muscle cells have an **external lamina**, but the lamina is absent at the sites of gap junctions. **Reticular fibers** are enmeshed within the substance of the external lamina, and they harness the contractile forces.

Using special stains, such as iron hematoxylin, reveals the slender longitudinal striations that represent aggregates of **myofilaments**. Additionally, **dense bodies** that act as Z disks are located intracellularly and along the cytoplasmic aspect of the sarcolemma. Smooth muscle cells usually aggregate in a sheet arranged so that individual muscle cells are packed tightly and their tapered ends fit in almost precisely among the wider regions of their neighbors.

ELECTRON MICROSCOPY OF SMOOTH MUSCLE

The sarcoplasm of smooth muscle cells at each pole of the nucleus houses mitochondria, sarcoplasmic reticulum, Golgi apparatus, and glycogen deposits. Myofilaments are also present, although they are not associated in the paracrystalline configuration as in striated muscle.

- The **thin filaments** are similar to those of striated muscle; however, instead of troponin, **caldesmon**, a protein that masks the active site of G actin, is associated with the thin filament.

- The **thick filaments** are composed of **myosin II** molecules, but instead of being lined up head to tail, the myosin heads protrude along the entire length of the thick filament. This arrangement allows contractions to occur for a longer time than in striated muscle, and the all-or-none law does not apply. It is possible for only a portion of the smooth muscle cell to contract.
- Intermediate filaments **vimentin** and **desmin** in unitary smooth muscle and **desmin** only in multiunit smooth muscle harness contractile forces generated by the myofilaments.
- Intermediate filaments and thin filaments are anchored into the **dense bodies**, structures composed of **α-actinin** and additional Z disk–associated molecules, that are located abutting the sarcolemma and interspersed within the sarcoplasm. Dense bodies form an interconnected complex that is responsible for the twisting of the smooth muscle cell on itself during contraction.
- A system of cholesterol and sphingolipid-rich **lipid rafts** abounds in the sarcolemma of smooth muscle cells. The lipid rafts, in association with **caveolin** proteins, form **caveolae**, small vesicles that function as primitive T tubules and induce the sarcoplasmic reticulum to release calcium into the sarcoplasm.

CONTROL OF SMOOTH MUSCLE CONTRACTION

Smooth muscle contraction depends on calcium levels within the sarcoplasm and the arrangement of **myosin II** whose **light meromyosin** portion contacts and masks the actin binding site of the S_1 moiety. Calcium ions enter the sarcoplasm via caveolae, from the sarcoplasmic reticulum, and through gated calcium channels of the sarcolemma. Four Ca^{++} ions bind to each calmodulin, and the calcium-calmodulin complex activates **MLCK** to phosphorylate the regulatory myosin light chain, which allows the S_1 moiety to release the light meromyosin; the myosin II molecule straightens out (see Fig. 8.11B) and aggregates with other myosin II molecules to form a thick filament. Calcium also binds to caldesmon to unmask the active site of the thin filament, the thin and thick filaments slide past each other, and muscle contraction occurs. Because in smooth muscle ATP hydrolysis occurs slowly, contraction is prolonged and uses less energy. When calcium is removed from the sarcoplasm, the calmodulin is no longer active, and MLCK also becomes inactive. The enzyme **myosin phosphatase** dephosphorylates the myosin light chain, myosin II folds on itself, and the thick myofilament becomes disassembled.

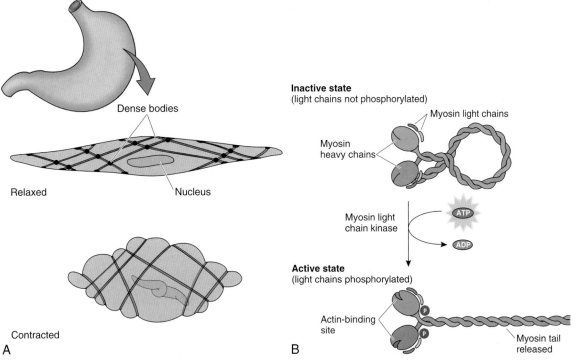

Figure 8.11 **A,** Smooth muscle cell in the relaxed and contracted states. **B,** Activation of the myosin molecule of smooth muscle. P, myosin light chain–bound phosphate. (**A,** *From Gartner LP, Hiatt JL: Color Textbook of Histology, 3rd ed. Philadelphia, Saunders, 2007, p. 182.* **B,** *Modified from Alberts B, Bray D, Lewis J, et al: Molecular Biology of the Cell. New York, Garland Publishing, 1994.*)

CLINICAL CONSIDERATION

LEIOMYOMA

Leiomyoma is a benign tumor of smooth muscle cells that occurs usually in blood vessels or in the wall of the digestive system, especially in the esophagus and small intestine, where it forms small nodules of interlaced smooth muscle cells. Leiomyomas of the gastrointestinal tract usually affect adults 30 to 60 years old and are of no major concern, unless they are painful or grow to be large enough to cause inability to swallow, obstruction of the lumen of the gastrointestinal tract, or intestinal strangulation. They usually can be treated by electrocautery or, if necessary, by surgical excision.

LEIOMYOSARCOMA

Leiomyosarcoma is an infrequent malignant tumor of smooth muscle cells that occurs in the walls of blood vessels. They are usually larger and not nearly as hard as leiomyomas, and may display necrotic and hemorrhagic regions. The smooth muscle cells are actively undergoing mitosis and form numerous fascicles. In most cases, the tumor spreads; metastasis may occur 10 to 15 years after the excision of the primary tumor, and prognosis for long-term survival of leiomyosarcoma patients is unfavorable.

9 NERVOUS TISSUE

The nervous system, with its hundreds of billions of **neurons** forming myriad intricate and complex interconnections among themselves and with an abundance of non–nervous system cells, functions as the communications and database center of the body. This communication center is based on the presence of **receptors** that receive information from outside and from inside the body and convey the data to processing centers. Here the newly received information is processed and compared with information stored in the database, and responses are formulated and conveyed to **effector organs** to perform the requisite actions. Neurons are supported physically and metabolically by non–nervous system cells, known as **neuroglia**.

The anatomic organization of the nervous system is as follows:

- The **central nervous system (CNS)** consists of the brain and spinal cord.
- The **peripheral nervous system (PNS)**, composed of 12 pairs of cranial and 31 pairs of spinal nerves and their respective ganglia, facilitates the ability of the nervous system to perform its plethora of functions.

The PNS is divided functionally into **sensory (afferent) components**, which perceive a stimulus and transmit it to higher centers for processing, and **motor (efferent) components**, which originate in either the brain or the spinal cord and transmit a motor nerve impulse to an effector organ (e.g., skeletal muscle, cardiac muscle, smooth muscle, gland). The motor component of the nervous system is subdivided further into the:

- **Somatic nervous system**, serving motor impulses exclusively to skeletal muscles of the body via a *single* neuron.

KEY WORDS
- **Neurons**
- **Neuroglia**
- **Nerve impulses**
- **Synapse**
- **Neurotransmitters**
- **Somatic nervous system**
- **Autonomic nervous system**
- **Meninges**

- **Autonomic nervous system**, serving motor impulses to cardiac muscle, smooth muscles, and glands via a *two-neuron system* with an autonomic ganglion interposed between the **preganglionic neuron** originating from the CNS and the **postganglionic neuron** originating in the autonomic ganglion. Additional neurons known as **neuroglial cells** serve in a supporting capacity to the impulse-transmitting neurons (Fig. 9.1).

Development of Nervous Tissue

Cytokines originating from the notochord stimulate ectoderm positioned above it to differentiate into **neuroepithelium**, which thickens into the **neural plate**. The margins of the neural plate initially fold to form the **neural groove** and eventually fuse with each other to form the cylindrical **neural tube**. The brain forms from the rostral end of the neural tube, whereas the spinal cord develops from its caudal end. Other structures of the nervous system, including neuroglia, neurons, choroid plexus, and ependyma, also arise from the neural tube. Arising from the right and left margins of the neural plate before their fusion, a thin strip of cells (**neural crest cells**) migrates away from the neural plate to give rise to the following structures:

- Sensory ganglia and autonomic ganglia and neurons originating in them
- Most of the mesenchyme and its derivatives in the head and anterior neck
- Odontoblasts
- Melanocytes
- Adrenal medulla chromaffin cells
- Arachnoid and pia mater cells
- Peripheral ganglia satellite cells
- Schwann cells

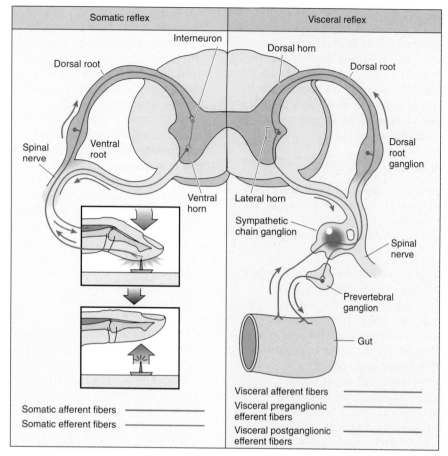

Figure 9.1 Comparison of somatic and autonomic reflexes. *(From Gartner LP, Hiatt JL: Color Textbook of Histology, 3rd ed. Philadelphia, Saunders, 2007, p 207.)*

CLINICAL CONSIDERATIONS

Because the nervous system develops early and is so complex, many abnormalities and congenital malformations may occur during embryogenesis. **Spina bifida** is a malformation resulting from an incomplete fusion of the neural tube in which the spinal cord and the spinal meninges may extend through the defect. **Spina bifida anterior** results from incompletely closed vertebrae. When severe, thoracic and abdominal viscera may be malformed.

When the anterior neuropore fails to close, there is an open cranial vault with an undeveloped brain. This developmental defect is known as **anencephaly** and is lethal.

Cortical cells that do not undergo proper migration may disrupt the normal functioning of nerve tissue called interneurons. This disruption may be responsible for **epilepsy**.

Hirschsprung's disease, or **congenital megacolon**, results from failure of neural crest cells to migrate into the wall of the forming distal colon. **Auerbach's plexus** of the enteric nervous system, which is responsible for innervating the distal colon, is absent, causing the colon to enlarge.

Nervous System Cells

Two separate groups of cells compose the nervous system. **Neurons** are functional nerve cells; they range in size from the smallest (5 μm) to the largest (150 μm) cell of the body and are responsible for conveying information to and away from the CNS. **Neuroglial cells** provide physical and metabolic support for the neurons.

STRUCTURE AND FUNCTION OF NEURONS

The typical neuron is composed of a **cell body (perikaryon** or **soma)** that consists of a nucleus surrounded by the perinuclear cytoplasm and two types of processes, several **dendrites**, and a single **axon** (Fig. 9.2).

- **Cell bodies** may be of different sizes and shapes, but in the CNS, most tend to be polygonal shaped, whereas cell bodies of the sensory ganglia are spherical. The cell body houses the nucleus, as well as various organelles, the most prominent of which are the rough endoplasmic reticulum (RER) (**Nissl body** of light microscopy), the large perinuclear Golgi apparatus, abundant mitochondria; and a well-developed system of microtubules, microfilaments, and neurofilaments. The microtubules sport **microtubule-associated protein 2 (MAP-2)**. The soma also houses inclusions such as **lipofuscin**, an age-related substance believed to be the indigestible remnants of lysosomal degradation; **melanin**, a dark brown pigment that may be the remnant of the synthesis of certain neurotransmitters (e.g., noradrenaline and dopamine); **secretory granules**, probably containing neurotransmitter substances; and **lipid droplets**.
- **Dendrites**, cell processes that receive stimuli originating from outside and inside the body, often form branches and may arborize to receive stimuli from multiple sources at the same time, which they transmit as an impulse toward the cell body. Neurons usually have several dendrites, each of which possesses organelles, but not Golgi, in their proximal regions. These processes are usually broader near the soma, but begin to taper at a distance. The neurofilaments of dendrites usually contact microtubules, which have MAP-2 associated proteins. As dendrites branch, they form numerous synapses and the dendrites of some neurons form small bulges, or spines, on their surface that provide larger surface areas for synapse formation.
- The cell body of a neuron possesses only a single **axon** that arises from a specialized region on the cell body called the **axon hillock**. An axon may extend long distances to provide motor supply to muscles and glands. The axon diameter varies and is related to the conduction velocity (i.e., as axon diameter increases, conduction velocity increases). The diameter is specific for the type of neuron, however. Although there is only one axon, it may give off branches at right angles, known as **collateral axons**, and as it approximates its target, it may arborize. Axons end in **axon terminals (end bulbs, end-foot, terminal boutons)** where they form **synaptic junctions (synapses)** with other cells.

  - The **axon hillock** is a specialized region of the cell body that occupies the opposite side of the cell body from where dendrites originate. The cytoplasm within the region of the axon hillock is devoid of RER, Golgi, ribosomes, and Nissl bodies but is rich in microtubules and neurofilaments perhaps regulating axon diameter.
  - On exiting the cell body, the axon's **initial segment** is without myelin and is termed the **spike trigger** zone where excitatory and inhibitory impulses are summed and evaluated to decide whether or not the impulse is to be transmitted.
  - Because the **axoplasm** (cytoplasm within the axon) is devoid of RER and polyribosomes, its maintenance is provided by the cell body. The axoplasm does possess, however, smooth endoplasmic reticulum (SER), abundant elongated mitochondria, microtubules with their associated protein **MAP-3**, and neurofilaments at the distal end.
  - **Oligodendroglia** in the CNS and **Schwann cells** in the PNS form a myelin sheath (white in color) that surrounds some axons. The CNS is divided into **white matter**, where most of the axons are myelinated, and **gray matter**, where most axons are not myelinated.
- Materials within the axoplasm and the cell body are ferried by a process called **axonal transport**, which occurs in two directions:
  - **Anterograde transport** conveys materials such as organelles, vesicles, actin, myosin, clathrin, and enzymes required for the synthesis of neurotransmitters in the axon terminal, toward the end-foot. The axon uses the motor protein **kinesin** for anterograde transport.
  - **Retrograde transport** conveys material, such as tubulin monomers and dimers, neurofilament subunits, enzymes, viruses, and molecules to be degraded, to the soma. The axon uses the motor protein **dynein** for retrograde transport.

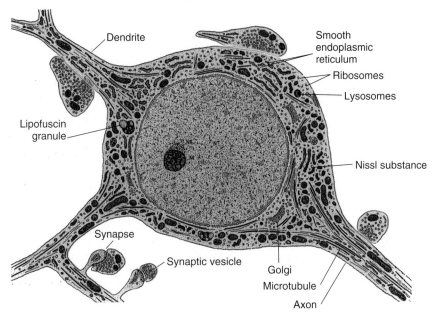

Figure 9.2 Ultrastructure of a neuron cell body. *(From Gartner LP, Hiatt JL: Color Textbook of Histology, 3rd ed. Philadelphia, Saunders, 2007, p 190.)*

CLINICAL CONSIDERATIONS

Certain viruses, such as herpes simplex and the rabies virus, employ retrograde axonal transport as a means of spreading from neuron to neuron within a chain. Also, toxins, such as *Clostridium tetani*—which causes tetanus—are spread in the same manner from the periphery to the CNS.

Most intracranial tumors are of neuroglial origin, and only rarely result from CNS neurons.

Neuroglial tumors include **benign oligodendrogliomas** and fatal **malignant astrocytomas**. Other intracranial tumors that arise from the connective tissues of the nervous system include **benign fibroma** and **malignant sarcoma**. **Neuroblastoma**, an extremely malignant tumor that attacks mainly infants and young children, is a PNS tumor located within the suprarenal gland.

NEURON CLASSIFICATION

The three categories of neurons are based on their **morphology** and the organization of their processes (Fig. 9.3):

- **Unipolar neurons (pseudounipolar neurons)** are located in the dorsal root ganglion and some ganglia of the cranial nerves. They possess only one process; however, that single process bifurcates into a peripheral branch that continues until it reaches the site it services and a central branch that gains entry to the CNS. The peripheral branch arborizes with receptor endings similar to a dendrite, and it functions as a receptor. The impulse passes to the central process, but bypasses the cell body.
- **Bipolar neurons** are found in the olfactory epithelium and in the ganglia of the vestibulocochlear nerve. They possess two processes—a dendrite and an axon.
- **Multipolar neurons** are ubiquitous, are generally motoneurons, and are located in the spinal cord and in the cerebral and cerebellar cortices. They possess several dendrites and one axon.

There are also three categories of neurons based on their **function**:

- **Sensory (afferent) neurons** are stimulated at their dendritic receptors at the periphery where they respond to external environmental stimuli, and from within the body where they respond to internal environmental stimuli and transmit the information to the CNS for processing.
- **Motor (efferent) neurons** originate in the CNS and transmit their impulses to other neurons, muscles, and glands.
- **Interneurons**, present solely within the CNS, function as intermediaries between sensory neurons and motoneurons; they establish and integrate the activities of neuronal circuits.

NEUROGLIAL CELLS

Neuroglial cells (Fig. 9.4) are at least 10 times more abundant than neurons, and although they cannot transmit nerve impulses, they have the essential function of providing support and protection for the neurons whose soma, dendrites, and axons they envelop. In contrast to neurons, neuroglial cells can undergo cell division. Neuroglial cells that function within the CNS include oligodendrocytes, microglia, astrocytes, and ependymal cells; Schwann cells are neuroglia cells in the PNS.

- **Oligodendrocytes** are of two types:
  - **Interfascicular oligodendrocytes** produce myelin, insulating axons of the CNS. A single oligodendrocyte may wrap several axons together in myelin.
  - **Satellite oligodendrocytes** surround the soma of large neurons and probably function to insulate them from unwanted contact.
- **Microglial cells** are small cells that originate in the bone marrow and serve as macrophages, belonging to the mononuclear phagocyte system. They reside in the CNS where they phagocytose debris and damaged cells and mount protection against viruses, microorganisms, and tumors. Additionally, they serve as antigen-presenting cells and secrete cytokines.
- There are two types of **astrocytes—protoplasmic astrocytes** located in the gray matter of the CNS and **fibrous astrocytes** located in the white matter. It has been proposed, however, that there is only a single type of astrocyte, and the presence of astrocytes in two different locations is responsible for their dissimilar characteristics. Both types of astrocytes possess intermediate filaments whose unique **glial fibrillar acidic protein** is a distinguishing characteristic of these cells. Astrocytes scavenge accumulated products, including ions and neurotransmitters and their metabolic remnants in their immediate area. Additional functions of astrocytes include repairing damage in the CNS, where they form scar tissue composed solely of cells; releasing glucose to nourish neurons of the cerebral cortex; and participating with the endothelial cells of blood vessels in the formation of the blood-brain barrier (BBB).
  - **Protoplasmic astrocytes** possess **pedicels** (vascular feet) contacting blood vessels. Others located adjacent to the pia of the brain or spinal cord possess pedicles that touch each other to form a thin layer that contact the pia mater, establishing the **pia-glial membrane**.
  - **Fibrous astrocytes** possess long processes that associate with blood vessels and pia mater, but contact is prevented by their basal lamina.

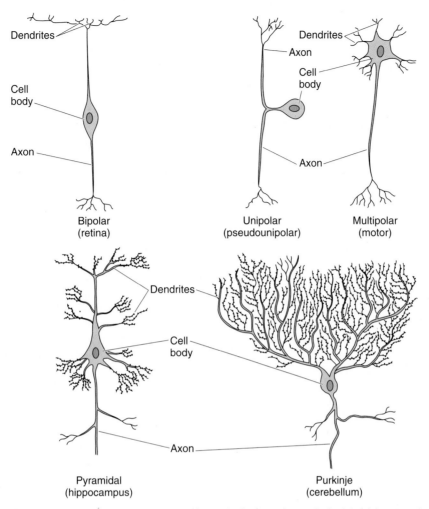

Figure 9.3 Types of neurons. *(From Gartner LP, Hiatt JL: Color Textbook of Histology, 3rd ed. Philadelphia, Saunders, 2007, p 189.)*

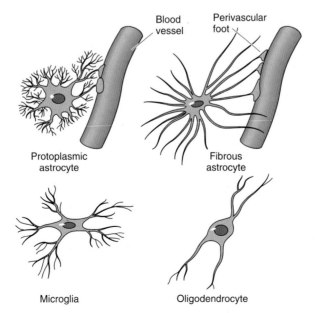

Figure 9.4 Types of neuroglial cells. *(From Gartner LP, Hiatt JL: Color Textbook of Histology, 3rd ed. Philadelphia, Saunders, 2007, p 193.)*

- **Ependymal cells** are cuboidal cells that line the ventricles of the brain and the central canal of the spinal cord. They also contribute to the formation of the **choroid plexus**, the structure responsible for the production of the **cerebrospinal fluid (CSF)**. Certain ependymal cells are ciliated, assisting in circulating the CSF, and others, known as tanycytes, have been implicated in the transfer of CSF to neurosecretory cells of the hypothalamus.

- **Schwann cells** arise from neural crest cells, and although they are considered neuroglial cells, they are located exclusively in the PNS (Fig. 9.5). Similar to oligodendrocytes, Schwann cells form a myelinated or unmyelinated sheath around axons, insulating them; however, in contrast to oligodendroglia, a single Schwann cell can myelinate only a single axon; however, several unmyelinated axons can be ensheathed by a single Schwann cell. The myelin sheath is the plasmalemma of the Schwann cell that is wrapped around the axon as many as 50 times. Thousands of Schwann cells line up side by side, and each wraps its plasma membrane around a small length of the axon. The region of the axon wrapped by one Schwann cell is known as the **internodal segment**. The region between two adjoining internodal segments lacks myelin and is referred to as the **node of Ranvier**. Because each Schwann cell has its own basal lamina, the axon at the node of Ranvier is covered by interdigitations of the Schwann cell processes and by the Schwann cell's basal lamina; thus, the axon is not exposed directly to its surrounding environment. Oligodendroglia do not form processes at the nodes of Ranvier; instead, the region of the node is occupied by the process of an astrocyte. (Fig. 9.6).

  - Although the axons of many neurons are myelinated in adults, not all axons are **myelinated** at the same time during **development**. Sensory nerves are not myelinated completely until several months after birth, whereas motor axons are almost completely myelinated at birth. In the CNS, the axons of some of the fiber tracts are not myelinated for the first few years of life.

  - **Myelination** is a complex and as yet incompletely understood process. The Schwann cell (or oligodendroglion in the CNS) membrane wraps around the axon, and during the wrapping process the cytoplasm is squeezed back into the cell body. The inner aspect of the plasmalemma comes very close to the inner aspect of the plasmalemma, and the outer aspect comes very close to the outer aspect, and this relationship is repeated with each turn of the wrapping.

  - Viewed with the electron microscope, the spiraling membrane presents a wider, darker line—the **major dense line** that indicates the contact between the two cytoplasmic aspects of the Schwann cell plasma membrane. The contact between the outer surfaces of the plasma membrane is noted as a thinner, **intraperiod line**. The major dense line and the intraperiod line alternate with one another. At very high resolution, a narrow gap is visible within the intraperiod line, known as the **intraperiod gap**; this is a very narrow **extracellular space** that permits communication between the axon and the milieu outside the myelin sheath. Naturally, only small ions are capable of traversing the intraperiod gap.

  - Certain regions of the myelin sheath have residual cytoplasm, and they appear as bleblike areas known as **Schmidt-Lanterman incisures**.

- The Schwann cell membrane that forms the myelin sheath is rich in **glycoproteins** and **sphingomyelin** and two essential protein components, **myelin protein zero (MPZ)** and **myelin basic protein (MBP)**. MPZ not only facilitates the process of myelin formation, but also assists in stabilizing the myelin sheath. MBP is also believed to help in maintaining the stability of the myelin sheath. MPZ is not present in myelin of the CNS; instead, another protein, **proteolipid protein (PLP)**, assumes its functions.

- The external aspects of the cell membranes (intraperiod lines) are held to each other by **tight junctions** that not only contain the usual proteins, **claudins** and **zonula occludens proteins**, but also contain **connexin 32 (Cx32)**.

- The region of the myelin sheath where the myelin wrapping ends farthest from the **axolemma** (axon membrane) is the **external mesaxon**.

- The region of the myelin sheath where the myelin wrapping ends closest to the axolemma is the **internal mesaxon**.

  - The **intraperiod gap** extends from the external to the internal mesaxon.

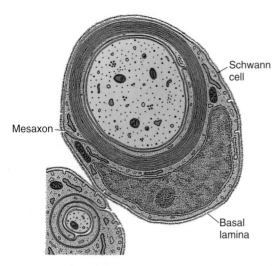

Figure 9.5 The fine structure of a myelinated nerve fiber and its Schwann cell. *(From Gartner LP, Hiatt JL: Color Textbook of Histology, 3rd ed. Philadelphia, Saunders, 2007, p 192.)*

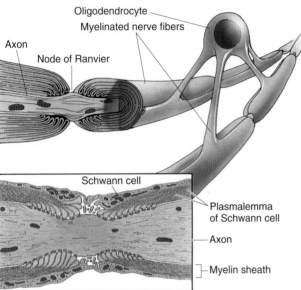

Figure 9.6 Diagrammatic representation of the myelin structure at the node of Ranvier of axons in the CNS and the PNS *(inset)*. *(From Gartner LP, Hiatt JL: Color Textbook of Histology, 3rd ed. Philadelphia, Saunders, 2007, p 197.)*

CLINICAL CONSIDERATIONS

Multiple sclerosis, a disease of demyelination within the CNS, is common. Individuals 15 to 45 years old are affected, and it is approximately 1.5 times more common in females. Regions of the CNS that are demyelinated include the cerebellum, white matter of the cerebrum, spinal cord, and cranial and spinal nerves. There are periods of multifocal inflammation accompanied by edema with demyelination of CNS axons. Each episode may lead to severe deterioration or malignancy or both within the affected nerves, and depending on areas affected, death may result within months. These attacks are followed by remissions lasting several months or decades. Each episode causes the patient to lose vitality. Multiple sclerosis is believed to be an inflammatory autoimmune disease resulting from the presence of an infectious agent.

Immunosuppressants combined with corticosteroids and anti-inflammatory treatment are the therapies of choice.

Radiation therapy involving the brain or spinal cord can lead to demyelination of the nerves in the pathway of the radiation beam. Also, the toxic substances used in **chemotherapy** can lead to demyelination of axons of the nervous system that may cause neurologic problems.

Guillain-Barré syndrome is an immune disorder resulting from recent respiratory or gastrointestinal infection. It produces inflammation and demyelination of peripheral nerves causing muscle weakness in the extremities. The onset is early and peaks within a few weeks. Early diagnosis with autoimmune globulin treatments and physical therapy are usually recommended.

Generation and Conduction of Nerve Impulses

The membranes of all cells are **polarized** electrically in such a fashion that the inner aspect of the membrane is less positive than the outer aspect because of the differential in ion concentrations, namely concentration of Na^+ and Cl^- ions is greater outside the cell than inside, and the concentration of K^+ ions is higher inside than outside the cell. This characteristic of cell membranes is accentuated in mammalian nerve cells, where the **resting potential** is -90 mV in large neurons, although it is less negative in smaller neurons and muscle fibers (Figs. 9.7 and 9.8). Neurons communicate by modulating the **membrane potential** by **depolarizing** and **repolarizing** the membrane, and in this fashion a wave of depolarization spreads along the processes of the neuron and is transmitted to another neuron, muscle cell, or the cell of a gland across a specialized junction known as the **synapse**. The axon plasma membrane possesses at least the following three ion channels and a Na^+-K^+ pump:

- **K^+ leak channels**, which permit K^+ to exit the cell along a gradient of potassium concentration resulting in a buildup of positive charges along the external aspect of the cell membrane. The K^+ leak channel establishes the resting membrane potential, although it is assisted in this to a very limited extent by **Na^+-K^+ pumps**.
- **Na^+-K^+ pumps** in the cell membrane, which pump three Na^+ ions out for every two K^+ ions it pumps into the cell.
- **Voltage-gated Na^+ channels**, which, if they are open, permit Na^+ ions to enter the cell. These channels open if the membrane is depolarized,

but the open state is unstable, and the channel becomes **inactivated** (i.e., it closes and cannot be opened again until the membrane is repolarized to its resting potential). This capability of this particular ion channel is due to its having two gates—a gate on its extracytoplasmic surface, the **activation gate**, and a second gate on its cytoplasmic surface, the **inactivation gate**. Although the activation gate remains open because of the voltage change, the inactivation gate closes, and Na^+ cannot pass through the ion channel, and the ion channel is said to be in its **refractory period**. Voltage-gated Na^+ channels can be:

- Closed (activation gate closed, inactivation gate open),
- Open (activation gate open, inactivation gate open), or
- Inactivated (refractory period—activation gate open, inactivation gate closed).
- **Voltage-gated K^+ channels**, which open—but do so slowly—when the membrane is depolarized, permitting an efflux of K^+ ions out of the neuron. These channels close when the membrane is repolarized.

Usually a neuron is stimulated at the axon's **spike trigger zone**. When this occurs, the membrane potential alters at that particular point, and the following sequence of events occurs:

1. Voltage-gated Na^+ channels **open** at the spike trigger zone, Na^+ ions enter the axon, and the preponderance of positive Na^+ ions at the internal aspect of the membrane reverses the membrane potential, and the membrane becomes **depolarized**.

Continued on p. 118

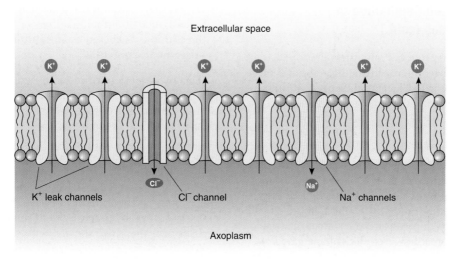

Figure 9.7 Schematic diagram of the establishment of the resting potential in a typical neuron. The K⁺ leak channels outnumber the Na⁺ and Cl⁻ channels; consequently, more K⁺ can leave the cell than Na⁺ or Cl⁻ can enter. Because there are more positive ions outside than inside the cell, the outside is more positive than the inside, establishing a potential difference across the membrane. Ion channels and ion pumps not directly responsible for the establishment of resting membrane potential are not shown. *(From Gartner LP, Hiatt JL: Color Textbook of Histology, 3rd ed. Philadelphia, Saunders, 2007, p 199.)*

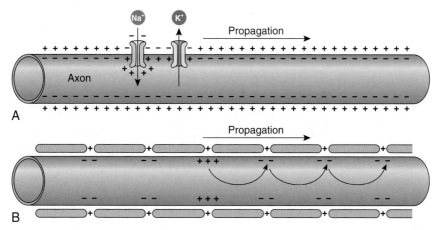

Figure 9.8 Schematic diagram of the propagation of an action potential in an unmyelinated (**A**) and myelinated (**B**) axon. *(From Gartner LP, Hiatt JL: Color Textbook of Histology, 3rd ed. Philadelphia, Saunders, 2007, p 200.)*

Generation and Conduction of Nerve Impulses (cont.)

2. The **voltage-gated Na⁺ channels** that opened at that point become **inactivated** for about 2 msec. The **voltage-gated K⁺ channels** open, K⁺ ions leave the axon at the spike trigger zone, and the region of the spike trigger zone is **repolarized** and even hyperpolarized for a fraction of a millisecond (Fig. 9.9).

3. Many of the Na⁺ ions that entered the axon in step 1 flow in both directions and would cause depolarization of the adjacent regions of the axon. This wave of depolarization would spread in both directions toward the soma and away from the soma; however, the **voltage-gated Na⁺ channels** toward the soma are in their **refractory period** and cannot open. **Propagation of the impulse (wave of depolarization)** cannot proceed in the direction of the soma (**retrograde propagation**); however, it can and does propagate away from the soma, toward the **axon terminals**.

4. The membrane voltage changes just described are known as an **action potential**; this is an *all-or-none* process that can occur 1000 times every second.

SYNAPSES

Synapses, specialized junctions where nerve cells communicate with other nerve cells or with effector cells (i.e., muscle cells or cells of glands), are of two types—**electric** and **chemical**. The former are gap junctions, but rarely occur in mammals with the exception of some regions in the CNS. The latter involve the release of a **neurotransmitter substance** into a specially adapted intercellular space known as a **synaptic cleft**, located between the plasmalemma of the end-foot of an axon (the **presynaptic membrane**) and a specialized region of the cell membrane (the **postsynaptic membrane**) of another neuron, muscle cell, or cell of a gland. Various types of synapses between two neurons are listed in Table 9.1 and are illustrated in Figure 9.10. The neurotransmitter substance released at the presynaptic membrane binds to receptors on the postsynaptic membrane, resulting in the opening of **receptor-associated ion channels**, which in turn results in the movement of ions through the lumen of the channel. If the ion movement causes a:

- Large enough depolarization of the postsynaptic membrane so that an action potential commences, the stimulus is known as an **excitatory postsynaptic potential**, or

- Hyperpolarization of the postsynaptic membrane so that an action potential does not commence, the stimulus is known as an **inhibitory postsynaptic potential**.

The presynaptic terminus, the end-foot, houses profiles of SER; mitochondria; and small, neurotransmitter-containing vesicles known as **synaptic vesicles**, 40 to 60 μm in diameter. These synaptic vesicles are clustered near the presynaptic membrane at and near the regions known as **active sites** because it is at these locations that the vesicles fuse with the presynaptic membrane and release their contents into the synaptic cleft. Synaptic vesicles that are at the active site are ready to release their contents, whereas vesicles near the active site are held in reserve by:

- The vesicle's transmembrane proteins **synapsin-I** and **synapsin-II**, which bind and immobilize the vesicles to actin filaments

- Phosphorylation of these two proteins, which release the synaptic vesicles from their attachment to the actin filaments allowing them to move to the active site.

Fusion of the synaptic vesicles at the active site with the presynaptic membrane is facilitated by the:

- Entry of Ca⁺⁺ ions into the end-foot via voltage-gated Ca⁺⁺ channels that opened because the action potential reached the end-foot plasmalemma

- Presence of Ca⁺⁺ ions in the cytoplasm that permit transmembrane proteins of the synaptic vesicle and presynaptic membrane **rab3A**, **synaptotagmin**, **synaptobrevin**, **syntaxin**, **SNAP-25** (soluble *N*-ethylmaleimide-sensitive fusion protein attachment protein-25), and **synaptophysin**, to interact with each other to complete the fusion process and allow the release of the neurotransmitter substances into the synaptic cleft

- Vesicle membrane that was added to the presynaptic membrane and is retrieved by endocytosis mediated by **clathrin coat**, a process facilitated by integral proteins **vesicle coat protein AP-2** and **synaptotagmin**. The retrieved membrane is ferried to the SER to be recycled.

The **postsynaptic membrane**, located across the synaptic gap from the presynaptic membrane, is thicker than the remaining membrane of the postsynaptic cell and houses receptors for the neurotransmitter released at the active site of the presynaptic neuron end-foot. The thickness of the postsynaptic membrane is usually indicative of its response to the neurotransmitter released.

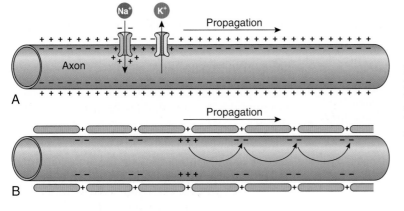

Figure 9.9 Schematic diagram of the propagation of an action potential in an unmyelinated (**A**) and myelinated (**B**) axon. *(From Gartner LP, Hiatt JL: Color Textbook of Histology, 3rd ed. Philadelphia, Saunders, 2007, p 200.)*

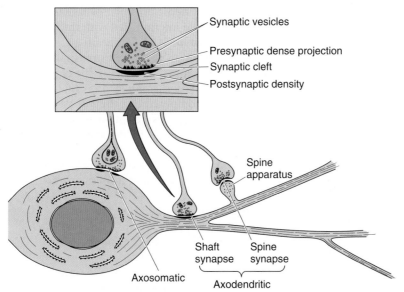

Figure 9.10 Schematic diagram of types of synapses. *(From Gartner LP, Hiatt JL: Color Textbook of Histology, 3rd ed. Philadelphia, Saunders, 2007, p 201.)*

Table 9.1 TYPES OF SYNAPSES BETWEEN TWO NEURONS

Type of Synapse	Regions of Neurons Involved
Axodendritic	Between axon and dendrite
Axosomatic	Between axon and soma
Axoaxonic	Between two axons
Dendrodendritic	Between two dendrites

CLINICAL CONSIDERATIONS

The bacterium *Clostridium botulinum* releases **botulinum toxin**, a neurotoxin that is exceptionally lethal in very small quantities (LD_{50} for intravenous administration is approximately 1 ng/kg). Although the toxin is heat sensitive and is denatured at 140° F, the bacterial spores remain viable and germinate under anaerobic conditions. The vegetative microorganisms release the toxin and usually, in improperly handled food or damaged canned food, the bacteria thrive. The toxin is a protease that specifically cleaves one of the fusion proteins (SNAP-25, syntaxin, or synaptobrevin) at myoneural junctions. The presence of cleaved fusion proteins prevents the fusion of synaptic vesicles with the presynaptic membrane and thwarts the release of acetylcholine, resulting in flaccid paralysis of the affected muscles. Death is usually due to the paralysis of the muscles of respiration, but the toxin takes effect over several days, and if recognized early enough death can be averted by artificial ventilation and the administration of available **botulinum antitoxins**.

Neurotransmitters (Signaling Molecules)

Neurotransmitters contact receptors on their target cells to initiate a specific response. Receptors are:

- **Fast-acting** (the process takes ≤1 msec) because they are coupled with ion channels, and the signaling molecules (first messenger system) activating them are known as **neurotransmitters**
- **Slow-acting** (the process can take several minutes) because they are coupled with G proteins, and the signaling molecules (activating a second messenger system) are known as **neuromodulators** or **neurohormones**

The more than 100 neurotransmitters/neurohormones may be categorized into three groups (Table 9.2):

- Small molecule transmitters (acetylcholine, amino acids, biogenic amines)
- Neuropeptides (opioid peptides, gastrointestinal peptides, hypothalamic releasing hormones, hormones stored in the neurohypophysis)
- Gases (nitric oxide and carbon monoxide)

Neurotransmitters may elicit different responses under different conditions, and the configuration of the postsynaptic receptor may dictate the effect of the neurotransmitter on the postsynaptic cell. Interneuronal synaptic communication usually requires multiple neurotransmitters or **volume transmission**, especially between brain cells, where neurotransmitters are located in the intercellular fluid between brain cells, resulting in activation of groups of cells that possess the proper receptors as opposed to activation of a single cell. Volume transmission is **slow acting** and is thought to apply to alertness, autonomic function, sensitivity to pain, and moods. In contrast, synaptic communication is **fast acting**.

Peripheral Nerves

Peripheral nerves containing sensory and motor nerve fibers are bundled together by nerve investments that permit observation with the unaided eye.

These bundles, known as **fascicles**, appear whitish because of the presence of myelin on many of those fibers.

CONNECTIVE TISSUE INVESTMENTS

Three separate, distinct connective tissue investments surround the nerves within the fascicle (Fig. 9.11):

- **Epineurium**, the outermost layer of the investments, completely surrounds the entire nerve and is continuous with the dura mater of the CNS. It is thickest at the origin of the nerve where it leaves the CNS, and becomes thinner as it gives off branches and eventually disappears. It is composed of dense, irregular collagenous connective tissue intermingled with thick elastic fibers. Collagen fibers of the sheath are organized in such a fashion as to prevent stretching.
- **Perineurium**, the middle layer of the connective tissue investments, surrounds individual nerve fascicles. It is composed of a thin, dense, irregular connective tissue with a few collagen fibers mixed with elastic fibers. The internal surface of the perineurium is lined by layers of epithelioid cells and a basal lamina separating the neuronal compartment from the connective tissue.
- **Endoneurium**, the innermost layer of the connective tissue investments, surrounds each nerve fiber individually. The endoneurium contacts Schwann cell basal lamina, isolating it from the perineurium and the Schwann cells. Near the terminus, it is only a few type III collagen fibers.

FUNCTIONAL CLASSIFICATION OF NERVES

Nerves are composed of sensory or motor fibers or both. The former, known as **afferent nerve fibers**, convey nerve signals from sensory receptors to the CNS for processing. The latter, known as **efferent nerve fibers**, originate in the CNS and convey motor impulses to effector organs. Mixed nerves are the most common type, and they carry afferent nerve fibers (sensory fibers) and efferent nerve fibers (motor fibers).

Table 9.2 COMMON NEUROTRANSMITTERS AND FUNCTIONS ELICITED BY THEIR RECEPTOR

Neurotransmitter	Compound Group	Function
Acetylcholine	Small molecule transmitter; not derived from amino acids	Myoneural junctions, all parasympathetic synapses, and preganglionic sympathetic synapses
Norepinephrine	Small molecule transmitter; biogenic amine; catecholamine	Postganglionic sympathetic synapses (except for eccrine sweat glands)
Glutamic acid	Small molecule transmitter; amino acid	Presynaptic sensory and cortex: most common excitatory neurotransmitter of CNS
GABA	Small molecule transmitter; amino acid	Most common inhibitory neurotransmitter of CNS
Dopamine	Small molecule transmitter; biogenic amine; catecholamine	Basal ganglia of CNS; inhibitory or excitatory, depending on receptor
Serotonin	Small molecule transmitter; biogenic amine	Inhibits pain; mood control; sleep
Glycine	Small molecule transmitter; amino acid	Brainstem and spinal cord; inhibitory
Endorphins	Neuropeptide; opioid peptide	Analgesic; inhibit pain transmission?
Enkephalins	Neuropeptide; opioid peptide	Analgesic; inhibit pain transmission?

From Gartner LP, Hiatt JL: Color Textbook of Histology, 3rd ed. Philadelphia, Saunders, 2007, p 204.

CLINICAL CONSIDERATIONS

Huntington's chorea, a hereditary disease, begins as painful joints, then flicking of the joints of the extremities. It progresses to flinging of the joints, including distortions accompanied by dementia and motor dysfunction. The onset of the disease is in the third and fourth decades. It is thought to be the result of the loss of the cells producing γ-aminobutyric acid (GABA), an inhibitory neurotransmitter. The dementia is thought to be related to loss of the cells secreting acetylcholine.

Parkinson's disease, the second most common neurodegenerative disease, is defined by resting tremor, slow voluntary movements, rigidity, and a mask-like face. The disease is due to the loss of dopaminergic neurons from the substantia nigra, resulting in the absence of dopamine in the brain. Several therapies have been developed and administered, but most provide only temporary relief without checking the death of dopaminergic neurons. Grafting of genetically modified cells to secrete dopamine that would establish new connections to certain cells in the brain where dopamine is needed is presently under study. One current therapy, **deep brain stimulation** (a pacemaker type of therapy), involves implanting electrodes in the thalamus and the globus pallidus, which reduces rigidity and tremors and increases balance.

CONDUCTION VELOCITY

Nerve conduction velocity is directly related to the degree of myelination (Table 9.3). Ions may access the plasma membrane only at the nodes of Ranvier in myelinated nerves because myelin present at the internodes insulates the plasma membrane from being available for ion exchange, and voltage-gated Na^+ channels are concentrated at the nodes of Ranvier. Action potentials jump from one node to the next, a process called **saltatory conduction**. Unmyelinated fibers, covered by only one layer of Schwann cell plasma membrane, are essentially uninsulated from the outward movement of excess Na^+ ions, and voltage-gated Na^+ channels are distributed along the entire length of the axonal plasma membrane. The conduction process, known as **continuous conduction**, is not only slower, but also requires more energy.

Somatic Motor and Autonomic Nervous Systems

Skeletal muscles receive **somatic motor innervation** via single efferent neurons whose cell bodies lie within the CNS. Smooth muscles, cardiac muscle, and glands receive **autonomic motor innervation** via a two-neuron chain where the soma of the first neuron is in the CNS, and the soma of the second neuron is located in an autonomic ganglion in the PNS.

- The **somatic motor nervous system** (Fig. 9.12) is composed of **spinal motor nerves** from the ventral horn of the spinal cord and **cranial motor nerves** serving skeletal muscles from motor nuclei of certain cranial nerves. As spinal motor nerves leave the CNS, they travel in spinal nerves to the muscle and synapse at the motor end plate. Cranial nerves leave the cranial vault and pass via branches of a cranial nerve to synapse on the motor end plate of the skeletal muscle.

- The **autonomic nervous system** (see Fig. 9.12) is an involuntary motor system serving smooth muscle, cardiac muscle, and glands. In contrast to the somatic motor system, the autonomic nervous system requires two neurons to reach the effector organs. The first motoneuron in the chain, the **preganglionic neuron**, originates in the CNS, and its axon seeks an **autonomic ganglion** located outside the CNS, where it synapses on multipolar cell bodies of **postganglionic neurons** located within the ganglion. Axons of the postganglionic neurons exit the ganglion and terminate on an **effector organ** (smooth muscle, cardiac muscle, or gland). Postganglionic synapses on the effector organs are more generalized than that of the somatic motor system because the neurotransmitter spreads out over a wider area with a more extensive effect. Additionally, muscles activated to contract may convey the stimulation to adjacent muscles via gap junctions.

Table 9.3 CLASSIFICATION OF PERIPHERAL NERVE FIBERS

Fiber Group	Diameter (μm)	Conduction Velocity (m/sec)	Function
Type A fibers—heavily (myelinated)	1–20	15–120	High-velocity somatic efferent fibers; also those that register acute pain, temperature, touch, pressure, and proprioception
Type B fibers—less myelination	1–3	3–15	Moderate-velocity fibers: visceral afferents; preganglionic autonomic fibers
Type C fibers—no myelination	0.5–1.5	0.5–2	Slow-velocity fibers: postganglionic autonomics; chronic pain

From Gartner LP, Hiatt JL: Color Textbook of Histology, 3rd ed. Philadelphia, Saunders, 2007, p 206.

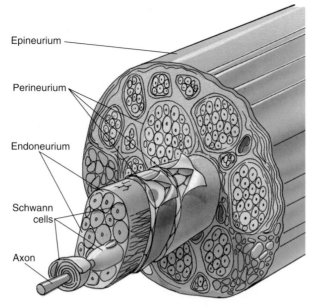

Figure 9.11 Structure of a nerve bundle. *(From Gartner LP, Hiatt JL: Color Textbook of Histology, 3rd ed. Philadelphia, Saunders, 2007, p 205.)*

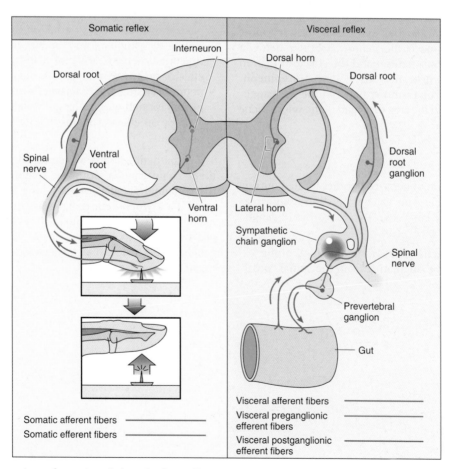

Figure 9.12 Comparison of somatic and visceral reflexes. *(From Gartner LP, Hiatt JL: Color Textbook of Histology, 3rd ed. Philadelphia, Saunders, 2007, p 207.)*

Somatic Motor and Autonomic Nervous Systems (cont.)

Autonomic innervation is subdivided into two functionally different divisions: the sympathetic nervous system and the parasympathetic nervous system. Broadly defined, the sympathetic system is regarded to be vasoconstrictor in function, whereas the parasympathetic system is regarded to be secretomotor in function.

- The **sympathetic nervous system** functionally prepares the body for *flight or fight* by slowing down visceral activity; dilating the pupils; increasing blood pressure, heart rate, and respiration; and increasing blood flow to skeletal muscles (Fig. 9.13).
- The **parasympathetic nervous system** functionally prepares the body for *rest and digest* by increasing visceral functions; constricting the pupils; decreasing blood pressure, heart rate, and respiration; and decreasing blood flow to skeletal muscles (see Fig. 9.13).

The neurotransmitter between the preganglionic and postganglionic neurons in the sympathetic and parasympathetic nervous systems is **acetylcholine**, and acetylcholine is the neurotransmitter between the postganglionic neuron and the effector organ in the parasympathetic nervous system. **Norepinephrine** is the neurotransmitter between the postganglionic neuron and the effector organ in the sympathetic nervous system.

Ganglia

An accumulation of nerve cell bodies located outside the CNS with the same general function is known as a **ganglion** (see Fig. 9.13). Two categories of ganglia exist:

- **Sensory ganglia** are associated with all of the sensory nerves originating from the spinal cord and with cranial nerves V, VII, IX, and X. Sensory ganglia associated with the spinal cord are called **dorsal root ganglia**, whereas sensory ganglia associated with the cranial nerves are identified by specific names related to the nerve. Sensory ganglia contain **unipolar neurons**. The endoneurium of the axon becomes continuous with the connective tissue surrounding the ganglion. Specialized receptors surrounding the terminals of peripheral nerves are able to transduce the various stimuli, initiating an action potential, which is passed directly to the brain or spinal cord for processing.
- **Autonomic ganglia** are associated with purely motor function. Preganglionic cell bodies of **parasympathetic neurons** are located in the brain and sacral spinal cord, whereas cell bodies of the **sympathetic neurons** are located in certain segments of the thoracic and lumbar spinal cord. The axons of the **preganglionic motoneurons** seek their ganglia where they synapse on **postganglionic motor cell bodies**. Axons of postganglionic neurons may rejoin the peripheral nerve of their origin to reach their effector organs. Many postganglionic parasympathetic fibers located in the head, on exiting the ganglia, join branches of the trigeminal nerve (CN V) for distribution to effector organs. Postganglionic parasympathetic neurons arising from **Meissner's** or **Auerbach's plexus** located within the gut wall simply synapse on effector organs that lie in close proximity.

Sympathetic ganglia are confined to the sympathetic chain ganglia along the spinal column or to the collateral ganglia located along the abdominal aorta. Parasympathetic ganglia associated with cranial nerves are located within the head (except for ganglia belonging to CN X), whereas parasympathetic ganglia associated with sacral nerves are located in the organ that they serve.

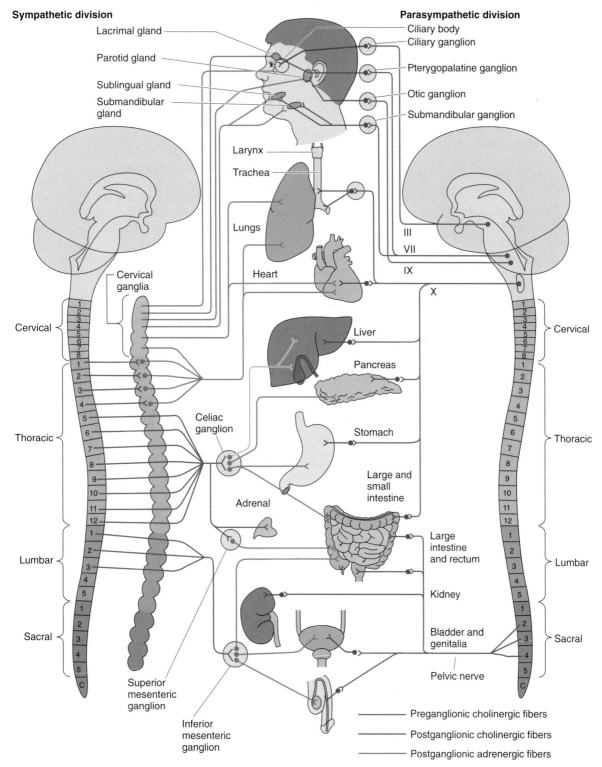

Sympathetic division

Parasympathetic division

Lacrimal gland

Parotid gland

Sublingual gland

Submandibular gland

Ciliary body

Ciliary ganglion

Pterygopalatine ganglion

Otic ganglion

Submandibular ganglion

Larynx

Trachea

Lungs

Heart

III

VII

IX

X

Cervical ganglia

Cervical

Thoracic

Lumbar

Sacral

Celiac ganglion

Adrenal

Superior mesenteric ganglion

Inferior mesenteric ganglion

Liver

Pancreas

Stomach

Large and small intestine

Large intestine and rectum

Kidney

Bladder and genitalia

Pelvic nerve

Cervical

Thoracic

Lumbar

Sacral

Preganglionic cholinergic fibers

Postganglionic cholinergic fibers

Postganglionic adrenergic fibers

Figure 9.13 Autonomic nervous system. *Left,* Sympathetic division. *Right,* Parasympathetic division. *(From Gartner LP, Hiatt JL: Color Textbook of Histology, 3rd ed. Philadelphia, Saunders, 2007, p 209.)*

The brain and spinal cord are composed of:

- **White matter**, which consists mostly of myelinated nerve fibers along with some unmyelinated fibers and neuroglial cells. The abundant myelin covering the axons gives it the white color.
- **Gray matter**, which consists of accumulations of neuronal cell bodies and their dendrites along with unmyelinated axons. The gray color indicates the absence of myelin.

The twisted, intertwined collection of axons, dendrites, and processes of neuroglial cells composes the **neuropil**. Localized collections of nerve bodies in the white matter are known as **nuclei**. Within the brain, gray matter is located on the periphery, whereas white matter is located deeper; in the spinal cord, gray matter is located deep to the white matter. In cross section of the spinal cord, the gray matter forms the letter *H*, and in its center is the **central canal**, a small foramen lined with **ependymal cells** that contains **CSF**. Central processes of sensory neurons terminate on **interneuron** cell bodies in the **dorsal horns**, the superior aspects of the vertical bars of the H. Interneuron axons terminate on motoneuron cell bodies in the inferior vertical bars of the H, the **ventral horns**. Axons of the motoneurons exit the spinal cord by passing out the ventral roots.

MENINGES

The meninges represent the three connective tissue coverings of the brain and spinal cord identified as the outer layer, the **dura mater**; an intermediate **arachnoid**; and the innermost layer, the **pia mater** (Fig. 9.14).

1. **Dura mater**, the outermost layer of the meninges, is different in the brain than in the spinal cord. The **cranial dura mater** is composed of dense connective tissue consisting of two separate components:
   - An outer **periosteal layer** closely adhered to the bony cranium, serving also as the periosteum of the inner aspect of the skull. It is highly vascularized and contains osteoprogenitor cells, fibroblasts, and bundles of type I collagen.
   - The innermost layer of the dura, the **meningeal layer**, which presents dark-staining fibroblasts possessing long processes, fine collagen fibers organized in sheets, and is vascularized by small arteries. The innermost

region of the meningeal layer, the **border cell layer**, consists of a thin layer of fibroblasts enveloped by an unstructured extracellular matrix lacking collagen fibers that extends into the meningeal layer.

The **spinal dura mater** is not represented in layers because it does not adhere to the vertebral canal as a periosteal layer. Rather, the spinal dura mater forms a complete tube surrounding the spinal cord beginning at the foramen magnum and ending at the second sacral segment. Along this tract, spinal nerves pierce the spinal dura, and the space between the bony vertebral canal and the dura, the **epidural space**, is filled with epidural fat and a venous plexus.

2. The avascular **arachnoid** consists of two layers:
   - One is a flat sheetlike layer that lies against the dura mater.
   - The second layer is formed of sparse, loosely organized modified fibroblasts (**arachnoid trabecular cells**) interspersed with a few fibers of collagen and some elastic fibers from **trabeculae** that contact the pia mater.
   - The space between the flat sheet contacting the dura and the trabeculae contacting the pia is known as the **subarachnoid space**.
   - Blood vessels course through the arachnoid as they progress from the dura on their way to the pia mater, but they are isolated from the arachnoid and from the **subarachnoid space** by a sheet of fibroblasts derived from the arachnoid. The subarachnoid space is a real space filled with CSF, but the subdural space, located between the dura and the sheetlike layer of the arachnoid that contacts the dura, is only a potential space. Specialized regions of the arachnoid, known as **arachnoid villi**, extend into the dural venous sinuses and translocate CSF from the subarachnoid space into these dural sinuses.

3. The innermost layer of the meninges, the **pia mater**, is composed of flattened fibroblasts, mast cells, macrophages, and lymphocytes, and is described as being closely apposed to the brain and spinal cord. The pia is separated from the actual brain tissue, however, by a thin membrane composed of **neuroglial processes** that adhere to the thin reticular and elastic fibers of the pia and form a physical barrier at the periphery of the CNS. A sheath of pial cells covers the rich vascular supply of the pia, which is replaced by neuroglial cells as these vessels penetrate the nervous tissue.

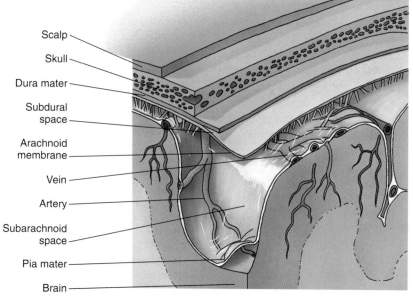

Scalp

Skull

Dura mater

Subdural space

Arachnoid membrane

Vein

Artery

Subarachnoid space

Pia mater

Brain

Figure 9.14 The skull and the layers of the meninges covering the brain. *(From Gartner LP, Hiatt JL: Color Textbook of Histology, 3rd ed. Philadelphia, Saunders, 2007, p 212.)*

CLINICAL CONSIDERATIONS

Tumors of the meninges, known as **meningiomas**, are most often slow-growing and benign. They produce possibly serious clinical manifestations, however, such as brain compression or increasing intracranial pressure.

Meningitis, an inflammation of the meninges, may be caused by bacteria or by viruses that have gained access to the CSF. Viral meningitis is not very dangerous; however, bacterial meningitis is not only a very hazardous condition, but it is also highly contagious. The pathogen may gain initial entry through the nose, ear, or throat, and can be spread by the exchange of respiratory secretions via coughing and kissing. The onset of meningitis is characterized by fever, stiff neck, nausea, and vomiting. Meningitis is diagnosed by the examination of the CSF obtained by lumbar puncture, and an antibiotic regimen is used to treat the disease. Vaccines are now available for protecting against some of the common bacteria that cause meningitis.

The **blood-brain barrier (BBB)** is exceedingly discriminating in permitting passage of substances from the bloodstream into the CNS. It prevents most therapeutic drugs, many antibiotics, toxins, and certain neurotransmitters including dopamine from entering the neural tissue. Perfusion of a hypertonic solution of mannitol may alter the tight junctions of the BBB sufficiently for a short time permitting the passage of therapeutic drugs. Another method of bypassing the BBB is the binding of the therapeutic drug to antibodies against **transferrin receptors** located in the endothelial cells of the capillaries, facilitating their transport into the CNS.

Certain diseases or conditions that affect the CNS, such as stroke, tumors, and infections, alter the BBB by reducing its functionality and permitting the entry of toxic substances and unwanted metabolites into the neural tissue.

The subarachnoid space is a real space filled with CSF, but the **subdural space**, located between the dura and the sheetlike layer of the arachnoid that contacts the dura, is only a potential space. It may become a real space after injury, however, when bleeding forces the two layers apart; this condition is called a **subdural hemorrhage**.

BLOOD-BRAIN BARRIER

Endothelial cells of the **continuous capillaries** located in neural tissues form tight junctions with each other, establishing the **blood-brain barrier (BBB)**, which limits the ability of blood-borne material to enter the confines of the CNS.

- Certain molecules, such as O_2, CO_2, water, and small lipids, can easily pass through the BBB.
- Most other substances, such as glucose, nucleosides, and amino acids, have to be transported by carrier proteins and ion channels that are specific for them.
- Still other materials pass through this barrier by the use of **receptor-mediated transport**.

The BBB is reinforced by **astrocytes** whose processes form **end-feet** that completely surround the basal lamina of the capillaries located in the CNS. The cylindrical sheath fashioned by these end-feet form the **perivascular glia limitans**. Astrocytes also function in transporting metabolites from the capillaries to the neurons and in scavenging K^+ ions and neurotransmitters from the extracellular spaces surrounding the neurons and their processes.

CHOROID PLEXUS

The **choroid plexus**, composed of tufts of highly vascularized pia mater surrounded by cuboidal ependymal cells, project into the ventricles of the brain and produce approximately 50% of the CSF. It is unknown where in the brain the remaining half of the CSF is produced. CSF fills the ventricles of the brain, the central canal of the spinal cord, and the subarachnoid spaces.

Cerebrospinal Fluid

The **CSF** is a clear, protein-poor but electrolyte-rich fluid that has a scant amount of lymphocytes and other cells (Table 9.4). Because CSF is formed on a continuous basis of 0.2 to 0.6 mL/min and is transferred into the dural venous sinuses by the arachnoid villi at the same rate, its formation and resorption acts as a pump that facilitates its circulation through the ventricles of the brain, central canal of the spinal cord, and subarachnoid spaces. This fluid functions in supporting the metabolic activities of the CNS, and by acting as a shock absorber diminishes sudden forces that may act on the brain and spinal cord.

CEREBRAL CORTEX

The cerebrum consists of two hemispheres whose periphery is composed of gray matter, the **cerebral cortex**, which overlies the thick layer of white matter located deeper within the cerebrum. The cerebral cortex is folded into elevated areas called **gyri** that are separated from each other by depressions called **sulci**.

- The cerebrum has a plethora of functions, including memory, learning, integration of sensory input, analysis of information, initiation of motor response, and thought processing.
- The cerebral cortex is composed of six horizontally arranged layers; the neurons in each layer possess distinct morphologic characteristics specific to that layer (Table 9.5).
- The outermost layer lies just deep to the overlying pia mater, and the sixth layer contacts the white matter of the cerebral cortex.
- All of the layers contain specific neurons and neuroglia.

Table 9.4 COMPARISON OF SERUM AND CEREBROSPINAL FLUID (CSF)

Constituent	Serum	CSF
White blood cells (cells/mL)	0	0–5
Protein (g/L)	60–80	Negligible
Glucose (mMol/L)	4–5.5	2.1–4
Na$^+$ (mMol/L)	135–150	135–150
K$^+$ (mMol/L)	4–5.1	2.8–3.2
Cl$^-$ (mMol/L)	100–105	115–130
Ca^{++} (mMol/L)	2.1–2.5	1–1.4
Mg^{++} (mMol/L)	0.7–1	0.8–1.3
pH	7.4	7.3

From Gartner LP, Hiatt JL: Color Textbook of Histology, 3rd ed. Philadelphia, Saunders, 2007, p 215.

Table 9.5 LAYERS OF THE CEREBRAL CORTEX

Layer	Layer Name	Neuron Cell Types*
1	Molecular	Horizontal cells
2	External granular	Tightly packed granule cells
3	External pyramidal	Large pyramidal cells
4	Internal granular	Pyramidal cells, small granule cells; thin layer, high cell density
5	Internal pyramidal	Large pyramidal cells; low cell density
6	Multiform	Martinotti cells

*All layers house neuroglia.

CLINICAL CONSIDERATIONS

Because CSF is produced in a continuous fashion, blockage of the ventricles or less than optimal functioning of the arachnoid villi results in enlargement of the ventricles, a condition known as **hydrocephalus**. This disorder has severe consequences because the excess CSF in the enlarged ventricles exerts pressure on the brain. Because the fontanelles and the bony sutures in the skull are not yet fused in fetuses and neonates, this condition results in enlargement of the head, mental impairment, malfunctioning muscles, and eventual death without treatment.

Alzheimer's disease, the most common neurodegenerative disease, affecting about 5 million individuals in the United States, results in dementia that is progressive and terminal. It is usually diagnosed in individuals older than 65 years, although the onset may have occurred years earlier. The most common early symptom is memory loss followed by confusion, irritability, aggression, and mood swings. Later symptoms include breakdown of language, long-term memory loss, decline of senses, general withdrawal, loss of bodily functions, and finally death. Although the cause is not clearly understood, it is characterized by the loss of neurons and synapses mainly within the cerebral cortex followed by gross atrophy of the individual cerebral lobes. Autopsies have shown that patients with Alzheimer's disease develop amyloid plaques and neurofibrillary tangles within the brain that, as they continue to expand, involve a greater number of neurons, rendering them nonfunctional.

CEREBELLAR CORTEX

The **cerebellum** comprises two lateral hemispheres and a central, connecting portion, known as the **vermis**. The peripheral layer of the cerebellum, the **cerebellar cortex**, is composed of gray matter that overlies the deeper white matter. The cerebellar cortex is responsible for maintaining balance during all phases of posture and coordinates voluntary muscle activity and muscle tone. The cerebellar cortex has three separate layers:

- **Molecular layer**—composed mainly of dendrites of Purkinje cells and unmyelinated axons from the granular layer, and some stellate cells and basket cells
- **Purkinje cell layer**—composed of large Purkinje cells (unique to the cerebellum) whose arborized dendrites are observed in the molecular layer, whereas their myelinated axons project into the white matter
- **Granular layer**—composed of crowded nuclei of small granule cells and glomeruli (cerebellar islands) representing synapses between axons entering the cerebellum and the resident granule cells.

Purkinje cells have only an **inhibitory output**, and they process and integrate simultaneous information from hundreds of thousands of excitatory and inhibitory synapses before forming a response. Purkinje cells release only GABA as their neurotransmitter substance, and they are the only cells of the cerebellum whose processes and responses extend outside the cerebellum.

Nerve Regeneration

Although there is some evidence that certain neurons may undergo proliferation, it is *generally* believed that most neurons and nerves within the CNS that have been destroyed by trauma cannot regenerate because they do not undergo proliferation. Damage to neurons and their processes within the CNS is permanent. Peripheral nerves that have been damaged are able to repair the damage, however, via a series of events known as the **axon reaction** (Fig. 9.15).

AXON REACTION

Reaction to the damage involves changes in three specific areas of the neuron: **local changes**, **anterograde changes**, and **retrograde changes**. Although some of the reactions to the damage occur quickly, most of the changes, repair, regeneration, and restoration of function take weeks to months to complete.

- **Local reaction** occurs at the site of the injury. If the axon is severed, the cut ends draw back from each other, and the axolemma covers the cut ends, diminishing the escape of axoplasm. Macrophages and fibroblasts invade the site of injury and release signaling molecules. The macrophages, aided by Schwann cells, begin to phagocytose the damaged tissue.
- **Anterograde reaction** involves the degeneration that occurs to the part of the axon that is between the site of the injury and the end-feet.
  - Within 7 days of the injury, the end-foot becomes swollen, and as it begins to degenerate, it loses its contact with the postsynaptic membrane. The remains of the end-foot become phagocytosed by the proliferating Schwann cells that migrate into the region of the former synapse.
  - The region of the axon and its myelin sheath, located between the injury site and the former synaptic cleft, become fragmented, a process known as **wallerian degeneration**. Schwann cells cease to form myelin, and instead begin to phagocytose the remnants of the distal axon and its myelin sheath; the basal lamina of the endoneurium remains intact
  - Schwann cells continue to reproduce, and the newly produced cells form a **Schwann tube** enveloped by the endoneurially derived basal lamina.
- **Retrograde reaction** and **regeneration** involves the portion of the neuron located between the site of injury and the soma within the CNS.
  - The injured neuron undergoes **chromatolysis**: its Nissl bodies diffuse, its nucleus shifts location, its soma enlarges, and the neuron manufactures macromolecules that are used for the regeneration of the damaged axon.
  - The proximal axon end begins to develop numerous **axon sprouts**, one of which finds the endoneurium to travel down the **lumen of the Schwann tube**; the other axon sprouts degenerate, and their remnants are phagocytosed by macrophages and Schwann cells.
  - The axon sprout lengthens within the Schwann tube, guided and promoted by factors produced by the Schwann cells, fibroblasts, and macrophages; growing at 3 to 4 mm/day, the axon sprout reaches the postsynaptic membrane and re-establishes synaptic contact.

If the Schwann tube is **blocked** by scar tissue, and the growing axon cannot penetrate its lumen, regeneration most likely would not occur. Consequently, the postsynaptic cell also atrophies in a development known as **transneuronal degeneration**, indicating that the neuron exerts a **trophic influence** on the cell with which it synapses.

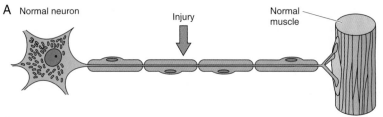

A Normal neuron

Injury

Normal muscle

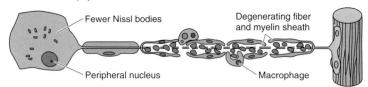

B 2 weeks after injury

Fewer Nissl bodies

Degenerating fiber and myelin sheath

Peripheral nucleus

Macrophage

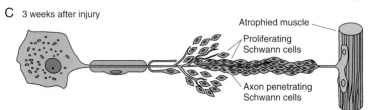

C 3 weeks after injury

Atrophied muscle

Proliferating Schwann cells

Axon penetrating Schwann cells

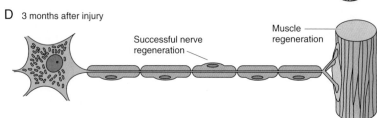

D 3 months after injury

Successful nerve regeneration

Muscle regeneration

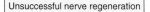

Unsuccessful nerve regeneration

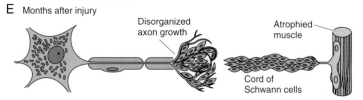

E Months after injury

Disorganized axon growth

Atrophied muscle

Cord of Schwann cells

Figure 9.15 Schematic diagram of nerve regeneration. **A,** Normal neuron. **B–D,** Appearance 2 weeks (**B**), 3 weeks (**C**), and 3 months (**D**) after injury. **E,** Appearance several months after injury of neuron with unsuccessful nerve regeneration. *(From Gartner LP, Hiatt JL: Color Textbook of Histology, 3rd ed. Philadelphia, Saunders, 2007, p 217.)*

CLINICAL CONSIDERATIONS

Until more recently, it was thought that regeneration within the CNS was impossible for many reasons, including the presence of macrophages called *microglia,* which phagocytose injured cells very quickly, and the cleared space is rapidly filled with a mass of glial cells forming a **glial scar**. There are **neuronal stem cells** in the CNS that may be stimulated to proliferate, however, giving rise to new neurons that assume the functions of the cells that were lost because of injury. More recent investigations involving stem cells, **neuronal plasticity**, nerve growth factor, nerve growth inhibitors, and **neurotrophins** offer hope of repairing and reversing the results of spinal cord injuries.

10 BLOOD AND HEMATOPOIESIS

The average human possesses approximately 5 L of **blood**, a red, somewhat thick fluid with a pH of 7.4. Blood is pumped by the heart through the vessels of the circulatory system, transporting nutrients; signaling molecules, electrolytes, and oxygen to the cells of the body; and ferrying waste products and carbon dioxide away from those same cells to be eliminated by the organs designed for those tasks. Additionally, specific cells and formed elements of the blood travel in the bloodstream to perform their functions inside the bloodstream, or when they reach their destination, they leave the circulatory system and enter the connective tissue compartment to carry out their particular duties. Blood also functions in regulating the osmotic and acid-base balance and temperature of the body. Because blood is a fluid, it has a protective mechanism of **coagulation**, driven by platelets, which minimizes blood loss in case of damage to blood vessels.

When 100 mL of blood is centrifuged in a heparinized test tube, it separates into its cells and formed elements and its fluid component, the **plasma**.

- The bottom 44 mL is composed of packed **erythrocytes** (red blood cells [RBCs]).
- The **buffy coat**, 1 mL composed of **leukocytes** (white blood cells [WBCs]), sits on top of the erythrocytes.
- On top of the leukocytes lies 55 mL of plasma.

The 44% of RBCs represents the **hematocrit**, the total erythrocyte volume.

Blood cells and platelets have natural life spans and must be replenished daily to maintain a constant number of each particular cell type in the circulating population. The process of this continuous renewal is known as **hematopoiesis (hemopoiesis)**.

Blood

PLASMA

Plasma constitutes 55% of blood volume, of which:

> **KEY WORDS**
> - **Plasma**
> - **Erythrocytes**
> - **Agranulocytes**
> - **Granulocytes**
> - **Stem cells**
> - **Progenitor cells**
> - **Precursor cells**
> - **Hematopoietic growth factors**

- 90% is water,
- 9% is proteins, and
  - 1% is electrolytes, nutrients, and dissolved gases.

The protein composition of plasma is presented in Table 10.1. The protein-poor fluid component of plasma leaves small venules and capillary beds to enter the connective tissue compartment where it is known as **extracellular fluid** (interstitial tissue fluid). The protein albumin exerts a colloid osmotic pressure within the vascular system that is responsible for keeping fluid within the vascular system and limiting the extracellular fluid volume.

When blood coagulates, some of the proteins and factors that are present in plasma are depleted during the clotting process. The straw-colored fluid that remains, **serum**, is a protein-rich remnant of plasma lacking fibrinogen.

FORMED ELEMENTS

The formed elements of blood are erythrocytes, leukocytes, and cell fragments known as platelets (Fig. 10.1). Special techniques and stains are used for the microscopic study of blood cells.

- Usually a drop of blood or bone marrow is spread on a glass slide and permitted to air dry.
- The slide is dipped in absolute methanol and air dried again.
- The slide is stained with **Wright** or **Giemsa** modification of the **Romanovsky-type stain**, which was originally composed of a combination of eosin and methylene blue.
- The slide is rinsed quickly in water, air dried again, and may be placed under a coverslip or observed without a coverslip.

In this book, all descriptions of blood cells (with the exception of reticulocytes, discussed in the section on erythropoiesis) are based on colors achieved by the use of these stains.

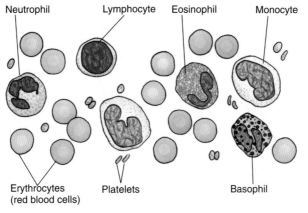

Figure 10.1 Formed elements of circulating blood. *(From Gartner LP, Hiatt JL: Color Textbook of Histology, 3rd ed. Philadelphia, Saunders, 2007, p 220.)*

Table 10.1 PROTEINS PRESENT IN PLASMA

Protein	Size	Source	Function
Albumin	60,000–69,000 Da	Liver	Maintains colloid osmotic pressure and transports certain insoluble metabolites
Globulins			
α-globulins and β-globulins	$80,000–1 \times 10^6$ Da	Liver	Transport metal ions, protein-bound lipids, and lipid-soluble vitamins
γ-globulin		Plasma cells	Antibodies of immune defense
Clotting proteins (e.g., prothrombin, fibrinogen, accelerator globulin)	Varied	Liver	Formation of fibrin threads
Complement proteins C1–C9	Varied	Liver	Destruction of microorganisms and initiation of inflammation
Plasma lipoproteins			
Chylomicrons	100–500 μm	Intestinal epithelial cells	Transport of triglycerides to liver
Very-low-density lipoprotein	25–70 nm	Liver	Transport of triglycerides from liver to body cells
Low-density lipoprotein	3×10^6 Da	Liver	Transport of cholesterol from liver to body cells

From Gartner LP, Hiatt JL: Color Textbook of Histology, 3rd ed. Philadelphia, Saunders, 2007, p 221.

Erythrocytes

Erythrocytes (RBCs) resemble biconcave disks and are the most numerous and smallest (7.2 μm in diameter) of the blood cells (see Fig. 10.1). There is a sex difference in the number of erythrocytes per unit volume: Women possess 4.5×10^6 RBCs per mm^3, and men possess 5×10^6 RBCs per mm^3. This number increases in both sexes if they live at higher elevations. In contrast to all other cells of the body, erythrocytes no longer possess organelles or a nucleus because they were extruded during their formation and before the time they entered circulation. Because of their shape, these cells have a high surface area-to-volume ratio, which assists in the performance of their function—carrying and exchanging O_2 for CO_2 and vice versa. To facilitate their ability to perform this function, these cells are packed with **hemoglobin**, and they possess the enzyme **carbonic anhydrase**. These cells preferentially:

- Release O_2 and pick up CO_2 in regions of low O_2 and high CO_2 tension—the tissues of the body
- Pick up O_2 and **release CO_2** in regions that are oxygen-rich and carbon dioxide–poor—the lungs

Erythrocyte Cell Membrane

The **cell membrane** of RBCs (Fig. 10.2) has the normal membrane composition of 40% phospholipids in the form of a bilayer, 10% carbohydrates, and 50% protein, which consists mostly of:

- **Glycophorin A**, one of the two transmembrane proteins, which forms part of the junctional complex of proteins that binds to spectrin
- Ion channels
- Carrier proteins, including the ion transporter **band 3 protein** that exchanges Cl^- and HCO_3^- ions across the cell membrane, permitting the erythrocyte to discharge CO_2 in the lungs
- Peripheral protein **band 4.1**, which binds glycophorin A to actin and tropomyosin

Supporting the plasmalemma is a network of **spectrin tetramers**, proteins that form hexagonal scaffolding beneath the plasma membrane with the assistance of **ankyrin**, which binds spectrin to band 3 protein. Additional support of the spectrin scaffolding is provided by the junctional complex of proteins composed of band 4.1 protein, actin,

adducin, tropomyosin, and glycophorin. The supporting network of proteins provides not only a great degree of flexibility for the erythrocyte, but also an amazing stability and capability to resist shearing forces. These cells live for approximately 120 days, and during that time they pass tens of thousands of times through narrow capillaries where they become distorted and subjected to powerful shearing forces, but when out of the confines of these channels they resume their normal shape.

The extracellular aspects of RBC plasmalemma sport inherited carbohydrate groups that are antigenic and must be taken into consideration during blood transfusions. The two principal antigens are **A** and **B antigens**, giving rise to four blood groups (Table 10.2). Additionally, 85% of the U.S. population has one of the three principal **Rh antigens** (**C**, **D**, and **E**), and these individuals are said to be Rh-positive, whereas the other 15% are Rh-negative (see Clinical Considerations).

Carbon Dioxide and Oxygen Transport

RBCs transport CO_2 and O_2 by two different mechanisms. Most of the **CO_2** is carried as HCO_3^- ions (formed by the action of **carbonic anhydrase** on H_2O and CO_2, forming H_2CO_3 that immediately dissociates into H^+ and HCO_3^-). In the lungs, where the CO_2 tension is low, HCO_3^- ions leave the RBC cytoplasm, and Cl^- ions enter via the ion exchanger **band 3 proteins** (the exchange is known as the **chloride shift**).

Oxygen is carried by the protein **hemoglobin**, a large tetramer. Each of the four polypeptide chains of hemoglobin is tightly bound to an iron-carrying **heme group**. Table 10.3 lists the major types of hemoglobin.

- The **globin** moiety of hemoglobin carries some CO_2 and is known as **carbaminohemoglobin**; it releases its CO_2 in areas of low CO_2 tension (the lungs).
- O_2, picked up in the oxygen-rich lungs, binds to the heme portion, and hemoglobin becomes known as **oxyhemoglobin** and is carried to oxygen-poor regions where it is easily released.
- The place of O_2 becomes occupied by **2,3-diphosphoglycerate**, and hemoglobin changes its name to **deoxyhemoglobin**.

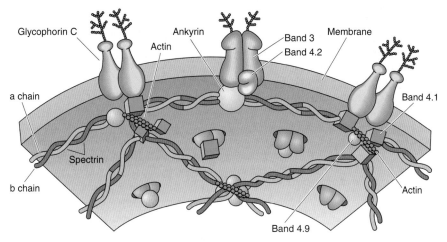

Figure 10.2 Erythrocyte cell membrane and associated proteins. *(From Gartner LP, Hiatt JL: Color Textbook of Histology, 3rd ed. Philadelphia, Saunders, 2007, p 224.)*

Table 10.2 ABO BLOOD GROUP SYSTEM

Blood Group	Antigens Present	Miscellaneous
A	Antigen A	
B	Antigen B	
AB	Antigens A and B	Universal acceptor
O	Neither antigen A nor B	Universal donor

From Gartner LP, Hiatt JL: Color Textbook of Histology, 3rd ed. Philadelphia, Saunders, 2007, p 224.

Table 10.3 MAJOR TYPES OF HEMOGLOBIN

Polypeptide Chains	Hemoglobin Type	Designation
$\alpha\alpha\gamma\gamma$	Fetal hemoglobin	HbF
$\alpha\alpha\beta\beta$	Adult hemoglobin (most common, 96%)	HbA$_1$
$\alpha\alpha\delta\delta$	Adult hemoglobin (rare, 2%)	HbA$_2$

CLINICAL CONSIDERATIONS

Erythroblastosis fetalis, a possibly deadly condition for the fetus, is due to an attack by the mother's immune system against the fetus' erythrocytes. During late pregnancy and at birth, it is possible for fetal blood to enter the mother's circulation. If the mother is Rh negative and the fetus is Rh positive, the mother forms antibodies against the Rh antigen. Initially, the mother produces IgM antibodies that are too large to cross the placental barrier, and there are no consequences for the fetus. Subsequent pregnancies may present complications if the fetuses are also Rh positive because the mother's immune system has switched isotypes; instead of continuing to form IgM, it forms IgG antibodies against the Rh antigen. IgG antibodies are smaller and can cross the placental barrier; they bind to the Rh antigens on the fetal erythrocytes and cause them to undergo hemolysis, killing the fetus. To circumvent this condition, the mother is given anti-Rh agglutinins after the birth of the first Rh-positive infant to mask the antigenic sites on the fetal blood cells and prevent the mother from mounting a full-fledged antigenic response against the Rh antigen.

The morphology of the erythrocyte is intimately related to its function; mutations that cause alterations in the normal shape of RBCs may cause some types of anemia. Alteration in the polypeptide chain of spectrin may reduce its binding capacity to band 4.1 protein, and the spectrin molecules are unable to form a proper support for the erythrocyte plasmalemma, resulting in a condition known as **hereditary spherocytosis**. These RBCs cannot carry enough oxygen, and they are fragile and have the propensity to be destroyed by the spleen, resulting in anemia.

Leukocytes

Leukocytes (WBCs) number only 6500 to 10,000 per mm³ of blood. They have no function within the confines of the circulatory system; they merely use it to reach their destination. When leukocytes arrive at their destination, they leave the capillaries or venules via **diapedesis** (migration between endothelial cells), enter the connective tissue compartment, and perform their function. There are two major categories of leukocytes (Table 10.4):

- **Agranulocytes**, leukocytes that do not possess specific granules
  - Lymphocytes
  - Monocytes
- **Granulocytes**, leukocytes that possess specific granules
  - Neutrophils
  - Eosinophils
  - Basophils

Lymphocytes

Lymphocytes, round cells with an acentric nucleus that occupies most of the cytoplasm, are only slightly larger than erythrocytes and form 20% to 25% of the WBC population (see Table 10.4). Although they are **agranulocytes**, meaning that they do not possess specific granules, they have some azurophilic granules, which on electron micrographs were shown to be lysosomes. There are three types of lymphocytes:

- **B cells** constitute 15% of the lymphocyte population and are responsible for the **humorally mediated immune response**. They enter an unknown region of the bone marrow to become immunologically competent. When antigenically stimulated, they become antibody-producing **plasma cells**.
- **T cells** form 80% of the lymphocyte population and are responsible for the **cell-mediated immune response**. They have to go to the thymic cortex to become immunologically competent.
- **Null cells** compose 5% of the lymphocyte population and are of two types: stem cells and natural killer (NK) cells.
  - Circulating **stem cells** can differentiate to form all blood cells and platelets of the blood.
  - **NK cells** are cytotoxic cells that do not require interaction either with the thymus or with T cells to perform their function.

Chapter 12 discusses the functions of B cells, T cells, and NK cells. Stem cells are discussed in detail later in this chapter.

Monocytes

Monocytes, round cells with a kidney-shaped nucleus, are the largest blood cells in the circulation (see Table 10.4). Electron microscopy shows that these cells are rich in lysosomes and that they have a small Golgi apparatus, usually ensconced in the nuclear indentation. A few days after they are released from the bone marrow into the circulation, they leave the bloodstream, enter the connective tissue compartment, and differentiate into **macrophages**, constituents of the **mononuclear phagocytic system**. Macrophages:

- Preferentially **phagocytose** dead and disrupted cells and invading pathogens, whether they are nonliving antigens or microorganisms
- **Release signaling molecules** that induce inflammatory responses and the proliferation of cells that act in the immune process
- Can fuse with each other to form a very large **foreign body giant cell** that can phagocytose the large substance if the particulate matter is too large for a single macrophage
- Become **antigen-presenting cells** that phagocytose antigens, break them down into smaller antigenic units known as **epitopes**, place them on their membrane bound **major histocompatibility complex antigens II (MHC II**, also known as **class II human leukocyte antigens [class II HLA]**), and present these protein fragments to immunocompetent cells

---

CLINICAL CONSIDERATIONS

Inflammation is the body's response to noxious stimuli, which may include physical or chemical insults or the invasion of the body by pathogens. The initial vascular response is known as **acute inflammation**, and it serves to eliminate the harmful agents and begin the process of healing. If the inflammation is protracted, it is referred to as **chronic inflammation** and entails the recruitment of monocytes, lymphocytes, plasma cells, and fibroblasts, which attempt to ameliorate the conditions causing the inflammation.

Table 10.4 LEUKOCYTES: FEATURES, CATEGORIES, AND FUNCTIONS

Features	GRANULOCYTES			AGRANULOCYTES	
	Neutrophils	Eosinophils	Basophils	Lymphocytes	Monocytes
No./mm^3	3500–7000	150–400	50–100	1500–2500	200–800
% WBCs	60–70	2–4	<1	20–25	3–8
Diameter (μm)					
Section	8–9	9–11	7–8	7–8	10–12
Smear	9–12	10–14	8–10	8–10	12–15
Nucleus	Three to four lobes	Two lobes (sausage-shaped)	S-shaped	Round	Kidney-shaped
Specific granules	0.1 μm, light pink*	1–1.5 μm, dark pink*	0.5 μm, blue-black*	None	None
Contents of specific granules	Type IV collagenase, phospholipase A$_2$, lactoferrin, lysozyme, phagocytin, alkaline phosphatase, vitamin B$_{12}$ binding protein	Aryl sulfatase, histaminase, β-glucuronidase, acid phosphatase, phospholipase, major basic protein, eosinophil cationic protein, neurotoxin, ribonuclease, cathepsin, peroxidase	Histamine, heparin, eosinophil chemotactic factor, neutrophil chemotactic factor, peroxidase, neutral proteases, chondroitin sulfate	None	None
Surface markers	Fc receptors, platelet-activating factor receptor, leukotriene B$_4$ receptor, leukocyte cell adhesion molecule-1	IgE receptors, eosinophil chemotactic factor receptor	IgE receptors	T cells: T cell receptors, CD molecules, IL receptors B cells: surface immunoglobulins	Class II HLA, Fc receptors
Life span	<1 wk	<2 wk	1–2 yr (in mice)	Few months to several years	Few days in blood, several months in connective tissue
Function	Phagocytosis and destruction of bacteria	Phagocytosis of antigen-antibody complex; destruction of parasites	Similar to mast cells to mediate inflammatory responses	T cells: cell-mediated immune response B cells: humorally mediated immune response	Differentiate into macrophage: phagocytosis, presentation of antigens

*Using Romanovsky-type stains (or their modifications).
CD, cluster of differentiation; HLA, human leukocyte antigen; IL, interleukin.
From Gartner LP, Hiatt JL: Color Textbook of Histology, 3rd ed. Philadelphia, Saunders, 2007, p 226.

Neutrophils

Neutrophils (polymorphonuclear leukocytes, polys) form approximately 60% to 70% of the WBC count (see Table 10.4). The nucleus of a young neutrophil has only two or three lobules, but nuclei of older cells become more lobulated, with each lobule connected to the main body nucleus (or to each other) by slim threads of chromatin. Frequently, nuclei of females display a small pouchlike bleb, or "drumstick," housing the **Barr body**—the **second X chromosome** that is believed to be inactive. The cell membrane of neutrophils displays **Fc receptor** and the **complement receptor** for C3b, and **L-selectin** and **integrins** that facilitate adhesion to the endothelial lining in preparation for **diapedesis**. The cytoplasm of neutrophils possesses three types of granules (see Table 10.4):

- **Specific granules**, which are small and house pharmacologic agents the cell uses to destroy microorganisms
- **Azurophilic granules (lysosomes)**, which contain hydrolytic and oxidative enzymes
- **Tertiary granules**, which house gelatinase, cathepsins, and certain glycoproteins

Chemotactic agents released by certain cells, such as mast cells, attract neutrophils to sites of acute inflammation, where they attack invading bacterial pathogens. To recognize the exit site from the blood vessel, endothelial cells, in response to **interleukin (IL)-1** and **tumor necrosis factor (TNF)** produced by connective tissue cells, display **intercellular adhesion molecules 1 and 2 (ICAM-1 and ICAM-2)**, to which the neutrophil integrins bind, stopping their travel in the bloodstream, and leave the blood vessel. To be able to enter the connective tissue and phagocytose the pathogenic bacteria:

- Tertiary granules release the enzyme **gelatinase**, which digests the basal lamina to ease diapedesis.
- Neutrophils release enzymes from their **specific granules** to kill bacteria that invaded the connective tissue.
- Neutrophils **phagocytose** bacteria using their membrane bound Fc and C3b receptors (Fig. 10.3A and B).
- **Azurophilic granules** release their enzymes into the bacteria-laden phagosomes (Fig. 10.3C).
- **Specific granules** release their enzymes into the bacteria-laden phagosomes that not only degrade

bacteria enzymatically, but also kill them by the formation of **superoxides** as reduced nicotinamide adenine dinucleotide phosphate (NADPH) oxidase acts on O_2, initiating a **respiratory burst** that includes the formation of **hypochlorous acid** and **hydrogen peroxide** (Fig. 10.3D).

Neutrophils die after they kill the invading pathogens and, with the dead bacteria and extracellular fluid, form **pus**.

Eosinophils

Eosinophils, composing 2% to 4% of the WBC population, are large round cells with a **bilobed nucleus**. Their cytoplasm is packed with large, eosinophilic **specific granules** and azurophilic granules that resemble the lysosomes of neutrophils (see Table 10.4). Their cell membrane displays IgG, IgE, and complement receptors, and receptors for eosinophil chemotactic factor, histamine, and leukotrienes. Eosinophils function in destroying parasites and phagocytosing and degrading antigen-antibody complexes. The specific granules of eosinophils have two regions:

- **Externum** houses various hydrolytic enzymes and cathepsins, peroxidase, and histaminase, which limits the inflammatory response (see Table 10.4).
- **Internum** houses **major basic protein (MBP)**, **eosinophil cationic protein (ECP)**, and eosinophil-derived neurotoxin. MBP and ECP form pores in the pellicles of parasites to permit hydrogen peroxide and superoxides formed by eosinophilic enzymes to reach and kill the parasites.

Basophils

Basophils form only 1% of the population of WBCs (see Table 10.4). Their cell membrane sports high-affinity receptors for IgE; they have an S-shaped nucleus, and their cytoplasm is packed with dark **specific granules** whose contents include histamine, heparin, eosinophil chemotactic factor, neutrophil chemotactic factor, peroxidase, neutral proteases, and chondroitin sulfate. Basophils also have **azurophilic granules** similar to those of eosinophils.

Although basophils probably are not related to mast cells, they have very similar functions because they both initiate **inflammatory responses**. Mast cell function is discussed in detail in Chapter 6.

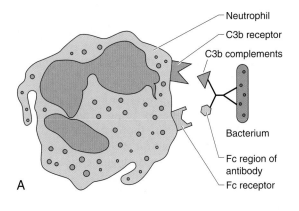

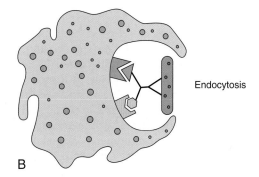

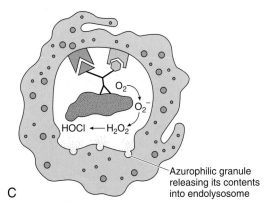

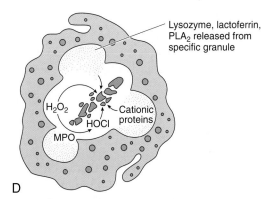

Figure 10.3 A–D, Process of bacterial phagocytosis using C3b and Fc receptors and their destruction by neutrophils. H_2O_2, hydrogen peroxide; HOCl, hypochlorous acid; MPO, myeloperoxidase; O_2^-, superoxide; PLA_2, phospholipase A_2. *(From Gartner LP, Hiatt JL: Color Textbook of Histology, 3rd ed. Philadelphia, Saunders, 2007, p 228.)*

CLINICAL CONSIDERATIONS

Mutations in the genes coding for ligands binding to selectins prevent leukocytes, such as neutrophils, from becoming marginated and from slowing down as they contact the luminal surfaces of endothelial cells. Normally, these ligands contact selectins displayed on the surface of endothelial cells; because these contacts are reversible, the leukocytes do not stop but merely slow down. This condition is known as **leukocyte adhesion deficiency I**. Macrophages in the connective tissue release IL-1 and TNF-α, which cause endothelial cells in the region of inflammation to express **ICAM-1** and **ICAM-2**. Two of the leukocyte integrins, **leukocyte function-associated antigen 1 (LFA-1)** and **macrophage-1 (Mac-1)**, adhere to ICAM-1 and ICAM-2, and the leukocytes come to a halt. **IL-8**, produced by inflammatory cells in the connective tissue, prompts the leukocytes to commit to diapedesis and leave the blood vessel to enter the connective tissue compartment. Individuals who present with mutations in the genes coding for the integrin molecules of the leukocytes have the condition known as **leukocyte adhesion deficiency I**, and some of their leukocytes cannot participate in the inflammatory response.

Mutations involving the gene that codes for the enzyme **NADPH oxidase** affect the ability of certain cells, such as neutrophils, to undergo respiratory burst response to pathogenic bacterial invasion of the connective tissue compartment. Although the neutrophils reach the area of infection and phagocytose the bacteria, they cannot destroy them quickly and efficiently enough to reduce their numbers to safe levels. Patients with this condition are mostly children, and they are said to have **hereditary deficiency of NADPH oxidase** and present with frequent bacterial infections.

Platelets

Platelets, cell fragments 2 to 4 μm in diameter (Fig. 10.4; see Table 10.4), are derived from megakaryocytes of the bone marrow and participate in the coagulation of blood and in the protection of damaged blood vessels. Platelets stay in the circulating blood for approximately 2 weeks and are then destroyed. Each platelet is discoid in shape and possesses a lighter periphery, the **hyalomere**, and a darker central region, the **granulomere**. Viewed with the electron microscope, platelets present a ring of 10 to 15 parallel microtubules, flanked by monomers of actin and myosin that encircle the platelet's perimeter. Two hyalomeres present two systems of cytoplasmic channels (Fig. 10.4):

- One that opens to the surface, a **surface opening tubular system**, that is an extension of the outer surface of the platelet, enhancing the surface area by a factor of 7 or 8
- One that does not open to the surface, the **dense tubular system**

The granulomere viewed with the electron microscope presents peroxisomes, mitochondria, glycogen granules, enzyme systems that facilitate platelet metabolism and adenosine triphosphate (ATP) production, and three types of granules whose contents are detailed in Table 10.5:

- **Alpha granules**
- **Delta granules**
- **Gamma granules (lysosomes)**

The function of platelets is to quench blood loss from damaged vessels by forming a clot to plug the defect in the vessel wall. When the endothelial lining is violated and platelets contact collagen, they become activated and attach to the damaged area, a process known as **platelet adhesion**, and to each other, known as **platelet aggregation**. The process of clot formation depends on the interaction of various factors derived from the plasma, platelets, and damaged tissue. An undamaged endothelial lining releases **nitric oxide** and **prostacyclins** to prevent platelet aggregation and **heparin-like molecule** and **thrombomodulin** to prevent coagulation. The process of blood clotting involves a sequence of factors that act in a cascade where the formation or activation of one factor induces the formation or activation of another factor. The entire complex sequence of these events is not presented in this textbook, but is well described in many textbooks of pathology. The principal steps in blood clotting are as follows:

- Damaged endothelium ceases to produce factors that prevent platelet aggregation and coagulation and releases **tissue thromboplastin**, **von Willebrand factor**, and the vasoconstrictor and endothelial cell mitosis stimulator **endothelin**.
- **Platelets** become **activated** because von Willebrand factor induces them to **adhere** to the **collagen** and **laminin** protruding into the lumen from the injured vessel wall, adhere to other platelets, and release the contents of their granules.
- **Adenosine diphosphate (ADP)** and **thromboplastin** released by the platelets increase their propensity to adhere to each other and cause the newly adhered platelets to degranulate.
- Plasmalemma of activated platelets produces arachidonic acid–derived **thromboxane A_2**, which constricts blood vessels and activates platelets.
- Platelets aggregate and acquire **platelet factor 3** on their plasma membrane, facilitating the precipitation of **coagulation factors**.
- In the presence of coagulation factors, **prothrombin** is converted to **thrombin**, a reaction catalyzed by thromboplastin derived from platelets and the damaged tissue.
- Thrombin converts **fibrinogen** to **fibrin**, a calcium requiring reaction.
- Fibrin monomers are cross-linked by **factor XIII** to form a **reticulum of clot** that, as it traps more blood cells and platelets, is transformed into a **thrombus (blood clot)**.
- Within 1 hour, **actin** and **myosin** monomers released by platelets coalesce to form **myofilaments** whose contraction reduces the size of the clot and pulls the cut edges of the vessel closer to each other, reducing leakage of blood from the damaged vessel further.
- When the endothelial lining is restored to normal, **plasminogen activator** converts **plasminogen** to **plasmin**, a protease that, in concert with **hydrolytic enzymes** derived from platelet **lambda granules**, dissolves the fibrin clot.

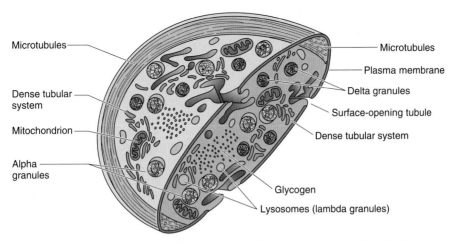

Figure 10.4 Anatomy of a platelet. *(From Gartner LP, Hiatt JL: Color Textbook of Histology, 3rd ed. Philadelphia, Saunders, 2007, p 233.)*

Table 10.5 PLATELET TUBULES AND GRANULES

Structure (Size)	Location	Contents	Function
Surface-opening tubule system	Hyalomere		Expedites rapid uptake and release of molecules from activated platelets
Dense tubular system	Hyalomere		Probably sequesters calcium ions to prevent platelet "stickiness"
Alpha granules (300–500 nm)	Granulomere	Fibrinogen, platelet-derived growth factor, platelet thromboplastin, thrombospondin, coagulation factors	Contained factors facilitate vessel repair, platelet aggregation, and coagulation of blood
Delta granules (dense bodies) (250–300 nm)	Granulomere	Calcium, ADP, ATP, serotonin, histamine, pyrophosphatase	Contained factors facilitate platelet aggregation and adhesion and vasoconstriction
Gamma granules (lysosomes) (200–250 nm)	Granulomere	Hydrolytic enzymes	Contained enzymes aid clot resorption

From Gartner LP, Hiatt JL: Color Textbook of Histology, 3rd ed. Philadelphia, Saunders, 2007, p 236.

CLINICAL CONSIDERATIONS

Vitamin K, a cofactor in the production of prothrombin and certain clotting factors, is frequently present at insufficient levels in newborns, and they are usually administered an injection of this vitamin to prevent them from dying of **hemorrhagic disease of the newborn**. Infants who are breastfed and have not been injected with vitamin K are particularly at risk for lacking sufficient levels of this vitamin. Adults who have conditions that impede fat absorption may also be subject to vitamin K deficiency, which manifests as excessive bleeding and frequent bruising. The administration of supplemental vitamin K usually alleviates the disorder.

Bone Marrow

Bone marrow (see Fig. 10.5), a gelatinous, extensively vascular, cell-rich connective tissue, occupies the marrow cavities of long bones and the intertrabecular spaces of spongy bones and provides a microenvironment that is conducive for **hematopoiesis**, formation of blood cells and platelets. In infants and young individuals, all marrow is hematopoietically active, and because most of the forming cells are erythrocytes, it is known as **red marrow**. As an individual approaches 20 years of age, much of the marrow housed in the diaphysis of long bones accumulates so much fat that it becomes hematopoietically inactive and is known as **yellow marrow**. The marrow's vascular supply arises from:

- **Arteries** that enter the marrow cavity via **nutrient canals**
- A system of large **sinusoids** that eventually deliver their blood into the **central longitudinal vein**, which delivers its blood into many **veins** that exit the marrow through nutrient canals.

In contrast to most veins, the veins of the marrow are smaller than their arterial counterparts, and hydrostatic pressure within the marrow is high enough to maintain the patency of the sinusoids. The marrow's vascular compartment comprises the blood vessels and sinusoids, and the interstices are populated by clusters of hematopoietic cells (**islands of hematopoietic cells**), constituting the **hematopoietic compartment**. The adluminal surfaces of the endothelial cells of the sinusoids are surrounded by a:

- **Basal lamina**
- Fine mesh of reticular fibers
- **Adventitial reticular cells** that contact the basal lamina, covering most of the sinusoidal surfaces

Cytoplasmic extensions of these adventitial reticular cells extend away from the sinusoids and establish contacts with cytoplasmic extensions of other adventitial reticular cells enclosing spaces that house **hematopoietic islands (hematopoietic cords)**. These clusters of hematopoietic cells are present in various stages of their development but most commonly are composed only of one specific cell lineage. In addition to the various maturing cells, **macrophages** are also present to destroy extruded nuclei, phagocytose discarded cytoplasm, and provide iron to cells of the erythrocytic series. Adventitial reticular cells control how much of the bone marrow volume is available for hematopoiesis; as they amass lipid in their cytoplasm, they increase in size and decrease the volume of the hematopoietic compartment.

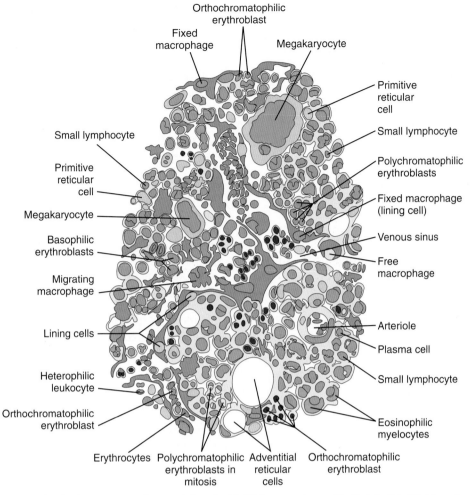

Figure 10.5 Diagram of rabbit bone marrow that was injected with lithium carmine and India ink. *(Modified from Fawcett DW: Bloom and Fawcett A Textbook of Histology, 12th ed. New York, Chapman & Hall, 1994, p 238.)*

HEMATOPOIESIS

Hematopoiesis has a prenatal and a postnatal component. **Prenatal hematopoiesis** begins around the 14th day of development and has four phases:

- The **mesoblastic phase** is initiated when **blood islands** form in the yolk sac; cells at the border of the blood island become endothelial cells, forming blood vessels, whereas most of the cells differentiate into **erythroblasts** that form nucleated **RBCs**.
- The **hepatic phase** replaces the mesoblastic phase at the end of the fifth week after fertilization; RBCs are still nucleated, and **leukocytes** begin to be formed at the eighth week after fertilization.
- The **splenic phase** begins during the fourth month of development, and the spleen and liver continue their hematopoietic function until parturition.
- The **myeloid phase** (**bone marrow phase**) starts around the sixth month of development and increases in importance as the fetus reaches

parturition; after birth, all hematopoiesis occurs in the bone marrow, although the liver and the spleen can resume hematopoiesis if necessary.

Postnatal hematopoiesis begins at birth and continues throughout the individual's life and produces an inordinate number of cells. An individual's bone marrow manufactures and replaces 1 billion blood cells every day through the process of hematopoiesis. **Stem cells**, the least differentiated of the hematopoietic cells, undergo cell division to form more differentiated cells, known as **progenitor cells**, which also proliferate to form **precursor cells** (Table 10.6). Stem cells and progenitor cells do not have histologic characteristics that differentiate them from one another. Precursor cells can be identified as belonging to a specific cell line, however, and each cell is identified by a specific name. Some precursor cells are able to proliferate, whereas others are postmitotic cells even though they continue to mature to become a circulating blood cell. The process of hematopoiesis is closely monitored and controlled by **cytokines** and **growth factors**.

Table 10.6 CELLS OF HEMOPOIESIS

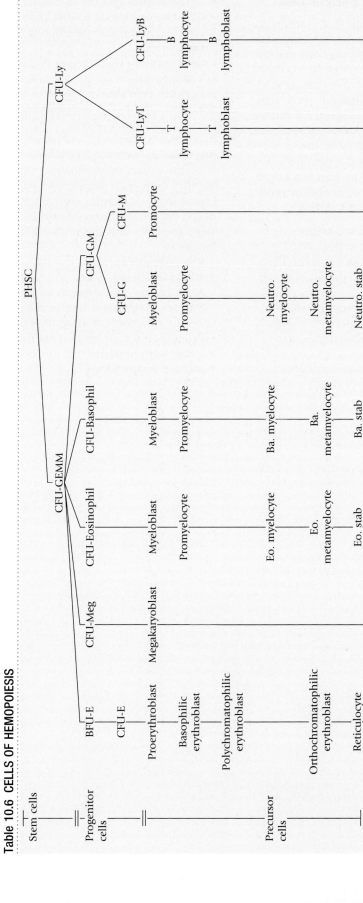

Ba., basophil; BFU, burst-forming unit (E, erythrocyte); CFU, colony-forming unit (E, erythrocyte); Eo., eosinophil; G, granulocyte; GEMM, granulocyte, erythrocyte, monocyte, mega-karyocyte; GM, granulocyte-monocyte; Ly, lymphocyte; LyB, B cell; LyT, T cell; M, monocyte; Meg, megakaryoblast; Neutro., neutrophil; PHSC, pluripotential hemopoietic stem cell. Modified from Gartner LP, Hiatt JL, Strum J: Histology. Baltimore, Williams & Wilkins, 1988.

Stem Cells, Progenitor Cells, and Precursor Cells

The antecedents of all blood cells and platelets are **stem cells**, known as **pluripotential hematopoietic stem cells (PHSCs)**, that reside in the bone marrow, forming approximately 0.1% of the entire nucleated cells of the marrow, and resemble lymphocytes. Although PHSCs seldom enter the cell cycle, occasionally they experience sudden spurts of mitotic activity, forming more PHSCs. Although stem cells are morphologically indistinguishable, they possess differing cell membrane markers that permit them to be recognized. PHSCs differentiate into two categories of stem cells (see Table 10.6) known as **multipotential hematopoietic stem cells (MHSCs)**:

- Colony-forming unit–granulocyte, erythrocyte, monocyte, and megakaryocyte cells (CFU-GEMMs) are responsible for the formation of progenitor cells that give rise to the myeloid cell lines.
  - **BFU-E (burst-forming unit–erythrocytes)** gives rise to **CFU-E** and then to erythrocytes.
  - **CFU-Meg** give rise to **megakaryocytes** that form platelets.
  - **CFU-Eosinophil** give rise to eosinophils.

- **CFU-Basophil** give rise to basophils.
- **CFU-GM** give rise to **CFU-G** and **CFU-M**, cells that give rise to neutrophils and monocytes.
- **Colony-forming unit–lymphocyte cells (CFU-Ly)** are responsible for the formation of **progenitor cells** that give rise to the lymphoid cells lines, CFU-LyT (T lymphocytes) and CFU-LyB (B lymphocytes).
- In contrast to stem cells and progenitor cells, **precursor cells** cannot regenerate themselves (i.e., they cannot produce more precursor cells), but they do possess definite histologic features permitting their identification as the predecessor of specific circulating blood cells (Fig. 10.6, see Table 10.6). The first precursor cell of each cell lineage is:
  - **Proerythroblasts**, which give rise to erythrocytes
  - **Megakaryoblasts**, which give rise to platelets
  - **Myeloblasts**—an exception to the rule because they are recognizable only as the precursors of neutrophils, eosinophils, or basophils
  - **Promonocytes**, which give rise to monocytes
  - **Naïve T lymphocytes**
  - **Naïve B lymphocytes**

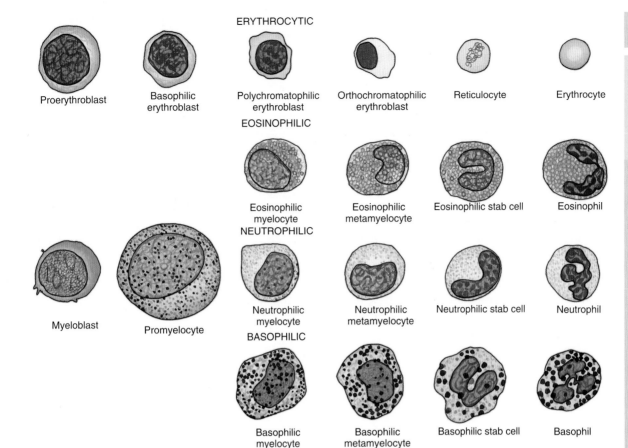

ERYTHROCYTIC

Proerythroblast | Basophilic erythroblast | Polychromatophilic erythroblast | Orthochromatophilic erythroblast | Reticulocyte | Erythrocyte

EOSINOPHILIC

Eosinophilic myelocyte | Eosinophilic metamyelocyte | Eosinophilic stab cell | Eosinophil

NEUTROPHILIC

Myeloblast | Promyelocyte | Neutrophilic myelocyte | Neutrophilic metamyelocyte | Neutrophilic stab cell | Neutrophil

BASOPHILIC

Basophilic myelocyte | Basophilic metamyelocyte | Basophilic stab cell | Basophil

Figure 10.6 Precursor cells of the erythrocytic and granulocytic series. *(From Gartner LP, Hiatt JL: Color Textbook of Histology, 3rd ed. Philadelphia, Saunders, 2007, p 240.)*

CLINICAL CONSIDERATIONS

Myelofibrosis is a condition in which fibroblasts of the bone marrow manufacture an abundance of fibrous connective tissue, instead of producing just slender collagen fibers to support the blood vessels, sinusoids, and blood islands of bone marrow. As more and more fibrous tissue is formed, the marrow becomes heavily inundated with this fibrous material, and the volume formerly available for hematopoiesis is reduced to such an extent that erythrocyte formation is reduced, and the patient becomes anemic. WBC formation may decrease or increase, whereas platelet formation decreases. This rare disorder, affecting 1 out of 50,000 people in the United States, is usually limited to individuals 50 to 70 years old.

Frequently, this disease has no known cause (idiopathic myelofibrosis), or it may accompany other bone marrow disorders or bone marrow infections. Many patients with this disease have been exposed to ionizing radiation or benzene. In

its early stages, myelofibrosis is asymptomatic and remains so until the patient becomes so anemic that he or she experiences a decline in energy levels, loses weight, and has weakness and general malaise. If the leukocyte and platelet counts are also depressed, the individual becomes susceptible to infection, petechiae, and hematomas. Because the bone marrow is incapable of sustaining normal hematopoiesis, the spleen and liver begin to assume the function of blood cell formation, and they both increase in size, causing abdominal pain. The only way to confirm that the patient has myelofibrosis is by obtaining a bone marrow biopsy specimen. Patients with this disorder may live for 10 years or more, but in certain cases the disease progresses rapidly (acute or malignant myelofibrosis). There is no cure for this condition, although bone marrow transplants have been successful in ameliorating the disease.

Hematopoietic Growth Factors
(Colony-Stimulating Factors)

Certain cells of the body produce numerous **gly-coproteins** that stimulate hematopoiesis. These **hematopoietic growth factors (colony-stimulating factors)** reach their target cells as endocrine hormones, paracrine hormones, or via cell-to-cell contact. Each of these factors stimulates a specific stem cell, progenitor cell, or precursor cell to proliferate or differentiate or both so that the level of a particular blood cell attains its normal concentration in the circulating blood (Table 10.7):

- **Steel factor (stem cell factor)**, **granulocyte-monocyte colony-stimulating factor**, **IL-3**, and **IL-7** induce PHSC, CFU-GEMM, and CFU-Ly to undergo mitosis to maintain their population density
- **Granulocyte colony-stimulating factor**, **monocyte colony-stimulating factor**, **IL-2**, **IL-5**, **IL-6**, **IL-11**, **IL-12**, **macrophage inhibitory protein-α**, and **erythropoietin** induce PHSC, CFU-GEMM, and CFU-Ly to give rise to progenitor cells (see Table 10.7).

Additionally, **colony-stimulating factors** induce unipotential precursor cells to form neutrophils, eosinophils, basophils, and monocytes; **erythropoietin** induces the formation of erythrocytes; and **thrombopoietin** induces the formation of platelets.

Steel factor, produced by stromal cells of the bone marrow, is expressed on the plasma membrane of these cells. For PHSC, CFU-GEMM, and CFU-Ly cells to become activated, they must contact the steel factor in the stromal cell plasmalemma. Hematopoiesis can occur only in areas where stromal cells express steel factor on their membranes. If hematopoietic cells are not contacted by hematopoietic growth factors, they enter into apoptosis, die, and are eliminated by macrophages.

Table 10.7 HEMATOPOIETIC GROWTH FACTORS

Factors	Principal Action	Site of Origin
Stem cell factor	Promotes hematopoiesis	Stromal cells of bone marrow
GM-CSF	Promotes CFU-GM mitosis and differentiation; facilitates granulocyte activity	T cells; endothelial cells
G-CSF	Promotes CFU-G mitosis and differentiation; facilitates neutrophil activity	Macrophages; endothelial cells
M-CSF	Promotes CFU-M mitosis and differentiation	Macrophages; endothelial cells
IL-1	In conjunction with IL-3 and IL-6, it promotes proliferation of PHSC, CFU-GEMM, and CFU-Ly; suppresses erythroid precursors	Monocytes; macrophages, endothelial cells
IL-2	Stimulates activated T cell and B cell mitosis; induces differentiation of NK cells	Activated T cells
IL-3	In conjunction with IL-1 and IL-6, it promotes proliferation of PHSC, CFU-GEMM, and CFU-Ly and all unipotential precursors (except for LyB and LyT)	Activated T cells and B cells
IL-4	Stimulates T cell and B cell activation and development of mast cells and basophils	Activated T cells
IL-5	Promotes CFU-Eo mitosis and activates eosinophils	T cells
IL-6	In conjunction with IL-1 and IL-3, promotes proliferation of PHSC, CFU-GEMM, and CFU-Ly; also facilitates CTL and B cell differentiation	Monocytes and fibroblasts
IL-7	Promotes differentiation of CFU-Ly; enhances differentiation of NK cells	Stromal cells
IL-8	Induces neutrophil migration and degranulation	Leukocytes, endothelial cells, and smooth muscle cells
IL-9	Induces mast cell activation and proliferation; modulates IgE production; promotes T helper cell proliferation	T helper cells
IL-10	Inhibits cytokine production by macrophages, T cells, and NK cells; facilitates CTL differentiation and proliferation of B cells and mast cells	Macrophages and T cells
IL-12	Stimulates NK cells; enhances CTL and NK cell function	Macrophages
γ-Interferons	Activate B cells and monocytes; enhance CTL differentiation; augment the expression of class II HLA	T cells and NK cells
Erythropoietin	CFU-E differentiation; BFU-E mitosis	Endothelial cells of peritubular capillary network of kidney; hepatocytes
Thrombopoietin	Proliferation and differentiation of CFU-Meg and megakaryoblasts	Unknown

BFU, burst-forming unit (E, erythrocyte); CTL, cytotoxic T cell; CFU, colony-forming unit (Eo, eosinophil; G, granulocyte; GEMM, granulocyte, erythrocyte, monocyte, megakaryocyte; GM, granulocyte-monocyte; Ly, lymphocyte; S, spleen); CSF, colony-stimulating factor (G, granulocyte; GM, granulocyte-monocyte; M, monocyte); IL, interleukin; NK, natural killer; PHSC, pluri-potential hematopoietic stem cell.

From Gartner LP, Hiatt JL: Color Textbook of Histology, 3rd ed. Philadelphia, Saunders, 2007, p 242.

Erythropoiesis, Granulocytopoiesis, Monocytopoiesis, and Lymphopoiesis

The formation of erythrocytes, **erythropoiesis**, requires two forms of progenitor cells to produce 2.5 × 10^{11} RBCs on a daily basis. If the number of RBCs in blood is less than the normal amount, endothelial cells of the kidney's peritubular capillary network and hepatocytes of the liver release erythropoietin. This factor, in concert with steel factor, IL-3, IL-9, and granulocyte-macrophage colony-stimulating factor, stimulates CFU-GEMM to differentiate into numerous BFU-E, which proliferate to form even more CFU-E cells. When these cells are formed, the kidney and liver cells cease the production of erythropoietin, and the low level of this factor induces the CFU-E to form **proerythroblasts**. The cells of the erythroblastic series and their properties are presented in Table 10.8.

The formation of granulocytes, **granulocytopoiesis**, depends on CFU-GM, which gives rise to two other progenitor cells: CFU-M, responsible for the monocyte formation, and CFU-G, responsible for neutrophil formation. Eosinophils and basophils arise from CFU-Eo and CFU-Ba. The factors IL-1, IL-6, and TNF-α induce the release of the growth factors granulocyte colony-stimulating factor, granulocyte-monocyte colony-stimulating factor, and IL-5, which function in stimulating the formation of neutrophils, eosinophils, and basophils. The first morphologically recognizable cell of the granulocytic precursors is the **myeloblast**, and the second is the **promyelocyte**. Neither myeloblasts nor promyelocytes possess specific granules, however, and all three granulocytes share these precursors. The next cell in the lineage has specific granules and can be recognized as a **neutrophilic**, **eosinophilic**, or **basophilic myelocyte**. The cells of the neutrophilic series are presented in Table 10.9.

The progenitor cell of **monocytopoiesis** is the bipotential **CFU-GM**, which gives rise to the unipotential **CFU-M**, from which promonocytes are derived. These give rise to monocytes that enter the circulation.

Platelets are derived from **CFU-Meg**, which give rise to **megakaryoblasts** that enlarge by undergoing **endomitosis**, where the cell undergoes mitosis without **cytokinesis** and gives rise to very large cells, known as **megakaryocytes**. These large cells lie next to sinusoids and extend their cytoplasm into the sinusoidal lumen. The cytoplasmic projections undergo fragmentation along demarcation channels and release proplatelets into the sinusoids. The proplatelets disperse into individual platelets and enter the circulation.

Lymphopoiesis begins with the stem cell **CFU-Ly**, which gives rise to the progenitor cells CFU-LyT and CFU-LyB. These cells give rise to naïve T cells (CFU-LyT) and naïve B cells (CFU-LyB).

Table 10.8 CELLS OF THE ERYTHROPOIETIC SERIES

Cell	Size (µm)	Nucleus* and Mitosis	Nucleoli	Cytoplasm*	Electron Micrographs
Proerythroblast	14–19	Round, burgundy-red; chromatin network is fine; mitosis	3–5	Gray-blue, peripheral clumping	Scant RER; many polysomes, few mitochondria; ferritin
Basophilic erythroblast	12–17	Same as above, but chromatin network is coarser; mitosis	1–2?	Similar to above but slight pinkish background	Similar to above; some hemoglobin is present
Polychromatophilic erythroblast	12–15	Round and densely staining; very coarse chromatin network; mitosis	None	Yellowish pink in bluish background	Similar to above but more hemoglobin is present
Orthochromatophilic erythroblast	8–12	Small, round, dense; eccentric or is being extruded; no mitosis	None	Pink in a slight bluish background	Few mitochondria and polysomes; much hemoglobin
Reticulocyte	7–8	None	None	Similar to mature RBC, but stained with cresyl blue; display bluish reticulum	Clusters of ribosomes; cell is filled with hemoglobin
Erythrocyte	7.5	None	None	Pink cytoplasm	Only hemoglobin

*Colors as appear using Romanovsky-type stains.
RER, rough endoplasmic reticulum.
From Gartner LP, Hiatt JL: Color Textbook of Histology, 3rd ed. Philadelphia, Saunders, 2007, p 246.

Table 10.9 CELLS OF THE NEUTROPHILIC SERIES

Cell	Size (μm)	Nucleus* and Mitosis	Nucleoli	Cytoplasm*	Granules	Electron Micrographs
Myeloblast	12–14	Round, reddish blue; chromatin network is fine; mitosis	2–3	Blue clumps in pale blue setting; cytoplasmic blebs at cell periphery	None	RER, small Golgi, many mitochondria and polysomes
Promyelocyte	16–24	Round to oval, reddish blue; chromatin network is coarse; mitosis	1–2	Bluish cytoplasm; no cytoplasmic blebs at cell periphery	Azurophilic granules	RER, large Golgi, many mitochondria, numerous lysosomes
Neutrophilic myelocyte	10–12	Flattened, acentric; chromatin network is coarse; mitosis	0–1	Pale blue cytoplasm	Azurophilic and specific granules	RER, large Golgi, numerous mitochondria, lysosomes, and specific granules
Neutrophilic metamyelocyte	10–12	Kidney-shaped, dense; chromatin network is coarse; no mitosis	None	Pale blue cytoplasm	Azurophilic and specific granules	Organelle population is reduced, but granules are as above
Neutrophilic band (stab; juvenile)	9–12	Horseshoe-shaped; chromatin network is very coarse; no mitosis	None	Pale blue cytoplasm	Azurophilic and specific granules	Same as above
Neutrophil	9–12	Multilobed; chromatin network is very coarse; no mitosis	None	Pale bluish pink	Azurophilic and specific granules	Same as above

*Colors as appear using Romanovsky-type stains (or their modifications).
RER, rough endoplasmic reticulum.
From Gartner LP, Hiatt JL: Color Textbook of Histology, 3rd ed. Philadelphia, Saunders, 2007, p 248.

11 CIRCULATORY SYSTEM

Cardiovascular System

The cardiovascular system is composed of a four-chambered heart divided into right and left atrial (receiving) chambers and right and left ventricular (discharging) chambers. The right side of the heart, containing the right atrium and right ventricle, comprises the pulmonary circuit delivering blood to the lungs for oxygenation and release of carbon dioxide. The oxygenated blood is returned to the left side (systemic circuit) of the heart and is pumped out of the left ventricle to be distributed to the tissues of the body.

The vessels constituting the cardiovascular system are:

KEY WORDS
• **Vessel tunics**
• **Arteries**
• **Arterioles**
• **Regulation of blood pressure**
• **Capillaries**
• **Veins**
• **Heart**
• **Lymph vessels**

- **Arteries** that originate at the heart and convey blood away from the heart; as these vessels arborize, their branches diminish in size the farther they are from the heart.
- **Veins** whose vessels return blood to the heart; the smallest vessels are farthest from the heart, and the largest vessels are closest to the heart.
- **Capillaries**, the smallest vessels with the thinnest walls, are interposed between the arterial and venous systems; they function in permitting the exchange of materials between cells and the bloodstream. Capillaries receive blood from the smallest arteries, the **arterioles** (and **metarterioles**), and deliver blood to the smallest veins, the **venules**.

BLOOD VESSEL TUNICS

The wall of arteries and veins is composed of three layers: **tunica intima**, **tunica media**, and **tunica adventitia** (Fig. 11.1).

- The innermost layer of the tunics, the **tunica intima**, is composed of a simple squamous epithelium and **endothelium** that lines the lumen of the vessel.

- Interposed between the endothelium and the **subendothelial connective tissue** is the **basement membrane**.
- In muscular arteries, the subendothelial connective tissue houses a few **smooth muscle cells**.
- The subendothelial connective tissue is surrounded by the **internal elastic lamina**, a perforated elastic membrane composed mostly of **elastin**.
- In cross sections of small vessels, such as a capillaries, one or two endothelial cells are able to encircle the lumen, whereas in large vessels, dozens of endothelial cells may be required to do the same.

- Endothelial cells provide a smooth, friction-free surface and secrete many substances, such as lamin; endothelin; types II, IV, and V collagen; nitric oxide (NO); and von Willebrand factor (vWF).
- On their luminal aspect, endothelial cell membranes sport angiotensin-converting enzyme and other enzymes that incapacitate numerous blood-borne agents, such as bradykinin, thrombin, prostaglandin, and serotonin.
- Lipoprotein lipase binds to the luminal aspect of endothelial cell membranes and cleaves lipoproteins.
- The thickest of the three coats, especially in arteries, is the **tunica media**, composed of multiple layers of smooth muscle cells, arranged in a helical configuration. The extracellular matrix of the tunica media contains elastic fibers formed by smooth muscle cells, types I and III collagen fibers, and ground substance. The outermost layer of the media, at least in large muscular arteries, houses slender elastic fibers composing the **external elastic lamina**. Instead of a tunica media, capillaries possess contractile cells known as **pericytes**.

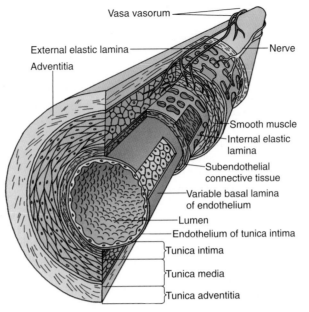

Vasa vasorum

External elastic lamina

Adventitia

Nerve

Smooth muscle

Internal elastic lamina

Subendothelial connective tissue

Variable basal lamina of endothelium

Lumen

Endothelium of tunica intima

Tunica intima

Tunica media

Tunica adventitia

Figure 11.1 A typical artery. *(From Gartner LP, Hiatt JL: Color Textbook of Histology, 3rd ed. Philadelphia, Saunders, 2007, p 252.)*

CLINICAL CONSIDERATIONS

A specific protein, **von Willebrand factor (vWF)**, which is a clotting factor, is produced by all endothelial cells; however, it is stored only within Weibel-Palade bodies of arteries. vWF facilitates the coagulation of blood as it attaches to platelets during the clotting process. von Willebrand's disease is an inherited bleeding disorder affecting clotting of the blood. It is usually caused by deficient or defective vWF.

An **aneurysm** is a ballooning out of the wall of an artery (or infrequently a vein) as a result of a weakness in the vessel wall. Aneurysms are usually related to aging as in atherosclerosis, or they may result from other conditions, such as Marfan syndrome, Ehlers-Danlos syndrome, or syphilis. Although aneurysms may occur in many arteries, the abdominal aorta is the most frequent site. If diagnosed in time, aneurysms may be repaired, but if an aneurysm is not discovered and it ruptures, a massive loss of blood occurs leading to death of the patient.

BLOOD VESSEL TUNICS (cont.)

- The outermost coat, the **tunica adventitia**, is a fibroelastic connective tissue that affixes blood vessels to the surrounding structures (Fig. 11.2).
  - In large blood vessels, the nutrients and oxygen present in the bloodstream are unable to percolate throughout the wall of the vessel; **vasa vasorum**, small arteries, enter the tunica adventitia, ramify throughout the wall of the vessel, and provide nutrients and oxygen for the cells located in the adventitia and the media. Vasa vasorum are more prominent in veins than in arteries.
  - The **nerve supply** of blood vessels also enters the tunica adventitia; the vasomotor nerves release the neurotransmitter **norepinephrine**, which diffuses to the smooth muscle cells of the tunica media. These are sympathetic vasomotor fibers that cause the smooth muscle cells to contract, and the wave of contraction is spread via gap junctions between neighboring smooth muscle cells, eliciting vasoconstriction.

ARTERIES

Arteries (Table 11.1) are large muscular blood vessels that gradually decrease in diameter as they carry blood away from the heart and deliver it into capillary beds. Although the definitions are not clear cut, there are three categories of arteries determined by their diameter, wall thickness, and other histologic features:

- Elastic (conducting) arteries are the largest.
- Arterioles are the smallest.
- Muscular (distributing) arteries range in size between the other two types.

Specialized Arterial Sensory Structures

Muscular arteries house specialized sensory organs, the **carotid sinus** and the **carotid body**, and the arch of the aorta houses a similar sensory structure, the **aortic body**.

- The **carotid sinus**, situated in the tunica adventitia of the internal carotid artery, is innervated by cranial nerve IX (glossopharyngeal

nerve), and because it monitors blood pressure, it acts as a **baroreceptor**. Information from the carotid sinus enters the vasomotor center where a response is formulated to preserve normal blood pressure.

- The **carotid body**, a small chemoreceptor organ well supplied with capillary beds, is situated at the bifurcation of the common carotid artery and is supplied by cranial nerves IX and X (glossopharyngeal and vagus nerves). It responds to changes in blood levels of CO_2, O_2, and H^+. Electron microscopic examination displays two types of cells that compose the carotid body:
  - The cytoplasm of **glomus cells (type I cells)** houses granules containing catecholamines and possesses cell processes that contact capillary endothelial cells and neighboring glomus cells.
  - Processes of **sheath cells (type II cells)** envelop the glomus cell processes and replace the Schwann cell sheath of naked nerve fibers that penetrate the glomus cell groups.
- The **aortic bodies**, present in the arch of the aorta, resemble the carotid bodies in morphology and function.

Regulation of Arterial Blood Pressure

Blood pressure is controlled by the **neural pathway** and by **biochemical pathways**.

- The **vasomotor center** of the brain, by controlling the neural pathway, is responsible for maintaining the proper blood pressure of 90–119/60–79 mm Hg, and it does so by causing the smooth muscle cells of the tunica media of blood vessels to be under a constant tonus.
  - If blood pressure decreases, the **sympathetic nervous system** increases muscle contraction by releasing the neurotransmitter norepinephrine.
  - If the blood pressure is too high, the **parasympathetic nervous system** decreases the tonus by releasing the neurotransmitter **acetylcholine**, which prompts the endothelial cells of the blood vessel to release **NO**. The smooth muscle cells of the tunica media relax when the NO reaches them.

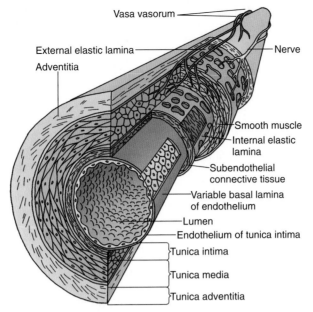

Figure 11.2 A typical artery. *(From Gartner LP, Hiatt JL: Color Textbook of Histology, 3rd ed. Philadelphia, Saunders, 2007, p 252.)*

Table 11.1 CHARACTERISTICS OF VARIOUS TYPES OF ARTERIES

Artery	Tunica Intima	Tunica Media	Tunica Adventitia
Elastic artery (*conducting*) (e.g., aorta, pulmonary trunk and arteries)	Endothelium with Weibel-Palade bodies, basal lamina, subendothelial layer, incomplete internal elastic lamina	40–70 fenestrated elastic membranes, smooth muscle cells interspersed between elastic membranes, thin external elastic lamina, vasa vasorum in outer half	Thin layer of fibroelastic connective tissue, vasa vasorum, lymphatic vessels, nerve fibers
Muscular artery (*distributing*) (e.g., carotid arteries, femoral artery)	Endothelium with Weibel-Palade bodies, basal lamina, subendothelial layer, thick internal elastic lamina	≤40 layers of smooth muscle cells, thick external elastic lamina	Thin layer of fibroelastic connective tissue, vasa vasorum not prominent, lymphatic vessels, nerve fibers
Arteriole	Endothelium with Weibel-Palade bodies, basal lamina, subendothelial layer not prominent, some elastic fibers instead of a defined internal elastic lamina	1–2 layers of smooth muscle cells	Loose connective tissue, nerve fibers
Metarteriole	Endothelium, basal lamina	Smooth muscle cells form precapillary sphincter	Sparse loose connective tissue

From Gartner LP, Hiatt JL: Color Textbook of Histology, 3rd ed. Philadelphia, Saunders, 2007, p 254.

Regulation of Arterial Blood Pressure (cont.)

- The kidneys and pituitary gland control the biochemical pathways.
  - The **kidneys** release the enzyme **renin** into the bloodstream. This enzyme cleaves circulating **angiotensinogen** into **angiotensin I**, which is converted into **angiotensin II**, a powerful constrictor of tunica media smooth muscles, by **angiotensin-converting enzyme**, present on the luminal plasma membrane of capillary endothelia.
  - The **pituitary** releases the potent vasoconstrictor **vasopressin (antidiuretic hormone)**.

Blood pressure is also modulated by the presence of **elastic membranes** in the large, muscular arteries, but especially by the ones in the elastic arteries.

- As the ventricles of the heart contract, they pump a large volume of blood into the aorta and pulmonary arteries, whose walls are richly endowed with elastic fibers and elastic membranes (**fenestrated membranes**). The vessel wall bulges, the elastic stretches and slowly returns to its normal size, and in this way the velocity of blood flow and blood pressure are not allowed to undergo rapid changes.

CAPILLARIES

Capillaries (Fig. 11.3) are the smallest blood vessels with the thinnest walls. They are composed of a simple squamous epithelium fashioned into a tube usually less than 50 μm in length and 8 to 10 μm in diameter. Where the endothelial cell meets itself, or other endothelial cells, in forming the tube, it overlaps itself and other cells forming a slight flap, the **marginal fold** that projects into the lumen. Endothelial cells also form **fascia occludentes (tight junctions)**. Interposed between arterioles and venules, capillaries form an anastomosing complex known as a **capillary bed**.

- Capillary endothelial cells are highly attenuated; they are less than 0.2 μm thick and their nuclei form bulges that project into the vessel's lumen.

- The cytoplasm possesses a scant amount of the normal organelles and intermediate filaments composed of **desmin** or **vimentin** or both.
- The abundance of **pinocytotic vesicles** associated with capillary plasmalemma is a distinguishing feature of capillaries.
- Capillaries form a **basal lamina** that coats their abluminal surface.
- **Pericytes**, contractile cells associated with capillaries and small venules, share the capillary's basal lamina, form gap junctions with the endothelial cells, and may act to regulate blood flow. Pericytes may also function as **regenerative cells** that assist in repairing damaged vessels.

Viewed with the electron microscope, three types of capillaries may be distinguished:

- **Continuous capillaries** are located in connective tissue, muscle, and nerve tissue, and modified continuous capillaries are located in the brain. Continuous capillaries contain numerous pinocytic vesicles, and their cell junctions are sealed with fasciae occludentes, so carrier-mediated transport is required for passage of amino acids, glucose, nucleosides, and purines. Although endothelial cells regulate the blood-brain barrier, astrocytes also have been shown to exert some influence.
- **Fenestrated capillaries**, located in endocrine glands, pancreas, and the intestines, possess **fenestrae (pores**, 60 to 80 nm in diameter) in their walls that are covered by a diaphragm. These pore/diaphragm complexes are situated at 50-nm intervals from each other, although they may be organized in clusters.
- **Sinusoidal capillaries**, located in bone marrow, spleen, liver, lymph nodes, and certain endocrine glands, are formed into amorphous channels (**sinusoids**) lined by endothelial cells that possess numerous large fenestrae without diaphragms. In some instances, the basal lamina and the endothelial wall may be discontinuous, facilitating a much freer exchange of materials between the blood and tissues.

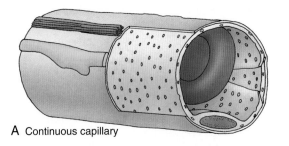

A Continuous capillary

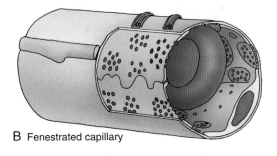

B Fenestrated capillary

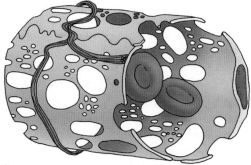

C Sinusoidal (discontinuous) capillary

Figure 11.3 A–C, Three types of capillaries. *(From Gartner LP, Hiatt JL: Color Textbook of Histology, 3rd ed. Philadelphia, Saunders, 2007, p 262.)*

CLINICAL CONSIDERATIONS

VASCULAR CHANGE

The largest arteries continue their growth to about age 25 with elastic laminae being continually added to the walls. Muscular arteries, beginning at middle age, display thickened walls with collagen and proteoglycan deposits resulting in reduced flexibility. Coronary vessels are the first to display aging signs, especially in the tunica intima. Changes are similar to those observed in arteriosclerosis.

ARTERIOSCLEROSIS

Arteriosclerosis is often associated with hypertension and diabetes. It is characterized by deposits of hyaline substance in the media walls of small arteries and arterioles (especially of the kidneys). Vessel rigidity results as the blood vessel walls become calcified.

ATHEROSCLEROSIS

Atherosclerosis is the most common cause of morbidity in vascular disease, characterized by deposits of noncellular yellowish lipid plaques (**atheromas**) in the intima, reducing the luminal diameter in the walls of the coronary arteries as well as in the walls of the largest arteries (e.g., carotid arteries), and also of the large arteries of the brain. Continued deposits can reduce luminal diameter and restrict blood flow to the region involved by 25 years of age. When this restricted blood flow occurs in the coronary vessels, referred pain may be the forerunner of heart attack and stroke.

Regulation of Blood Flow into a Capillary Bed

The regulation of blood flow into capillary beds is accomplished by arteriovenous anastomoses (AVA) and central channels (Fig. 11.4).

- **AVAs** bypass capillary beds; instead, there is a direct connection between the arterial and venous sides. The connecting vessel possesses three regions—an arterial end, a venous end, and an intermediate segment. The intermediate segment has a:
  - Thickened tunica media and modified smooth muscle cells in the subendothelial layer and
  - Rich adrenergic and cholinergic nerve supply controlled directly by the thermoregulatory center in the brain
- Blood flow is controlled by opening or closing these AVA shunts.
  - When the AVA shunt is closed, blood flows normally through the capillary bed.
  - When the shunt is open, blood bypasses the capillary bed.

Although AVAs are located throughout the body, they are especially common in the skin, where they function in thermoregulation.

- **Central channels** are composed of a metarteriole and its continuation, the thoroughfare channel.
  - **Metarterioles**, arising from arterioles, possess precapillary sphincters that, when open, allow the flow of blood into the capillary bed.
  - Blood from the capillary beds enters the **thoroughfare channels**; because these channels do not have sphincters, blood can always enter them, and from there blood is delivered into small venules.

Histophysiology of Capillaries

Physiologic studies of capillary permeability showed the presence of two types of pores in the walls of capillaries (Fig. 11.5): **small pores**, which probably represent slight gaps between epithelial cell junctions (9 to 11 nm in diameter), and **large pores**, which probably represent fenestrae and transport vesicles (50 to 70 nm in diameter).

- Small molecules can diffuse either through the entire thickness of the endothelial cell or through the intercellular junctions.

- Larger molecules are transported from the extracellular space into the lumen (or vice versa) via the use of **pinocytotic vesicles**, a process known as **transcytosis**.
- Other substances, such as those packaged in the Golgi apparatus of the endothelial cells, are delivered to the luminal aspect of the plasmalemma in **clathrin-coated vesicles**, where the cargo is exchanged for different cargo, which is transported to the abluminal aspect of the cell membrane to be released into the extracellular matrix.
- White blood cells leave the lumen via **diapedesis**: they penetrate either the endothelial cell or the endothelial cell junctions to enter the extracellular space. Frequently, diapedesis is facilitated by the presence of adhesion molecule receptors on the luminal aspect of the endothelial cells that are recognized by adhesion molecules expressed on leukocyte membranes.

The pharmacologic factors **histamine** and **bradykinin** increase capillary permeability, facilitating the egress of fluid from the vessel lumen and increasing the extracellular fluid volume. If the increase in extracellular fluid is substantial, it is referred to as **edema**.

The capillary endothelium also produces:

- Macromolecules destined for the extravascular environment, such as **laminin**, **fibronectin**, and **collagen (types II, IV, and V)**
- Substances that participate in the **clotting mechanism**, in the regulation of tunica media **smooth muscle tone**, and in **diapedesis** of neutrophils
- Pharmacologic agents, such as the vasodilator **prostacyclin**, which also impedes platelet aggregation
- **Enzymes** that degrade and inactivate norepinephrine, prostaglandins, serotonin, thrombin, and bradykinin
- **Enzymes**, such as **lipoprotein lipase**, that cleave lipoproteins and triglycerides into glycerol and fatty acids for storage in adipocytes and **angiotensin-converting enzyme** that converts the weak vasoconstrictor angiotensin I to the potent vasoconstrictor **angiotensin II**.

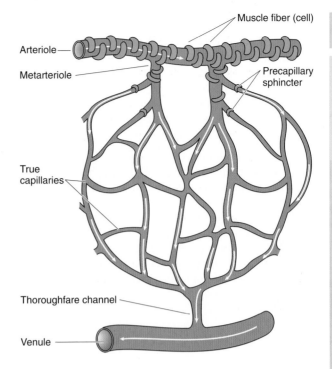

Arteriole

Muscle fiber (cell)

Metarteriole

Precapillary
sphincter

True
capillaries

Thoroughfare channel

Venule

Figure 11.4 Control of blood flow through a capillary bed. The central channel, composed of the metarteriole on the arterial side and the thoroughfare channel on the venous side, can bypass the capillary bed by closure of the precapillary sphincters. *(From Gartner LP, Hiatt JL: Color Textbook of Histology, 3rd ed. Philadelphia, Saunders, 2007, p 264.)*

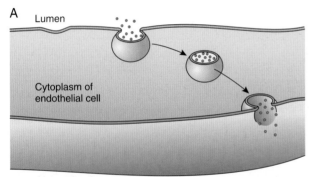

A

Lumen

Cytoplasm of
endothelial cell

Connective tissue

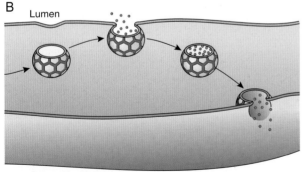

B

Lumen

Connective tissue

Figure 11.5 A–C, Methods of transport across capillary endothelia. *(Adapted from Simionescu N, Simionescu M: In Ussing H, Bindslev N, Sten-Knudsen O [eds]: Water Transport Across Epithelia. Copenhagen, Munksgaard, 1981.)*

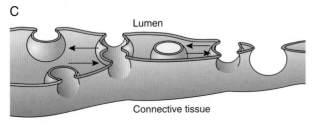

C

Lumen

Connective tissue

VEINS

Capillary beds deliver their blood to **venules**, from which the blood drains into **veins** of increasing size until it enters the atria of the heart. Because veins are low-pressure blood vessels, there are more veins than arteries, and their luminal diameter is greater such that they contain approximately 70% of the total blood volume.

- Veins and arteries are usually side by side, but the walls of veins are flattened because their walls are thinner, less elastic, and much less muscular.
- Although veins possess the same three tunics as arteries, the boundary between their tunica media and tunica intima is relatively indeterminate; the tunica media is reduced, but the tunica adventitia is increased in thickness.

- Veins are classified into three groups: venules, medium and small veins, and large veins (Table 11.2).

To thwart the reversal of blood flow, low-pressure, medium-sized veins—especially the veins of the lower extremity—possess **valves** that ensure a unidirectional flow of blood. Venous valves are:

- Composed of two leaflets derived from the tunica intima that project into the lumen
- Flimsy, but are reinforced by elastic and collagen fibers derived from the tunica intima
- Pressed against the luminal aspect of the vessel wall as blood flows toward the heart
- Flipped back into and blocking the lumen, like two hands cupped to hold water in the palms of the hands, resisting blood flow in the opposite direction

Table 11.2 CHARACTERISTICS OF VEINS

Type	Tunica Intima	Tunica Media	Tunica Adventitia
Large veins	Endothelium, basal lamina, valves in some, subendothelial connective tissue	Connective tissue, smooth muscle cells	Smooth muscle cells oriented in longitudinal bundles, cardiac muscle cells near their entry into the heart, collagen layers with fibroblasts
Medium and small veins	Endothelium, basal lamina, valves in some, subendothelial connective tissue	Reticular and elastic fibers, some smooth muscle cells	Collagen layers with fibroblasts
Venules	Endothelium, basal lamina (pericytes, postcapillary venules)	Sparse connective tissue and a few smooth muscle cells	Some collagen and a few fibroblasts

From Gartner LP, Hiatt JL: Color Textbook of Histology, 3rd ed. Philadelphia, Saunders, 2007, p 265.

CLINICAL CONSIDERATIONS

Varicose veins are superficial veins that have become enlarged and tortuous. Varicose veins are usually the result of aging as the walls of the veins have degenerated, or the muscles within the vein have lost their tone, or the venous valves have become incompetent. Varicose veins may also develop in the terminal end of the esophagus (esophageal varices) and at the terminal end of the anal canal (hemorrhoids).

HEART

The **heart** (Fig. 11.6), a highly modified blood vessel, possesses three layers: **endocardium** (corresponds to tunica intima); **myocardium** (corresponds to tunica media), composed of **cardiac muscle**; and **epicardium** (corresponds to tunica adventitia).

- **Endocardium** lines the lumen of the heart; because it is a continuation of the tunica intima of the blood vessels, it is composed of a simple squamous epithelium, which overlies a fibroelastic connective tissue with a scattered collection of fibroblasts. A deeper layer of dense connective tissue is richly supplied with elastic fibers and intermingled with smooth muscle cells. The deepest layer, the **subendocardial layer**, separating the endocardium from the myocardium, is composed of loose connective tissue with blood vessels, nerve fibers, and **Purkinje fibers**.
- **Myocardium**, the middle and most robust layer of the heart wall, is composed of cardiac muscle cells organized in spirals surrounding each of the four chambers of the heart. Cardiac muscle cells have various functions:
  - Joining the myocardium to the **fibrous skeleton** of the heart
  - Synthesizing and secreting hormones, such as **atrial natriuretic polypeptide**, **cardionatrin**, and **cardiodilatin**; these hormones function in maintaining fluid and electrolyte balance and reducing blood pressure
  - Generating and conducting impulses

- The generating and conducting impulses are performed by:
  - A specialized group of modified cardiac cells that form the **sinoatrial (SA) node** located in the right atrial wall at its junction with the superior vena cava. These nodal cells spontaneously depolarize, generating impulses to initiate a heart beat at approximately 70 beats/min.
  - The impulses generated spread over the atrial chambers of the heart and along pathways to the **atrioventricular (AV) node** located in the septal wall just superior to the tricuspid valve.
  - The modified cardiac muscle cells located in the AV node receive the impulses from the SA node and transmit the signals via the **AV bundle (bundle of His)** to the apex of the ventricular walls and branches of the AV bundles, known as **Purkinje fibers**, large, modified cardiac muscle cells, to transmit the impulses to cardiac muscle cells.
- Although the heartbeat is generated by these specialized cardiac muscle cells, the heart rate and stroke volume are moderated by the autonomic nervous system:
  - Sympathetic fibers increase the heart rate.
  - Parasympathetic innervation decreases the heart rate.

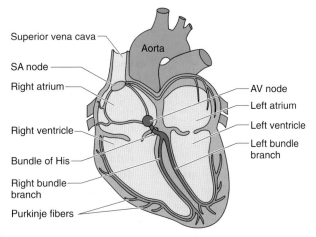

Figure 11.6 Diagram of the heart illustrating locations of the SA and VA nodes, Purkinje fibers, and bundle of His. *(From Gartner LP, Hiatt JL: Color Textbook of Histology, 3rd ed. Philadelphia, Saunders, 2007, p 267.)*

CLINICAL CONSIDERATIONS

Rheumatic heart disease results from being stricken with rheumatic fever during childhood. Rheumatic fever scars the valves resulting from fibrotic healing, causing them to lose their elasticity so that the valves can neither close properly (incompetence) nor open properly (stenosis). The most common valve affected is the bicuspid AV valve followed by the aortic valve.

Infections that engage the pericardial cavity are called **pericarditis**, and these may be severe enough to restrict the normal heartbeat as the pericardial cavity becomes burdened with fluid along with adhesions that develop between the serous layer of the pericardium and the epicardium.

Raynaud's phenomenon is a condition resulting in discolorations of the fingers or toes or both after exposure to changes in temperature (cold or hot) or emotional events. Skin discoloration results from abnormal spasms of the blood vessels and from a diminished blood supply to the local tissues. Initially, the digits involved turn white because of the diminished blood supply. The digits then turn blue because of prolonged lack of oxygen. Finally, the blood vessels reopen, causing a local "flushing" phenomenon, which turns the digits red. This three-phase color sequence occurs most often on exposure to cold temperature and is characteristic of Raynaud's phenomenon. Raynaud's phenomenon most frequently affects women, especially in the second, third, or fourth decades of life. Individuals can have Raynaud's phenomenon alone or as a part of other rheumatic diseases. The cause is unknown.

HEART (cont.)

- **Epicardium**, representing the outermost layer of the heart (**visceral pericardium**), consists of the **mesothelium**, a simple squamous epithelium, which overlies the subepicardial layer of loose, **fat-laden** connective tissue with its coronary vessels, nerves, and ganglia. Enclosing the entire heart and becoming continuous with the visceral pericardium on the great vessels entering and leaving the heart is the **parietal pericardium**, composed of an **inner serous layer** and an **outer fibrous layer**. The **pericardial cavity** located between visceral and parietal pericardium contains serous fluid to reduce friction between the two surfaces of the pericardium during the movement of the heart (Fig. 11.7).

The heart is the **pump** responsible for the circulation of blood throughout the body, and to accomplish that task it has four chambers—the two **atria**, which receive blood from the venous system, and the two **ventricles**, which propel the blood from the heart to circulate throughout the body. The four chambers are divided into two circuits: a pulmonary circuit and a systemic circuit (see Fig. 11.7).

- Blood received from the tissues of the body enters the **right atrium** and passes through the **right AV valve (tricuspid valve)** to enter the **right ventricle**.
- Blood is discharged from the right ventricle through the **semilunar valve** to enter the **pulmonary trunk**, and from here the deoxygenated blood goes to the **lungs** to be oxygenated.
- Oxygenated blood returning from the lungs enters the **left atrium**, and after passing through the **left AV valve** (**bicuspid valve**, also known as the **mitral valve**), it enters the **left ventricle**.
- From the left ventricle, the blood is discharged through another **semilunar valve** to enter the **aorta** for distribution to the tissues of the body.

Valves prevent the flow of blood back into the originating chamber.

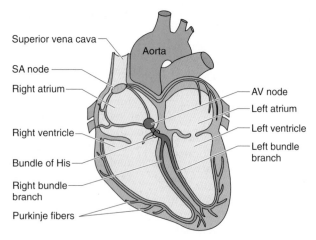

Figure 11.7 Diagram of the heart illustrating locations of the SA and VA nodes, Purkinje fibers, and bundle of His. *(From Gartner LP, Hiatt JL: Color Textbook of Histology, 3rd ed. Philadelphia, Saunders, 2007, p 267.)*

CLINICAL CONSIDERATIONS

Coronary heart disease affects about 14 million individuals in the United States. It develops when calcium and scar tissue build up in the coronary arteries that serve the myocardium. Over time, the plaque and calcium buildup results in atherosclerosis giving rise to narrowing of the coronary artery lumina so that the heart muscle does not receive enough blood. This condition causes chest pain and angina (referred pain down the left arm). When the artery becomes completely blocked, it may cause a myocardial infarction (heart attack) or cardiac arrest. Angioplasty is presently the treatment of choice for partially occluded arteries.

Lymphatic Vascular System

Lymph, the extracellular tissue fluid that bathes the interstitial tissue spaces of the body, is collected by blind-ended **lymphatic capillaries** (Fig. 11.8) located within the connective tissue compartments and is delivered to larger and larger vessels, eventually to be returned to the cardiovascular system via the two **lymphatic ducts** into veins at the root of the neck. Tributaries of the lymphatic system are located throughout the body except in the central nervous system, orbit, cartilage and bone, internal ear, and epidermis. The lymphatic vascular system is an open system; lymph does not circulate, and it is not propelled by a pump. Interposed at various intervals along the routes of the lymphatic vessels are **lymph nodes** through which the lymph is filtered.

- **Afferent lymphatic vessels** dispense the lymph to the lymph nodes containing abundant channels lined with endothelium and copious macrophages that clear the lymph of particulate matter.
- As the filtered lymph exits the lymph node, lymphocytes are introduced into the lymph, which is returned to the lymphatic vessel via **efferent lymphatic vessels**.

LYMPHATIC CAPILLARIES AND VESSELS

The blind-ended lymphatic capillaries, formed by a highly attenuated simple squamous epithelium, possess an incomplete basal lamina, and in the absence of tight junctions intercellular spaces are commonly present between the adjoining endothelial cells. The lumina of these delicate vessels are maintained open by **lymphatic anchoring filaments** (5 to 10 nm in diameter) that are inserted into the abluminal plasma membranes.

Lymph from the lymphatic capillaries drains into small and then medium-sized lymphatic vessels whose composition is similar to small veins but with larger lumina and thinner walls. Still larger lymphatic vessels possess a thin layer of elastic fibers and smooth muscle covered by elastic fibers blending into surrounding connective tissue. The two largest of the lymphatic vessels, the **right lymphatic duct** and the **thoracic duct**, which empty their contents into the venous system within the neck, are similar in composition to large veins, having the three defined tunics and possessing nutrient vessels similar to the vasa vasorum of arteries and veins.

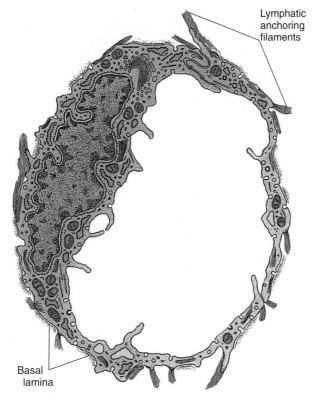

Lymphatic
anchoring
filaments

Basal
lamina

Figure 11.8 Diagram of ultrastructure of a lymphatic capillary. *(From Gartner LP, Hiatt JL: Color Textbook of Histology, 3rd ed. Philadelphia, Saunders, 2007, p 270.)*

CLINICAL CONSIDERATIONS

Lymphedema is an abnormal buildup of interstitial fluid that causes swelling, most often in the arms or legs. Lymphedema develops when lymph vessels or lymph nodes are missing, impaired, damaged, or removed. Primary lymphedema is rare and is caused by the absence of certain lymph vessels at birth, or it may be caused by abnormalities in the lymphatic vessels. Secondary lymphedema occurs as a result of a blockage or interruption that alters the lymphatic system. Secondary lymphedema can develop from an infection, malignancy, surgery, scar tissue formation, trauma, deep vein thrombosis, radiation, or other cancer treatment.

Cancerous tumor cells gain entry to the lymphatic system from the site of the primary tumor. During their travel within the lymphatic vessels, these tumor cells enter a lymph node where their spread may be hindered. The tumor cells may proliferate in the lymph node, however, and eventually leave to metastasize at a secondary site. It is incumbent on the surgeon to remove not only the cancerous growth but also to remove enlarged lymph nodes in the pathway and associated lymphatic vessels in an effort to prevent secondary spread of the cancerous cells by metastatic growth.

12 LYMPHOID (IMMUNE) SYSTEM

The **lymphoid system** protects against foreign invasions, such as macromolecules and microorganisms, and against virally altered cells. This system is composed of collections of nonencapsulated cells, known as the **diffuse lymphoid system**, and encapsulated collections of cells, **lymph nodes**, **tonsils**, **thymus**, and **spleen**.

Overview of the Lymphoid System

There are three **lines of defense** that the body has: the **epithelium**, which isolates the body from the external environment; the **epidermis**; and the various **mucosae**. These form physical obstacles that usually prevent foreign pathogens from gaining access to the sterile body compartments. These relatively thin barriers can be damaged by trauma, and some pathogens are able to penetrate them even if intact. Two additional lines of defense are innate (nonspecific) and adaptive (acquired) immune systems. In most cases, these systems can protect the body when these barriers have been violated.

INNATE IMMUNE SYSTEM

The more primitive and evolutionarily older but faster-responding **innate (natural) immune system** consists of complement, antimicrobial peptides, cytokines, macrophages, neutrophils, natural killer (NK) cells, and Toll-like receptors. This system is **nonspecific** and does not establish an immunologic memory of the agent that elicited its attack. Table 12.1 lists acronyms used in this chapter.

- **Complement**, an assortment of macromolecules circulating in the blood, precipitates in a specific sequence and forms a **membrane attack complex** on the cell membranes of pathogens that entered the bloodstream. Neutrophils and macrophages possess C3b receptors that induce these cells to phagocytose microorganisms bearing C3b on their surface.
- **Antimicrobial peptides**, such as **lysozyme** and **defensin**, not only kill microorganisms but also attract T cells and dendritic cells.

> **KEY WORDS**
> - **Innate immune system**
> - **Adaptive immune system**
> - **Immunoglobulins**
> - **T cells**
> - **B cells**
> - **MHC molecules**

- There are several categories of signaling molecules, collectively known as **cytokines**, based on their origin and functions:
  - Molecules manufactured by lymphocytes are **interleukins**.
  - Chemoattractants are **chemokines**.
  - Molecules that induce proliferation and differentiation are **colony-stimulating factors (CSFs)**.
  - Antiviral cytokines are known as **interferons**.
  - **Macrophages** are phagocytes that can recognize Fc portions of antibodies, C3b portions of complement, and carbohydrates that belong to microorganisms. They interact with T cells and B cells presenting antigens to them. Macrophages also induce proliferation of CFU-GM and CFU-G.
- Because **NK cells** participate in antibody-dependent cellular cytotoxicity, they resemble cytotoxic T lymphocytes (CTLs). In contrast to CTLs, NK cells do not have to go to the thymus to become cytotoxic cells. NK cells possess **killer-activating receptors** and **killer-inhibitory receptors**. The former, by recognizing the Fc portion of IgG antibodies, kill the cells to which the variable portion of IgG antibodies are attached, unless there are major histocompatibility complex type I molecules on the cell membranes of these cells.
- **Toll-like receptors**, integral proteins present in the plasmalemma of cells of the innate immune system, function when arranged in pairs. Some of these receptors are transmembrane proteins, whereas others are associated only with the cytoplasmic aspect of the cell membrane. Almost all Toll-like receptors induce the nuclear factor-κB pathway to initiate an intracellular response sequence culminating in the release of specific cytokines. Toll-like receptors also may activate an inflammatory response and launch a response involving T and B cells of the acquired immune system. Table 12.2 presents the putative functions of the various Toll-like receptors.

Table 12.1 ACRONYMS AND ABBREVIATIONS

Acronym/Abbreviation	Definition
ADDC	Antibody-dependent cellular cytotoxicity
APC	Antigen-presenting cell
BALT	Bronchus-associated lymphoid tissue
B lymphocyte	Bursa-derived lymphocyte (bone marrow–derived lymphocyte)
C3b	Complement 3b
CD	Cluster of differentiation molecule (followed by an Arabic numeral)
CLIP	Class II associated invariant protein
CSF	Colony-stimulating factor
CTL	Cytotoxic T lymphocyte (T killer cell)
Fab	Antigen-binding fragment of an antibody
Fc	Crystallized fragment (constant fragment of an antibody)
GALT	Gut-associated lymphoid tissue
G-CSF	Granulocyte colony-stimulating factor
GM-CSF	Granulocyte-macrophage colony-stimulating factor
HEV	High endothelial venule
IFN-γ	Interferon-γ
IL	Interleukin (followed by an Arabic numeral)
M cell	Microfold cell
MAC	Membrane attack complex
MALT	Mucosa-associated lymphoid tissue
MHC I and MHC II	Major histocompatibility class I molecules and class II molecules
MIIC vesicle	MHC class II–enriched compartment
NK cell	Natural killer cell
PALS	Periarterial lymphatic sheath
SIGs	Surface immunoglobulins
TAP	Transporter protein (1 and 2)
TCM	Central memory T cell
TCR	T cell receptor
TEM	Effector T memory cell
T_H cell	T helper cell (followed by an Arabic numeral)
TLRs	Toll-like receptors
T lymphocyte	Thymus-derived lymphocyte
TNF-α	Tumor necrosis factor-α
T reg cell	Regulatory T cell
TSH	Thyroid-stimulating hormone

From Gartner LP, Hiatt JL: Color Textbook of Histology, 3rd ed. Philadelphia, Saunders, 2007, p 274.

Table 12.2 TOLL-LIKE RECEPTORS AND THEIR PUTATIVE FUNCTIONS

Domains	Receptor Pair	Function
Intracellular and extracellular (on cell membrane)	TLR1–TLR2	Binds to bacterial lipoprotein; binds to certain proteins of parasites
	TLR2–TLR6	Binds to lipoteichoic acid of gram-positive bacterial wall and to zymosan
	TLR4–TLR4	Binds to LPS of gram-negative bacteria
	TLR5–?*	Binds to flagellin of bacterial flagella
	TLR11–?*	Host recognition of *Toxoplasmosis gondii*
Intracellular only	TLR3–?*	Binds to double-stranded viral RNA
	TLR7–?*	Binds to single-stranded viral RNA
	TLR8–?*	Binds to single-stranded viral RNA
	TLR9–?*	Binds to bacterial and viral DNA
	TLR10–?*	Unknown
	TLR12–?*	Unknown

*Currently, TLR partner is unknown.
LPS, lipopolysaccharide.
From Gartner LP, Hiatt JL: Color Textbook of Histology, 3rd ed. Philadelphia, Saunders, 2007, p 275.

ADAPTIVE IMMUNE SYSTEM

The **adaptive (acquired) immune system** is specific and composed of T and B lymphocytes (T and B cells) and antigen-presenting cells (APCs), although they also use the components of the innate immune system to perform their task of protecting the body. These cells not only release cytokines to communicate with each other, but also contact one another, and by recognizing particular membrane bound molecules, they induce specific responses in the other cells to combat foreign substances known as antigens. By definition:

- All **antigens** can interact with an antibody whether or not they can induce an immune response.
- An **immunogen** is a foreign substance that has the ability to initiate an immune response.

The cells of the adaptive immune system release cytokines, recruiting cells of the innate immune system to assist in the response against the invading antigens. The adaptive immune system is typified by the following four characteristics: **specificity**, **diversity**, **memory**, and ability to **distinguish between self and nonself**. There are two types of immune reactions mounted by the adaptive immune system:

- **Humoral immune response** uses immunoglobulins (**antibodies**) manufactured by differentiated B cells, known as **plasma cells**. Antibodies bind to and either inactivate the antigens or mark them for destruction by macrophages.
- **In cell-mediated immune response**, a specific category of T cells, **CTLs**, is induced to contact the foreign or virally altered cell and drive it into **apoptosis**.

The cells of the adaptive immune system develop in the **bone marrow** where B cells mature and develop into immunocompetent cells. T cells have to leave the bone marrow and enter the **thymic cortex**, however, to develop into immunocompetent cells. Immunocompetent B and T cells leave their **primary lymphoid organs** (bone marrow and thymus) to enter diffuse lymphoid tissue, lymph nodes, and the spleen—collectively known as **secondary lymphoid organs**. Here they search out and contact antigens.

CLONAL SELECTION AND EXPANSION

To be able to recognize and eliminate all the possible antigens and pathogens that one may contact in a lifetime, during embryogenesis about 10^{15} lymphocytes are established. Each lymphocyte has the property of recognizing a particular foreign antigen,

and each proliferates to form a cluster of identical cells, where each cluster is known as a **clone**. The members of each clone possess the same **membrane-bound antibodies** (surface immunoglobulins [sIgs]) or the same **T cell receptor (TCR)** for B cells and T cells, respectively. If the sIg or the TCR is against the macromolecules of the self, that clone is either eliminated during embryonic development (**clonal deletion**) or inactivated so that it cannot initiate an immune response (**clonal anergy**), protecting the individual from autoimmunity.

- First contact with a particular antigen elicits a slow, weak adaptive immune system response, the **primary immune response**, because the B and T cells have never met this antigen before and are considered to be **naïve (virgin) cells**.
- After contact, naïve cells proliferate and form **effector cells** (**plasma cells** for humoral response, and CTLs, T-helper [T_H] cells T_H1, T_H2, T_H17, and **CD regulatory T cells [T reg cells]** for cell-mediated immune response) that respond to and eliminate the antigen and **memory cells** that resemble naïve cells. Effector cells live for a long time (years), respond faster and more vigorously to a new challenge by the same antigen (**secondary immune response, anamnestic response**), and greatly increase the size of their clone (**clonal expansion**).

Immunoglobulins (Antibodies)

A special family of glycoproteins, known as **antibodies (immunoglobulins)**, is manufactured in enormous numbers by plasma cells and in small quantities by B cells (that place them on their cell membranes as sIgs, B cell receptors). A representative antibody (IgG) resembles the letter Y and is composed of four polypeptide chains (Fig. 12.1).

- Two long, identical **heavy chains**, secured to each other by disulfide bonds, form the stem and arms of the Y (where the arm and stem are held to each other by a hinge region).
- Two short, identical **light chains** participate in the formation of the arms of the Y, each held to its heavy chain by disulfide bonds.

Enzymatic cleavage of an antibody by papain occurs at the hinge region and forms an **Fc fragment**, the stem, whose amino acid sequence is constant, and two **Fab fragments** (antigen binding), each composed of a light chain and part of a heavy chain, whose distal portions are specific in their ability to bind *only one* particular **epitope** (the antigenic determinant region of an antigen). There are five different classes of immunoglobulins depending on various characteristic differences (Table 12.3).

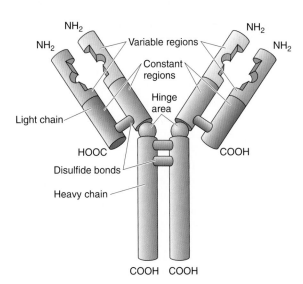

Figure 12.1 Drawing of a typical IgG. *(From Gartner LP, Hiatt JL: Color Textbook of Histology, 3rd ed. Philadelphia, Saunders, 2007, p 278.)*

Table 12.3 IMMUNOGLOBULIN ISOTYPES

Class and No. Units*	Cytokines†	Binds to Cells	Biological Characteristics
IgA 1 or 2	TGF-β	Temporarily to epithelial cells during secretion	Secreted into tears, saliva, lumen of the gut, and nasal cavity as **dimers**; individual units of the dimer are held together by **J protein** manufactured by plasma cells and protected from enzymatic degradation by a **secretory component** manufactured by the epithelial cell; combats antigens and microorganisms in lumen of gut, nasal cavity, vagina, and conjunctival sac; secreted into milk, protecting neonate with passive immunity; **monomeric** form in bloodstream; assists eosinophils in recognizing and killing parasites
IgD 1		B cell plasma membrane	Surface immunoglobulin; assists B cells in recognizing antigens for which they are specific; functions in the activation of B cells after antigenic challenge to differentiate into plasma cells
IgE 1	IL-4, IL-5	Mast cells and basophils	Reaginic antibody; when several membrane-bound antibodies are cross-linked by antigens, IgE facilitates degranulation of basophils and mast cells, with subsequent release of pharmacological agents, such as heparin, histamine, eosinophil and neutrophil chemotactic factors, and leukotrienes; elicits immediate hypersensitivity reactions; assists eosinophils in recognizing and killing parasites
IgG 1	IFN-γ, IL-4, IL-6	Macrophages and neutrophils	Crosses placenta, protecting fetus with passive immunity; secreted in milk, protecting neonate with passive immunity; fixes complement cascade; functions as **opsonin**; that is, by coating microorganisms, facilitates their phagocytosis by macrophages and neutrophils, cells that possess Fc receptors for the Fc region of these antibodies; participates in **antibody-dependent cell-mediated cytotoxicity** by activating NK cells; produced in large quantities during secondary immune responses
IgM 1 or 5		B cells (in monomeric form)	Pentameric form maintained by J-protein links, which bind Fc regions of each unit; activates cascade of the complement system; is the first isotype to be formed in the primary immune response

*A unit is a single immunoglobulin composed of two heavy and two light chains; IgA exists as a monomer and as a dimer.
†Cytokines responsible for switching to this isotype.
Fc, crystallizable fragment; IFN, interferon; IL, interleukin; NK, natural killer; TGF, transforming growth factor.

CELLS OF THE ADAPTIVE AND INNATE IMMUNE SYSTEMS

The adaptive and innate immune systems rely on the following cells: B cells, T cells, macrophages and their subtype APCs, and NK cells.

B Lymphocytes (B Cells)

B cells develop and become immunocompetent in the bone marrow. These cells manufacture IgM and IgD antibodies and insert their Fc end into their plasmalemma (**sIgs**) so that the Fab end projects into the external milieu. The Fc portion is affixed to the cell membrane by two transmembrane proteins, Igβ and Igα, that, when the sIg contacts an epitope, transduce that information intracellularly, starting a sequence of steps whose consequence is:

- **Activation** of the B cell, whose responsibility is the **humorally mediated immune system**.
- Activated B cells **proliferate** to form plasma cells and B memory cells.
  - Memory cells are responsible for clonal expansion.
  - Plasma cells manufacture IgM and then switch to a different isotype (Table 12.4).

Certain polysaccharides, such as peptidoglycans of bacterial membranes, are thymic-independent antigens because they can initiate a humoral immune response without T cell intermediaries. Only IgM antibodies are produced, however, and B memory cells are not formed.

T Lymphocytes (T Cells)

T cells develop in the bone marrow but have to enter the cortex of the thymus to express the necessary plasmalemma-bound molecules to become immunocompetent (see later in the section on the thymus). In contrast to B lymphocytes, T cells:

- Possess **TCRs** rather than sIgs.
  - TCRs resemble antibodies in that their constant region is embedded in the plasmalemma, and their variable region, projecting into the intercellular space, binds to epitopes.
- Do not recognize epitopes unless APCs proffer it to them.

- Express **cluster of differentiation proteins (CD molecules)** on their plasmalemma (Table 12.5).
  - About 200 different CD molecules have been identified. The **TCR complex**, consisting of TCR, CD3, and either CD4 or CD8, recognizes and binds to epitopes presented by APCs.
- Are able to act only in their immediate vicinity.
- Ignore nonprotein antigens.
- Recognize epitopes only if they are associated with one of the two classes of **MHC molecules** of APCs. These molecules are genetically determined and are unique to each individual, characterizing the *self*.
  - MHC class I are on the cell membranes of nucleated cells.
  - MHC class II (and MHC class I) are on the cell membranes of APCs.

T cells can become **activated** only if they recognize not only the epitope but also the MHC molecule. If the T cell does not recognize the MHC molecule, it cannot mount an immune response; therefore, T cells are said to be **MHC-restricted**. T lymphocytes are classified into three broad categories:

- Naïve T cells
- Memory T cells
- Effector T cells

Naïve T cells are immunologically competent and have CD45RA molecules on their plasmalemma, but have not as yet been challenged immunologically. When they are challenged, they proliferate to form memory and effector T lymphocytes.

Memory T cells possess CD45R0 molecules on their plasmalemma and are of two types: **central memory T cells (TCMs)**, whose cell membrane sports CR7⁺ molecules, and **effector memory T cells (CR7⁻ cells, TEMs)**, which do not have CR7 molecules on their surface. These cells establish the immunologic memory of the immune system. TCMs reside in the paracortex of lymph nodes where they bind to APCs, inducing the APCs to release IL-12. This cytokine causes TCMs to proliferate and form TEMs. The newly formed TEMs travel to the site of inflammation, differentiate into **effector T cells**, and respond to the antigenic challenge.

Table 12.4 ISOTYPE SWITCHING FROM IgM

Switch to	Cytokine from T_H Cell	Microorganism	Function
IgE	IL-4, IL-5	Parasitic worms	Attach to mast cells
IgG	IL-6, IFN-γ	Bacteria and viruses	Opsonizes bacteria, fixes complement, induces NK cells to kill virally altered cells (ADCC)
IgA	TGF-β	Bacteria and viruses	Secreted onto mucosal surface

ADCC, antibody-dependent cellular cytotoxicity; IL, interleukin; IFN, interferon; NK, natural killer; TGF, transforming growth factor.

Table 12.5 SELECTED SURFACE MARKERS INVOLVED IN THE IMMUNE PROCESS

Protein	Cell Surface	Ligand and Target Cell	Function
CD3	All T cells	None	Transduces epitope–MHC complex binding into intracellular signal, activating T cell
CD4	T helper cells	MHC II on APCs	Coreceptor for TCR binding to epitope–MHC II complex, activation of T helper cell
CD8	Cytotoxic T cells and suppressor T cells	MHC I on most nucleated cells	Coreceptor for TCR binding to epitope–MHC I complex; activation of cytotoxic T cell
CD28	T helper cells	7 on APCs	Assists in the activation of T helper cells
CD40	B cells	CD40 receptor molecule expressed on activated T helper cells	Binding of CD40 to CD40 receptor permits T helper cell to activate B cell to proliferate into B memory cells and plasma cells

APC, antigen-presenting cell; CD, cluster of differentiation molecule; MHC, major histocompatibility complex; TCR, T cell receptors.
From Gartner LP, Hiatt JL: Color Textbook of Histology, 3rd ed. Philadelphia, Saunders, 2007, p 281.

CLINICAL CONSIDERATIONS

IgM is the first antibody to be formed by B cells until T_H cells instruct them to switch to IgG synthesis. Individuals who have defective **CD40 ligands** are unable to switch isotypes and have excess blood levels of IgM, a condition known as **hyper-IgM syndrome**, resulting in humoral immunodeficiency–induced chronic infections.

All nucleated cells possess **MHC I molecules**, and these have to be recognized by CTLs to mount an immune response. Many tumor cells and virally altered cells stem the synthesis of MHC I molecules to avoid being recognized and destroyed by CTLs. NK cells are able to destroy these cells, however, because they do not need to recognize MHC I molecules.

Effector T Cells

Effector memory T cells give rise to **effector T cells**, three different groups of immunocompetent cells that have the ability to mount an immune response. The three categories are T_H cells, **CTLs** and **T killer cells**, and **T reg cells**.

All T_H cells display **CD4 molecules** on their plasmalemma and have the ability to work with cells that belong to the innate and the adaptive immune systems. T_H cells also function in activating CTLs to kill foreign and virally altered cells and in activating B cells to differentiate into plasma cells to form antibodies. There are four subcategories of T_H cells (a fifth one was placed into the T reg cell category), and they all secrete various cytokines (Table 12.6):

- **T_H0 cells**, precursors of the other three classes of T_H cells, are able to release many cytokines.
- **T_H1 cells**:
  - Direct responses against pathogens that invade the cytosol.
  - Initiate cell-mediated immune responses.
  - Secrete IL-2, which induces mitosis in CD4 and CD8 T cells and CTL cytotoxicity.
  - Secrete IFN-γ, which induces macrophages to destroy phagocytosed microorganisms and activates NK cells. Macrophages secrete IL-12, which causes formation of more T_H1 cells and restrains production of T_H2 cells.
  - Secrete tumor necrosis factor-β, which promotes acute inflammation by neutrophils.
- **T_H2 cells** function in prompting humoral responses against parasites and infection of the mucosa and secrete:
  - IL-4, which encourages B cells to switch to IgE production for allergic responses and, with IL-10, impedes the development of T_H1 cells.
  - IL-5, which prompts eosinophil formation.
  - IL-6, which encourages formation of T and B cells to battle asthma and systemic lupus erythematosus.
  - IL-9 which augments mast cell responses and T_H2 cell proliferation

  - IL-13, which encourages B cell formation and retards formation of T_H1 cells.
- **T_H17 cells secrete IL-17** and boost neutrophil response by facilitating their recruitment; they also develop from naïve T cells if IL-6 and transforming growth factor-β are present.
- **CTLs**, in contrast to T_H cells, have **CD8 molecules** on their plasmalemma. The TCRs of CTLs binds to epitopes on the plasma membranes of foreign, virally altered tumor cells; additionally, CTLs:
  - Insert **perforins** into the target cell plasmalemma, inducing creation of pores in the membrane.
  - Secrete **granzymes** that enter the target cell's cytosol through the newly formed pores, driving the cell into **apoptosis**.
  - Possess **CD95L (death ligand)** on their plasmalemma and bind to and activate **CD95 (death receptor)** on the target cell membrane, inducing the cascade of apoptotic death in the target cell.
- **T reg cells** also have CD4 molecules on their plasmalemma and function in suppressing the immune response. The two categories of T reg cells, which may function together to curtail autoimmune responses, are:
  - **Natural T reg cells**, which stem an immune response in a non–antigen-specific fashion by binding to APCs.
  - **Inducible T reg cells** (previously known as T_H3 cells), which secrete IL-10 and TGF-β to prevent the formation of T_H1 cells.
- In contrast to the other T cells, **natural T killer cells** are able to respond against lipid antigens that APCs with CD1 molecules on their cell surface present to them. Natural T killer cells are similar to NK cells in that they can be activated without intermediate steps, although only after they spent time in the thymic cortex where they become immunocompetent. These cells release IL-4, IL-10, and IFN-γ.

Table 12.6 ORIGIN AND SELECTED FUNCTIONS OF SOME CYTOKINES

Cytokine	Cell Origin	Target Cell	Function
IL-1a and IL-1b	Macrophages and epithelial cells	T cells and macrophages	Activate T cells and macrophages
IL-2	T_H1 cells	Activated T cells and activated B cells	Promotes proliferation of activated T cells and B cells
IL-4	T_H2 cells	B cells	Promotes proliferation of B cells and their maturation to plasma cells; facilitates switch from production of IgM to IgG and IgE
IL-5	T_H2 cells	B cells	Promotes B cell proliferation and maturation; facilitates switch from production of IgM to IgE
IL-6	Antigen-presenting cells and T_H2 cells	T cells and activated B cells	Activates T cells; promotes B cell maturation to IgG-producing plasma cells
IL-10	T_H2 cells	T_H1 cells	Inhibits development of T_H1 cells and inhibits them from secreting cytokines
IL-12	B cells and macrophages	NK cells and T cells	Activates NK cells and induces the formation of T_H1-like cells
TNF-α	Macrophage	Macrophages	Self-activates macrophages to release IL-12
	T_H1 cells	Hyperactive macrophages	Stimulates hyperactive macrophages to produce oxygen radicals, facilitating bacterial killing
IFN-α	Cells under viral attack	NK cells and macrophages	Activates macrophages and NK cell
IFN-β	Cells under viral attack	NK cells and macrophages	Activates macrophages and NK cells
IFN-γ	T_H1 cells	Macrophages and T cells	Promotes cell killing by cytotoxic T cells and phagocytosis by macrophages

IL, interleukin; IFN, interferon; NK, natural killer; T_H, T helper; TNF, tumor necrosis factor.
From Gartner LP, Hiatt JL: Color Textbook of Histology, 3rd ed. Philadelphia, Saunders, 2007, p 284.

CLINICAL CONSIDERATIONS

Occasionally, the immune system develops a dysfunction, as in **Graves' disease**, in which the thyroid follicular cells' receptors for thyroid-stimulating hormone are no longer recognized as part of the self. Instead, these receptors become viewed as if they were antigens. Conditions where the self is viewed as if it were foreign are known as **autoimmune diseases**. Antibodies bind to the TSH receptors, causing the follicular cells to secrete an overabundance of thyroid hormone. Patients with Graves' disease present with an enlarged thyroid gland and exophthalmos (protruding eyeballs).

Major Histocompatibility Complex Molecules

MHCs, located on the surface of APCs, including virally attacked and virally altered cells, function in holding short peptides cleaved from antigens, known as **epitopes**, that are presented to T cells. MHC molecules of every individual differ from MHC molecules of other individuals; T cells can recognize the **self**. There are two types of MHC molecules:

- **MHC I** presents epitopes (8 to 12 amino acids long) cleaved from proteins made by the cell (**endogenous protein**); all nucleated cells, including APCs, manufacture MHC I molecules.
- **MHC II** presents epitopes (13 to 25 amino acids long) cleaved from phagocytosed proteins (**exogenous proteins**); only APCs manufacture MHC II molecules.

Loading Major Histocompatibility Complex I Molecules

Proteasomes cleave **endogenous proteins** into **epitopes** 8 to 12 amino acids in length. The epitopes, transferred into the rough endoplasmic reticulum by **transporter proteins**, TAP1 and TAP2, are bound to MHC I, and the complex is transferred to the Golgi apparatus for packaging and transport. The MHC I–epitope complex is transported to the plasma membrane of the cell to be presented to CTLs, which determine whether or not the cell has to be destroyed. If the cell is producing viral protein, it is driven into apoptosis; if the cell is producing *self* proteins, the cell is allowed to live.

Loading Major Histocompatibility Complex II Molecules

- **Exogenous proteins** phagocytosed by macrophages and APCs are cleaved into increasingly smaller fragments in early and late endosomes (13 to 25 amino acids long).
- Simultaneously, these cells synthesize **MHC II molecules** on their rough endoplasmic reticulum in whose lumen the MHC II molecule temporarily binds **class II–associated invariant protein** (**CLIP**).
- MHC II–CLIP complex enters the Golgi apparatus to be packaged and delivered to MIIC vesicles (MHC II–enriched compartment) that also receives epitopes from late endosomes.

- Within the MIIC vesicle, CLIP is exchanged for the epitope, and the MHC II–epitope complex is delivered to the cell membrane for insertion.
- APCs and macrophages present the MHC II–epitope complex to T_H cells, which determine whether to mount an immune response.

Antigen-Presenting Cells

There are two types of **APCs**:

- Members of the mononuclear phagocyte system, such as macrophages and dendritic cells
- B cells and thymic epithelial reticular cells

APCs phagocytose and process antigens, load the epitopes on MHC II molecules, place the complex on their plasma membrane, and present the complex to T cells. APCs release cytokines such as IL-1, IL-6, IL-12, and TNF-α, which affect the immune response and a host of other signaling molecules that function outside the immune system.

Interaction Among Lymphoid Cells

To mount an immune response, **lymphoid cells interact** with one another and examine each other's surface molecules. If the molecules of the presenter cell are not recognized, the lymphocyte to which they are presented is driven into apoptosis. If the molecules are recognized, the lymphocyte that recognizes them becomes **activated**—that is, it proliferates and differentiates. For activation to occur:

- The **epitope** must be recognized.
- A **costimulatory signal** (either released or membrane bound) must be recognized.

T_H2 Cell–Mediated Humoral Immune Response

For all thymus-dependent antigens, B cells internalize and disassemble their antigen-sIg complex, load the MHC II, and place the MHC II–epitope complex on its plasmalemma to present it to a T_H2 cell (Fig.12.2).

- **Step 1**: T_H2 cell recognizes the epitope with its TCR and the MHC II with its CD4 molecule.
- **Step 2**: T_H2 cell's CD40 receptor and CD28 molecule have to bind to the B cell's CD40 molecule and CD80 molecule, resulting in the formation of **B memory cells** and **plasma cells**.

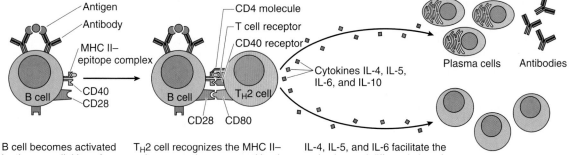

B cell becomes activated by the cross-linking of surface antibodies by the antigen. B cell places MHC II–epitope complex on its surface.

T_H2 cell recognizes the MHC II–epitope complex presented by the B cell, using its TCR and CD4 molecules. Additionally, the T_H2 CD40 receptor binds to the CD40 molecule on the B cell plasmalemma and CD28 binds to CD80.

Binding of CD40 to CD40 receptor causes proliferation of B cells. The T_H2 cell releases cytokines IL-4, IL-5, IL-6, and IL-10. Binding of CD28 of B cell to CD80 of T_H2 cell activates more T_H2 cells.

IL-4, IL-5, and IL-6 facilitate the activation and differentiation of B cells into B memory cells and antibody-forming plasma cells. IL-10 inhibits the proliferation of T_H1 cells.

Figure 12.2 Activation of B cells by T_H2 cells to produce B memory cells and antibody-forming plasma cells. The humoral response to thymus-independent antigens and the interaction with T_H2 cells are not required. *(From Gartner LP, Hiatt JL: Color Textbook of Histology, 3rd ed. Philadelphia, Saunders, 2007, p 285.)*

CLINICAL CONSIDERATIONS

Acquired immunodeficiency syndrome (AIDS) is caused by human immunodeficiency virus (HIV), which has the ability to bind to the CD4 molecules of T_H cells. After binding to the CD4 molecules, the virus introduces its core into the T_H cell, debilitating it. As the virus increases in number and infects additional T_H cells, the number of T_H cells diminishes, and the patient is unable to mount an immune response and succumbs to opportunistic infections.

T$_H$1 Cell–Mediated Killing of Virally Transformed Cells

The ability of a **CTL** to kill a virally transformed cell depends on two conditions:

1. It must receive signaling molecules from an activated T$_H$1 cell.
2. It must be bound to the **same APC** that is in the process of activating the T$_H$1 cell (Fig. 12.3).

- **Activation of the T$_H$1 cell** occurs when the following two steps are achieved:
  - **Step 1**: T$_H$1 cell TCR and CD4 molecules must be able to bind to the epitope–MHC II complex of the APC, inducing the APC to place a **B7 molecule** on its plasmalemma.
  - **Step 2**: T$_H$1 cell's CD28 molecule has to bind to the APC's B7 molecule, and the T$_H$1 cell releases IL-2, IFN-γ, and TNF.
- **Activation of the CTL** occurs when the following two steps are achieved:
  - **Step 1**: CTL's CD8 molecule and TCR must recognize the APC's **epitope–MHC II complex**, and the CTL's CD28 molecule must bind to the APC's **B7 molecule**.
  - **Step 2**: T$_H$1 cell releases IL-2, which must bind to the IL-2 receptor of the CTL. The activated CTL proliferates because of the influence of IFN-γ.

The activated CTLs bind, via TCR and CD8, to the epitope–MHC I complex of the virally transformed cells and kill the transformed cells by:

- Inserting perforins into the transformed cells' plasmalemma, which cause the formation of large pores through which the components of the cytosol leak out of the cell
- Inserting perforins into the transformed cells' plasmalemma and releasing granzymes into the cytosol, driving the cell to apoptosis
- Alternatively, the CTL's **Fas ligand (CD95L molecule, death ligand)** can bind with the transformed cells' **Fas protein (CD95, death receptor)**, which drives the transformed cells to **apoptosis**.

T$_H$1 Cells Assist Macrophages in Killing Phagocytosed Bacteria

Macrophages have to be activated by T$_H$1 cells before they can destroy bacteria that they phagocytosed. This process requires that first the T$_H$1 cell become activated; the activated T$_H$1 cell then instructs the macrophage to destroy the bacteria in its phagosomes (Fig. 12.4). The activation of the T$_H$1 cell requires two steps:

- **Step 1**: T$_H$1 cell's CD4 molecule and TCR have to recognize the epitope–MHC II complex of the macrophage.
- **Step 2**: T$_H$1 cell activates itself by expressing IL-2 receptors and releasing IL-2, which binds to the newly expressed receptors and induces mitotic activity of the T$_H$1 cells.

The newly formed, **activated T$_H$1 cells** bind to the macrophages with bacteria in their phagosomes.

- **Step 1**: T$_H$1 cell's CD4 molecule and TCR have to recognize the epitope–MHC II complex of the macrophage, and the T$_H$1 cell releases IFN-γ.
- **Step 2**: Macrophage is activated by IFN-γ and releases TNF-α, which also binds to the macrophage; these two signaling molecules initiate the destruction of the phagocytosed bacteria by the formation of oxygen radicals.

Lymphoid Organs

Lymphoid organs are of two types:

- **Primary (central) lymphoid organs** (fetal liver, postnatal bone marrow, and thymus), where lymphocytes become immunocompetent
- **Secondary (peripheral) lymphoid organs** (lymph nodes, spleen, postnatal bone marrow, and mucosa-associated lymphoid tissue [MALT]), where immunocompetent cells can interact with other cells and with antigens to initiate an immune response against pathogens and antigens

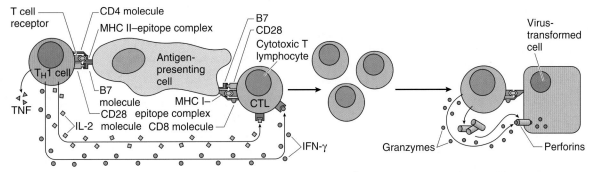

T_H1 cell TCR binds to MHC II–epitope complex of antigen-presenting cell. The CD4 molecule of the T_H1 cell recognizes MHC II. These two events cause the APC to express B7 molecules on its surface, which bind to CD28 of the T_H1 cell, causing it to release IL-2, IFN-γ, and TNF.

The same APC also has **MHC I–epitope** complex expressed on its surface that is bound by a CTL's CD8 molecule and T-cell receptor. Additionally, the CTL has CD28 molecules bound to the APC's B7 molecule. The CTL also possesses IL-2 receptors, which bind the IL-2 released by the T_H1 cell, causing the CTL to undergo proliferation, and IFN-γ causes its activation.

The newly formed CTLs attach to the MHC I–epitope complex via their TCR and CD8 molecules and secrete **perforins** and **granzymes**, killing the virus-transformed cells. Killing occurs when granzymes enter the cell through the pores established by perforins and act on the intracellular components to drive the cell into apoptosis.

Figure 12.3 Activation of CTLs by T_H1 cells. The T_H1 cell and the CTL must be complexed to the same APC. *(From Gartner LP, Hiatt JL: Color Textbook of Histology, 3rd ed. Philadelphia, Saunders, 2007, p 286.)*

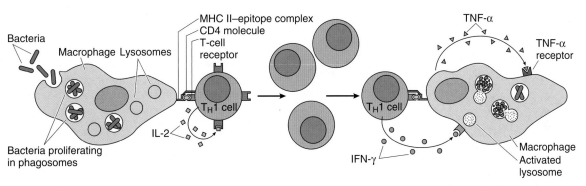

T_H1 cell's TCR and CD4 molecules recognize the MHC II–epitope complex presented by a macrophage that was infected by bacteria. The T_H1 cell becomes activated, expresses IL-2 receptors on its surface, and releases IL-2. Binding of IL-2 results in proliferation of the T_H1 cells.

The newly formed T_H1 cells contact infected macrophages (TCR and CD4 recognition of MHC II–epitope complex) and release interferon-γ (IFN-γ). IFN-γ activates the macrophage to express TNF-α receptors on its surface as well as to release TNF-α. Binding of IFN-γ and TNF-α on the macrophage cell membrane facilitates the production of oxygen radicals by the macrophage resulting in killing of bacteria.

Figure 12.4 Activation of macrophages by T_H1 cells. *(From Gartner LP, Hiatt JL: Color Textbook of Histology, 3rd ed. Philadelphia, Saunders, 2007, p 287.)*

THYMUS

The **thymus**, a small endodermally derived organ located in the superior mediastinum, is divided into two **lobes** by its connective tissue **capsule** and functions in educating T cells to become immunocompetent. Although around the time of puberty the thymus begins to **involute** (degenerate) and becomes infiltrated by adipocytes, it is still functional in adults. Each lobe of the thymus is subdivided into incomplete lobules so that each lobule has its individual **cortex**, but shares the **medulla** with other lobules (Fig. 12.5).

The **thymic cortex** is occupied by numerous lymphocytes whose large nuclei and scant cytoplasm impart a dark, basophilic image in histologic sections. Immunoincompetent **T cell precursors** from the bone marrow enter the cortex of the thymus to proliferate and become immunocompetent T cells. To do this, they must contact various **epithelial reticular cells** of the cortex and develop some and eliminate other surface markers.

- **T cell precursors** from the bone marrow enter the corticomedullary junction of the thymus and migrate into the **outer cortex**, where they are known as **thymocytes**.
- **Notch-1 receptors** on the thymocyte plasmalemma receive signaling molecules from the cortical epithelial reticular cells, causing them to become committed to the **T cell lineage**.
- Thymocytes begin to express some **T cell markers**—CD2, but not CD3-TCR complex and not CD4 or CD8—therefore, they are known as **double negative thymocytes**.
- As the double negative thymocytes move deeper into the cortex (nearer the medulla), they **express**, and then **suppress**, other proteins on their surface.
- These double negative thymocytes express **pre–T cell receptors** (pre-TCRs) that cause the cells to proliferate.
- These newly formed thymocytes express CD4 and CD8 molecules and become known as **double positive thymocytes**.
- The double positive thymocytes rearrange their genes coding for the **variable region of their TCR** and express a low level of the CD3-TCR complex on their surface.
- The double positive thymocytes that express low levels of CD3-TCR on their surface are tested by cortical epithelial reticular cells to see if they can recognize **self-MHC–self-epitope complexes**.
  - Most double positive thymocytes (about 90%) do not recognize these complexes and are driven into apoptosis, and cortical macrophages phagocytose the dead cells.
  - Some double positive thymocytes (10%) recognize these complexes and are allowed to

mature, express higher levels of TCRs, and stop expressing both CD4 and CD8 molecules.

- When the T cells express either CD4 or CD8, they are known as **single positive thymocytes**, and they leave the cortex to enter the thymic medulla.
- Single positive thymocytes contact **medullary epithelial reticular cells** and **dendritic cells** that challenge them to see if the thymocytes recognize self-epitopes that were not presented to them in the cortex.
  - **Single positive thymocytes** that would mount an attack against the self are driven into **apoptosis** in the medulla, and the dead cells are eliminated by medullary macrophages (**clonal deletion**).
  - **Single positive thymocytes** that would not initiate an immune response against the self are allowed to leave the thymus to populate secondary lymphoid organs as **naïve T cells**.

Epithelial Reticular Cells

There are six types of **epithelial reticular cells**, three in the cortex and three in the medulla:

- Type I cells isolate the cortex from the connective tissue capsule and trabeculae and form a sheath around blood vessels of the cortex.
- Type II cells are located in the midcortex and surround islands of thymocytes; they present self-antigens, MHC I molecules, and MHC II molecules to thymocytes.
- Type III cells are located at the corticomedullary junction, they present self-antigens, MHC I molecules, and MHC II molecules to thymocytes.
- Type IV cells are located in the medulla at the corticomedullary junction; they assist type III cells in isolating the cortex from the medulla.
- Type V cells form the architectural framework of the medulla.
- Type VI cells form **thymic (Hassall's) corpuscles**, release **thymic stromal lymphopoietin** that promotes clonal deletion, and assist in driving single positive T cells into apoptosis.

Some individuals who are born without a thymus, a condition known as **DiGeorge's syndrome**, are unable to generate T cells and are incapable of mounting a cell-mediated immune response. Because T_H cells are required in the initiation of most humorally mediated immune responses, these patients are mostly immunoincompetent. As long as patients with DiGeorge's syndrome are protected from infection, they can survive; however, most die of infections, or because many of these patients are also born without parathyroid glands, they die of **calcium tetani** (severe **hypocalcemia**).

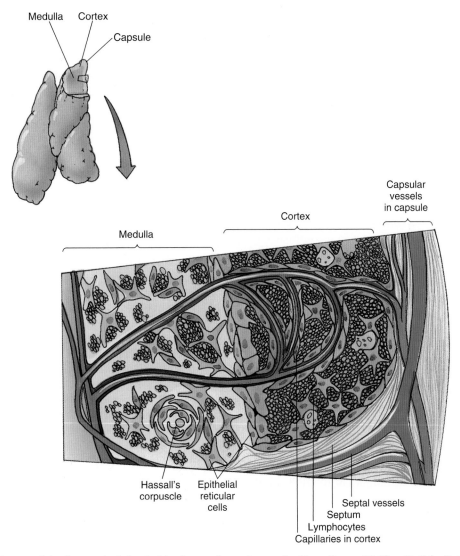

Figure 12.5 Diagram of the thymus depicting its histology and vascular supply. *(From Gartner LP, Hiatt JL: Color Textbook of Histology, 3rd ed. Philadelphia, Saunders, 2007, p 288.)*

CLINICAL CONSIDERATIONS

The blood supply of the thymus first gains entry into the medulla and forms a capillary bed at the junction of the cortex and the medulla. Branches of these capillaries enter the cortex and immediately become surrounded by a sheath of type I epithelial reticular cells that are held to one another by fasciae occludentes. These epithelial reticular cells form the **blood thymus barrier** in the thymic cortex, which ensures that macromolecules carried in the bloodstream cannot enter the cortex and interfere with the immunologic development of T cells. The endothelial cells of the cortical capillaries and the type I epithelial reticular cells possess their own basal lamina, which adds support to the barrier. The space between the epithelial sheath and the endothelium is patrolled by macrophages that destroy macromolecules that manage to escape from the capillaries. The cortex of the thymus drains into the venous network of the medulla.

LYMPH NODES

Lymph nodes are usually small, bean-shaped structures (≤3 cm in diameter) with a convex surface and a concave surface (hilum) invested by a connective tissue **capsule** (Fig. 12.6) that is usually embedded in **adipose tissue**. Deep to the capsule, the parenchyma is subdivided into:

- An outer **cortex**, housing B cells that form primary and secondary lymphoid nodules
- A middle **paracortex**, housing T_H cells
- Deeper **medulla**, whose predominant cells are lymphocytes, plasma cells, and macrophages

The capsule on the convex aspect sends **trabeculae** into the cortex, subdividing it into incomplete compartments; as the trabeculae continue into the paracortex and the medulla, they become more tortuous and less definite (see Fig. 12.6). Lymph nodes house T cells, B cells, dendritic cells, macrophages, and APCs, and function in clearing lymph and initiating immunologic reactions against foreign antigens. Lymph enters the lymph node via **afferent lymph vessels** that pierce the convex surface and whose valves prevent the lymph from flowing out of the node. The lymph percolates through the node and exits, via **efferent lymph vessels**, which also have valves to prevent the lymph from reentering the node at the hilum. Arteries enter and veins leave the lymph node at the hilum; these vessels use trabeculae to penetrate the parenchyma of the node. In the paracortex, the veins form **high endothelial venules (HEVs)**.

The incomplete compartments of the **cortex of a lymph node** are bounded superiorly by the connective tissue **capsule** and laterally by **trabeculae** derived from the capsule (see Fig. 12.6). As the afferent lymph vessels pierce the capsule, they deliver their lymph into the **subcapsular sinus**, from which the lymph travels into **paratrabecular sinuses** that follow the trabeculae and deliver their lymph into the very tortuous **medullary sinuses** that are drained by **efferent lymph vessels**. These lymphatic sinuses are lined by simple squamous **endothelial cells**, and their lumina are spanned by an interdigitating complex of **stellate reticular cells** that not only slow the flow of lymph but also are used as scaffoldings by **macrophages** that phagocytose antigenic particulate matter.

The cortical **compartments** display dark, spherical secondary or primary lymphoid nodules.

- **Secondary nodules** (see Fig. 12.6) are formed as a reaction to an antigenic stimulation, and they actively produce B cells (**centroblasts**) that have not as yet expressed sIgs. Proliferation of these cells occurs initially in the dark zone and later in the light zone of the central, clear area (the **germinal center**); the centroblasts displace the resting B cells, pushing them away to form the dense **mantle (corona)** that fashions a cap over the germinal center toward the subcapsular sinus. Additional cells that are located in a secondary follicle are:
  - **Migrating dendritic cells**, such as **Langerhans cells** of the skin, are bone marrow–derived and are distributed throughout the body; when they detect foreign antigens, they migrate to the nearest lymph node to initiate an immune response.
  - **Follicular dendritic cells** are not derived from bone marrow and reside in the lymph node; they present antigens to **centrocytes**, newly formed B cells that have expressed sIgs. Follicular dendritic cells force B cells with improper sIgs into apoptosis and permit the other B cells to differentiate into **B memory cells** and **plasma cells**, which enter the medulla and leave the lymph node.
  - **Reticular cells** synthesize type III collagen (reticular fibers), which forms the architectural framework of lymph nodes.
  - **Macrophages** destroy apoptotic cells.
- **Primary nodules** (see Fig. 12.6) are resting nodules in that they do not have germinal centers or a mantle until B cells that were activated by T helper cells at the border of the cortex and paracortex migrate into the primary nodule to form a germinal center, transforming the primary into a secondary nodule.

The **paracortex** (see Fig. 12.6) is the T cell–rich region of the lymph node. Here HEVs permit the entry of B and T cells into the lymph node. B cells migrate to the cortex, and T cells remain in the paracortex.

The **medulla** (see Fig. 12.6) is composed of medullary sinusoids, trabeculae, and **medullary cords**, structures formed by reticular fibers, reticular cells, and macrophages, and B cells and plasma cells that were formed in secondary lymphoid follicles.

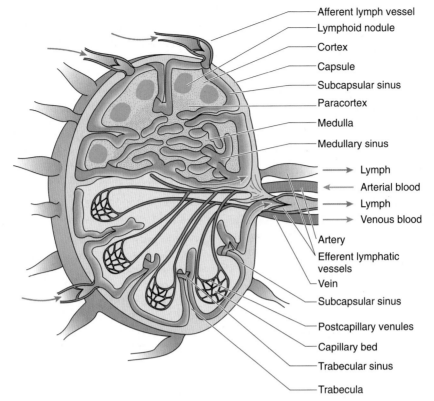

Figure 12.6 Diagram of a typical lymph node. *(From Gartner LP, Hiatt JL: Color Textbook of Histology, 3rd ed. Philadelphia, Saunders, 2007, p 291.)*

Labels in figure:
- Afferent lymph vessel
- Lymphoid nodule
- Cortex
- Capsule
- Subcapsular sinus
- Paracortex
- Medulla
- Medullary sinus
- Lymph
- Arterial blood
- Lymph
- Venous blood
- Artery
- Efferent lymphatic vessels
- Vein
- Subcapsular sinus
- Postcapillary venules
- Capillary bed
- Trabecular sinus
- Trabecula

CLINICAL CONSIDERATIONS

In a healthy individual, **lymph nodes** are too soft to be able to be palpated. If the patient has a regional infection, however, the lymphocytes of the node draining that particular area proliferate; the node swells, becomes hard and painful, and may be palpated with ease. Each area of the body is drained by a series of lymph nodes that are connected to one another by lymph vessels. This formation of chains of lymph nodes is frequently responsible for the spread of infections or the metastasis of malignancy from one part of the body to another. As **lymph** percolates throughout the sinusoids of the lymph node, macrophages remove approximately 99% of foreign or undesirable particulate matter by phagocytosing it.

APCs that contacted antigens make their way to the lymph node nearest to their location, present the MHC-epitope complex to T helper cells, and initiate an immune response. When in the lymph node, these APCs are known as **migrating dendritic cells**.

Antigens that enter the lymph node via the afferent lymph vessels are picked up by **follicular dendritic cells**, which present the epitope to

resident lymphocytes. When the antigen is recognized, a B cell becomes activated at the interface of the paracortex and cortex, it migrates into a primary lymphoid nodule, and begins to undergo rapid mitosis, forming a **germinal center**, transforming the **primary** into a **secondary lymphoid nodule**. If the **activated B cells** express improper sIgs, they are driven into **apoptosis** by the follicular dendritic cells; if they present proper sIgs, they are permitted to continue to differentiate into **B memory cells** and **plasma cells**. The newly differentiated cells migrate into the medulla of the lymph node and form **medullary cords**. Approximately 90% of the plasma cells leave the lymph node via the efferent lymph vessels and migrate to the **bone marrow**, where they manufacture and release antibodies until they die. The remaining 10% of plasma cells stay in the medullary cord and manufacture antibodies until they also die. Most B memory cells also leave their lymph node of origin to seed other **secondary lymphatic organs**, where they set up small **clones** in case the same antigen invades the body again. A few B memory cells remain in their lymph node of origin and establish a small clone there.

SPLEEN

The **spleen** has a dense, irregular, and collagenous connective tissue **capsule** that is covered by the peritoneum, a simple squamous epithelium. The largest lymphoid organ, the spleen has a convex surface and a concave area, the **hilum**, where the capsule sends connective tissue **trabeculae**, bearing blood vessels and nerve fibers into the substance of the spleen. Attached to the capsule and the trabeculae is a three-dimensional complex of **type III collagen fibers** with their associated **reticular cells** that form the physical framework of the spleen. In contrast to lymph nodes, the spleen is not divided into a cortex, paracortex, and medulla; instead, it comprises **white pulp**, the **marginal zone**, and **red pulp** (sporting an abundance of tortuous sinusoids) that are intermingled (Fig. 12.7) to serve the **functions** of the spleen:

- Filtering blood and destroying senescent erythrocytes
- Forming T and B cells and mounting immune responses
- Hematopoiesis in the fetus and, if the need arises, in adults

Vascular Supply of the Spleen

The large artery supplying the spleen, the **splenic artery**, forms several branches before it enters the substance of the spleen at its **hilum** (Figs. 12.7 and 12.8).

- The vessels travel via trabeculae as **trabecular arteries** that provide numerous, ever smaller branches in correspondingly smaller trabeculae.
- When the arteries are 200 μm or smaller in diameter, they leave their respective trabeculae, and their tunica adventitia unravels and becomes mired in a sheath of T cells, known as the **periarterial lymphatic sheath (PALS)**. The artery occupying the center of the PALS is referred to as the **central artery**.
- As the central artery becomes smaller in diameter, it loses its PALS, and it forms a series of small, straight arterioles that parallel each other as they enter the red pulp, known as the **penicillar arteries**, each of which has three sections:
  - Pulp arteriole
  - Sheathed arteriole that possesses a coat of macrophages (Schweigger-Seidel sheath)
  - Terminal arterial capillary, which delivers blood directly into a sinusoid (closed

circulation) or into the red pulp tissue in the vicinity of a sinusoid (open circulation) or, as believed by most investigators, in open and closed circulations.
- **Veins of the pulp** (see Fig. 12.8) receive blood from the sinusoids and are drained by larger veins that accompany arteries of corresponding sizes in trabeculae that lead the larger veins to the hilum, where they form the large splenic vein.

White Pulp, Marginal Zone, and Red Pulp

The three components of the spleen are white pulp, marginal zone, and red pulp.

- **White pulp** is the sheath of **T lymphocytes**, the **PALS**, whose center is delineated by the **central artery**. Often a **lymphoid nodule**, composed of B cells, is formed within the PALS so that the T cells surround a spherical accumulation of B cells. If the nodule is responding to an immunologic challenge, a **germinal center** is also present. In the spleen, as in lymph nodes, T and B cells occupy prescribed regions (see Figs. 12.7 and 12.8).
- **Marginal zone**, a region approximately $\frac{1}{10}$ mm wide, is the interface between the white pulp and red pulp (see Fig. 12.7). The cells of the marginal zone are **interdigitating dendritic cells (APCs)**, **macrophages**, **plasma cells**, **T cells**, and **B cells**. Additionally, small sinusoids, **marginal sinuses**, abound in this region. Capillaries, derived from the central artery, enter the red pulp for a short distance, recur, and empty into the marginal sinuses.
- The **red pulp** (see Figs. 12.7 and 12.8) is composed of vascular spaces, the **sinusoids**, surrounded by the stroma of the red pulp, the **splenic cords**, consisting of a network of reticular fibers that are invested by **stellate reticular cells** to prevent the collagen fibers from contacting the extravasated blood that percolates through its interstices and precipitating the **coagulation** cascade. The endothelial cells of the sinusoids are unusual in that they are fusiform cells whose longitudinal axes parallel the long axis of the sinusoids. The endothelium is quite leaky with wide spaces between adjacent cells through which blood cells can easily escape from the lumen into the splenic cords. Sparse, threadlike **reticular fibers**, coated with discontinuous **basal lamina**–like material, wrap around the endothelial lining of the sinusoids.

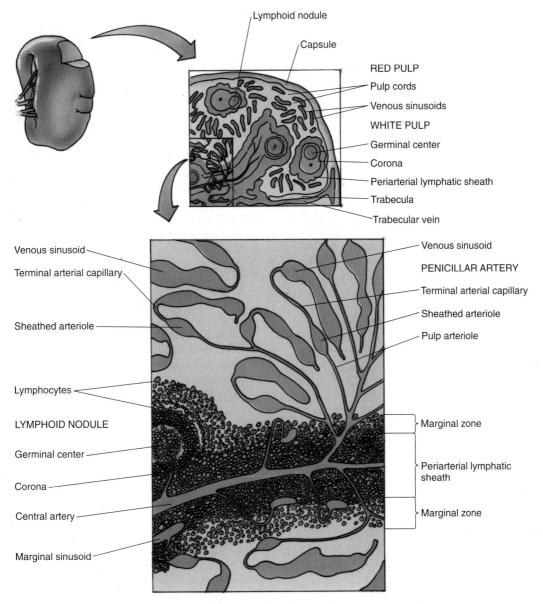

Figure 12.7 Diagram of the spleen. *(From Gartner LP, Hiatt JL: Color Textbook of Histology, 3rd ed. Philadelphia, Saunders, 2007, p 294.)*

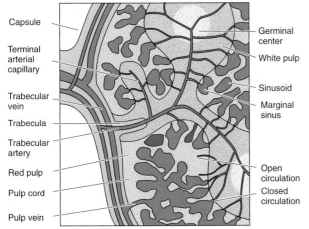

Figure 12.8 Diagram of the closed and open circulation in the spleen.

SPLEEN (cont.)

The functions of the spleen are intimately interconnected with the design of its **vascular supply**.

- The first region where blood entering the spleen contacts the splenic parenchyma is at the **marginal sinusoids**, where **APCs** search for antigens, and **macrophages** attack microorganisms traveling in the bloodstream. **T** and **B cells** leave the bloodstream through the walls of the marginal sinusoids and enter the **PALS** and the **lymphoid nodules**.
- At the **marginal zone, interdigitating dendritic cells** present their MHC-epitope complex to **T cells. B cells** recognize **thymus-independent antigens** to initiate an immune response; they differentiate into plasma cells, most of which migrate to the bone marrow and make antibodies.
- Material that is not eliminated in the marginal zone enters the sinusoids of the **red pulp** to be eliminated there by **macrophages**. This material includes old platelets and senescent erythrocytes. Old erythrocytes are recognized because they lose sialic acid residues and have galactose moieties on their cell membranes.

MUCOSA-ASSOCIATED LYMPHOID TISSUE

The mucosae of the respiratory, digestive, and urinary tracts display nonencapsulated clusters of lymphoid nodules and lymphocyte infiltrations known as **MALT**; examples are **gut-associated lymphoid tissue (GALT)**, **bronchus-associated lymphoid tissue (BALT)**, and **tonsils**.

- **Lymphoid follicles** located all along the mucosa of the **alimentary canal**, known as **GALT**, are composed of B cells with a peripheral association of T cells. The most prominent GALT is located in the mucosa of the ileum, known as **Peyer's patches** (Fig. 12.9A). Arterioles supplying Peyer's patches are drained by veins, some of which are **HEVs** that permit the exit of lymphocytes and macrophages from their lumina (Fig. 12.9B–D).

- **M cells (microfold cells)**, associated with Peyer's patches, trap antigens from the lumen of the gut and transfer these unprocessed antigens to APCs present in Peyer's patches.
- **BALT** is similar in morphology and function to GALT except that these follicles are located in the mucosa of the respiratory tract.

Tonsils

Tonsils, a collection of partially encapsulated **lymphoid nodules** (palatine, pharyngeal, lingual, and numerous very small tonsils), are located at the entrance of the **oral pharynx**, protecting it from inhaled antigens. In the presence of an antigenic challenge, lymphocytes become activated and proliferate, enlarging the affected tonsil.

- The paired **palatine tonsils**, ensconced between the palatoglossal and palatopharyngeal folds, are covered by a stratified squamous epithelium and present about a dozen deep **crypts** that may house food and other debris and microorganisms and desquamated epithelial cells. The parenchyma of the palatine tonsils has numerous **lymphoid nodules**, some with germinal centers. The deep aspect of the palatine tonsils possesses a dense fibrous **capsule**.
- The unpaired **pharyngeal tonsil**, located in the nasal pharynx, is similar to the palatine tonsil except it has a respiratory epithelium covering it and shallow infoldings, called **pleats** instead of crypts, and its **capsule** is thinner. When the pharyngeal tonsil is inflamed, it is known as the **adenoid**.
- The **lingual tonsils**, located on the dorsal aspect of the posterior one third of the **tongue**, are covered by a **stratified squamous epithelium** that dips into the numerous **crypts** whose floor receives the **posterior mucous minor salivary glands**. The deep aspect of the lingual tonsils possesses a thin capsule. The parenchyma of the lingual tonsils is composed of **lymphoid nodules**, many of which display **germinal centers**.

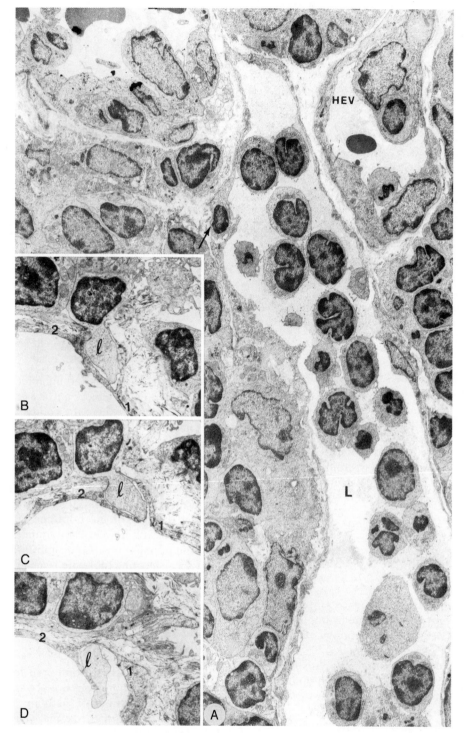

Figure 12.9 Transmission electron micrographs. **A,** ALPA vessel (L) of the interfollicular area full of lymphocytes that has an intraendothelial channel that includes lymphocytes (*arrow*) in the endothelial wall (×3000). **B–D,** Ultrathin serial sections that document various stages through an intraendothelial channel composed of one (1) and two (2) endothelial cells (×9000). ℓ, lymphocyte. *(From Azzali G, Arcari MA: Ultrastructural and three-dimensional aspects of the lymphatic vessels of the absorbing peripheral lymphatic apparatus in Peyer's patches of the rabbit. Anat Rec 258:76, 2000.)*

13 ENDOCRINE SYSTEM

The maintenance of homeostasis and the control of the metabolic activity of certain organs and organ systems are under the control of the autonomic nervous system and of the **endocrine system**. The former acts rapidly by releasing neurotransmitter substances in the immediate environment of the organ system being controlled, whereas the latter acts more slowly and at a distance by releasing **hormones**—messenger molecules that use the bloodstream to reach their destination. Nonetheless, these two separate systems function together in orchestrating the body's metabolic activities. The endocrine system is composed of:

> **KEY WORDS**
> - **Hormones**
> - **Pituitary gland**
> - **Hypothalamohypophyseal tract**
> - **Thyroid gland**
> - **Parathyroid glands**
> - **Suprarenal cortex**
> - **Suprarenal medulla**
> - **Pineal body**

- Richly vascularized **glands**—the pituitary, thyroid, parathyroid, and suprarenal glands and the pineal body
- Clusters of endocrine cells, such as the **islets of Langerhans** in the pancreas
- Individual endocrine cells scattered among the epithelial lining of the gastrointestinal tract and respiratory tract (**diffuse neuroendocrine system cells**).

Hormones

Hormones are classified into three categories based on their chemical nature:

- **Proteins and polypeptides**, such as insulin and luteinizing hormone (LH), are hydrophilic and bind to cell surface receptors on the extracellular surface of the plasma membrane.
- **Amino acid derivatives**, such as thyroxine and norepinephrine, are hydrophilic and bind to cell surface receptors on the extracellular surface of the plasma membrane.
- **Steroid and fatty acid derivatives**, such as estrogens and androgens, are hydrophobic and bind to intracellular receptors in the cytosol.

The binding of a hormone to its receptor (either to **cell surface receptors** or to **intracellular receptors**) initiates **signal transduction**, the process of cellular reaction to the hormone. Signal transduction by cell surface receptor binding activates:

- Protein kinase, which activates regulatory proteins, such as adenylate cyclase, to form the **second messenger**, **cyclic adenosine monophosphate**. Other systems form different second messengers, such as cyclic guanosine monophosphate, phosphatidylinositol derivatives, calcium ions, and sodium ions
- **G proteins**, which activate a second messenger system
- Catalytic receptors, which activate protein kinases to initiate a phosphorylation cascade

Signal transduction by intracellular receptor binding is achieved by entry into the nucleus of the **hormone receptor complex**, where the complex binds to the DNA in the vicinity of a promoter site, initiating messenger RNA (mRNA) transcription with eventual translation of the mRNA to form the requisite protein.

If the amount of hormone released is insufficient to initiate signal transduction, a **positive feedback** is generated by the target cell to ensure the release of a larger quantity of the hormone. Activation of a target cell occurs, however, that initiates not only the requisite response but also an **inhibitory response**, whereby a signaling molecule is generated that activates a **feedback mechanism** that shuts down the endocrine gland/cell, preventing it from releasing more of the hormone.

Pituitary Gland (Hypophysis)

The **pituitary gland (hypophysis)**, responsible for the production of numerous hormones, is suspended from the hypothalamus of the brain and is housed in the sella turcica of the cranial vault (Fig. 13.1). This small gland, the size of a pea, is derived from two separate sources:

- The **neurohypophysis** is an evagination of the diencephalon.
- The **adenohypophysis** is an outpocketing of the oral cavity (Rathke's pouch).

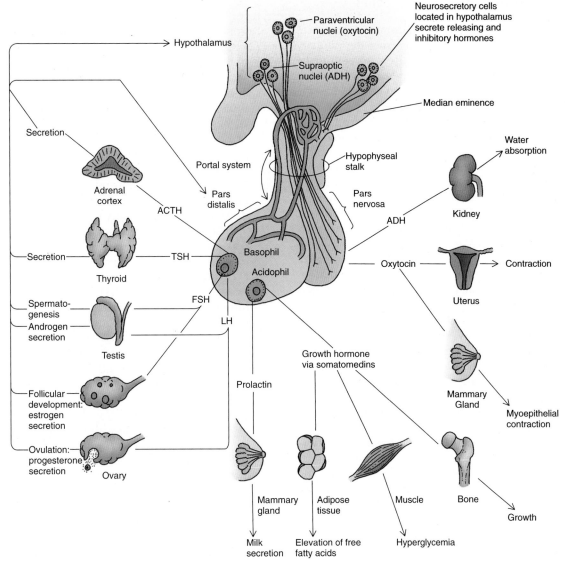

Figure 13.1 The pituitary gland and its target organs. ACTH, adrenocorticotropic hormone; ADH, antidiuretic hormone; FSH, follicle-stimulating hormone; TSH, thyroid-stimulating hormone. *(From Gartner LP, Hiatt JL: Color Textbook of Histology, 3rd ed. Philadelphia, Saunders, 2007, p 305.)*

Table 13.1 DIVISIONS OF THE PITUITARY GLAND

Adenohypophysis (Anterior Pituitary)	Neurohypophysis (Posterior Pituitary)
Pars distalis (pars anterior)	Median eminence
Pars intermedia	Infundibulum
Pars tuberalis	Pars nervosa

Pituitary Gland (Hypophysis) (cont.)

Nerve fibers and neurotransmitter substances derived from the hypothalamus enter the pituitary and its vascular supply, respectively, to coordinate the release of the hormones produced by or stored in the pituitary. The hypophysis is subdivided into the **adenohypophysis (anterior pituitary)** and the **neurohypophysis (posterior pituitary)**, each of which has its own subdivision (Table 13.1). Residual cells of Rathke's pouch remain inserted between the adenohypophysis and the neurohypophysis as colloid-filled vesicles. The infundibulum is enveloped by a sheath of endocrine cell, known as the **pars tuberalis**. The pituitary receives its blood from **superior** and **inferior hypophyseal arteries**, branches of the internal carotid arteries.

The two superior hypophyseal arteries vascularize the infundibulum and the pars tuberalis, and arborize to form the **primary capillary plexus** (composed of fenestrated capillaries) of the **median eminence**. The inferior hypophyseal arteries predominantly serve the posterior pituitary. The primary capillary bed is drained by the hypophyseal portal vein, which delivers its blood into the **secondary capillary bed** (also composed of fenestrated capillaries) that permeates the anterior pituitary.

Axons derived from neurons of the hypothalamus terminate in the region of the primary capillary bed and release their **hypothalamic neurosecretory hormones** (**releasing** or **inhibitory hormones**), which find their way into the primary capillary bed. The hypophyseal portal veins deliver the neurosecretory hormones into the secondary capillary bed, which permeates the substance of the anterior pituitary. The hypothalamus is able to regulate the activity of the anterior pituitary by releasing hormones (factors), listed in Table 13.2.

ADENOHYPOPHYSIS (ANTERIOR PITUITARY)

The adenohypophysis, arising from Rathke's pouch, has three regions—the pars distalis, pars intermedia, and pars tuberalis (Fig. 13.2).

- The capsule of the **pars distalis** sends reticular fibers into the substance of the gland fibers that support the parenchymal cells and the sinusoidal capillaries of the secondary capillary bed. The parenchymal cells of the pars distalis are of two types: (1) cells whose secretory granules take up histologic stains, known as **chromophils**, and (2) cells whose secretory granules do not take up histologic stains, known as **chromophobes**. The granules of certain chromophils are preferentially stained by acidic dyes, **acidophils**, whereas the granules of other chromophils stain with basic dyes, **basophils**.
  - **Acidophils**, the most abundant cells of the pars distalis, are of two types: **somatotrophs**, which secrete **somatotropin**, a growth hormone, and **mammotrophs**, which secrete **prolactin**, the hormone that fosters the development of mammary glands in a gravid woman and lactation to nourish the newborn.
  - **Basophils** are located at the periphery of the pars distalis. Three subtypes are represented: (1) **corticotrophs**, which secrete **adrenocorticotropic hormone (ACTH)** and **lipotropic hormone**; (2) **thyrotrophs**, which secrete **thyrotropin**; and (3) **gonadotrophs**, which secrete **follicle-stimulating hormone (FSH)** and **luteinizing hormone (LH)**.
  - **Chromophobes** possess little cytoplasm, possess few secretory granules, and do not take up histologic stains. These cells are probably chromophils that have released the contents of their secretory granules, although some investigators suggest that they may be stem cells. The most prominent cells of the pars distalis are the **folliculostellate cells**, whose function is unknown.
- The **pars intermedia (zona intermedia)**, located between the pars anterior and the pars nervosa, houses colloid-filled cysts derived from Rathke's pouch and clusters of basophils that produce **pro-opiomelanocortin**. The hormones **α-melanocyte-stimulating hormone (α-MSH)**, **β-endorphin**, **corticotropin**, and **lipotropin** all are formed by the cleaving of this prohormone. In contrast to lower animals, in humans, α-MSH induces prolactin release and is known as **prolactin-releasing factor**.
- The **pars tuberalis** partially envelops the stalk of the pituitary. Although it is not described as secreting any hormones, some of its cells contain FSH and LH.

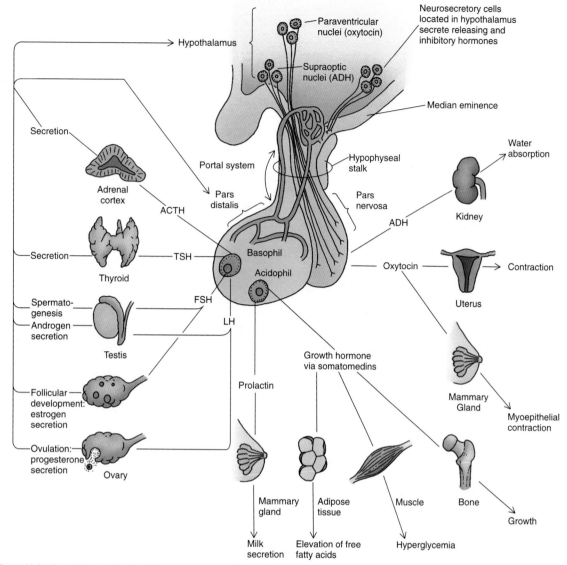

Figure 13.2 The pituitary gland and its target organs. *(From Gartner LP, Hiatt JL: Color Textbook of Histology, 3rd ed. Philadelphia, Saunders, 2007, p 305.)*

Table 13.2 RELEASING HORMONES OF THE HYPOTHALAMUS AND THEIR FUNCTIONS

Releasing Hormone	Function
Thyroid-stimulating hormone (TSH)–releasing hormone	Release of thyroid stimulating hormone
Corticotropin-releasing hormone	Release of adrenocorticotropin
Somatotropin-releasing hormone	Release of somatotropin (growth hormone)
Luteinizing hormone (LH)–releasing hormone	Release of LH and FSH
Prolactin-releasing hormone	Release of prolactin
Prolactin-inhibitory factor	Inhibits prolactin secretion

NEUROHYPOPHYSIS

The **neurohypophysis** (posterior pituitary gland) develops from the hypothalamus and is divided into three regions (Figs. 13.3 and 13.4): **median eminence**, **infundibulum**, and **pars nervosa**. The entire neurohypophysis may be considered to be a prolonged extension of the hypothalamus. The **hypothalamohypophyseal tract** is composed of unmyelinated axons of neurosecretory cells located in the two nuclei of the hypothalamus:

- **Supraoptic**
- **Paraventricular**

The neurosecretory cells of these nuclei manufacture **antidiuretic hormone (ADH, vasopressin)** and oxy-tocin and the carrier protein **neurophysin** to which these hormones are bound (Fig. 13.5).

Pars Nervosa

The hypothalamohypophyseal tract terminates in the **pars nervosa**, and these axons are supported by **pituicytes**, glia-like cells characteristic of this region of the pituitary gland. The hormones **ADH** and **oxytocin** are stored in their active state in varicosities of the axons, known as **Herring bodies**, and are released, on demand, in the vicinity of the fenestrated capillary bed established by the two inferior hypophyseal arteries (Tables 13.2 and 13.3).

CLINICAL CONSIDERATIONS

Pituitary adenomas represent the common tumors of the anterior pituitary gland. Because the pituitary gland is confined within the hypophyseal fossa of the sphenoid bone, its growth and enlargement impinges on its normal function of hormone production in the pars distalis. When left untreated, these tumors may erode the bone and other neural tissues.

Diabetes insipidus may be related to lesions in the hypothalamus or pars nervosa or both that reduce production of ADH, leading to renal dysfunction in which the urine cannot be concentrated. As a result, an individual with diabetes insipidus drinks enormous quantities of water and may secrete 20 L of urine per day (polyuria).

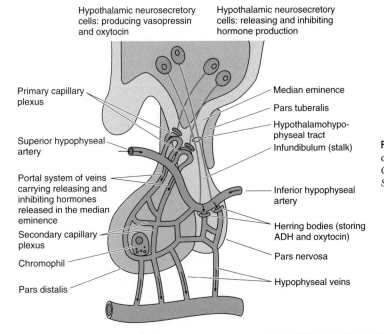

Hypothalamic neurosecretory cells: producing vasopressin and oxytocin

Hypothalamic neurosecretory cells: releasing and inhibiting hormone production

Primary capillary plexus

Superior hypophyseal artery

Portal system of veins carrying releasing and inhibiting hormones released in the median eminence

Secondary capillary plexus

Chromophil

Pars distalis

Median eminence

Pars tuberalis

Hypothalamohypo-physeal tract

Infundibulum (stalk)

Inferior hypophyseal artery

Herring bodies (storing ADH and oxytocin)

Pars nervosa

Hypophyseal veins

Figure 13.3 The pituitary gland and its circulatory system. *(From Gartner LP, Hiatt JL: Color Textbook of Histology, 3rd ed. Philadelphia, Saunders, 2007, p 306.)*

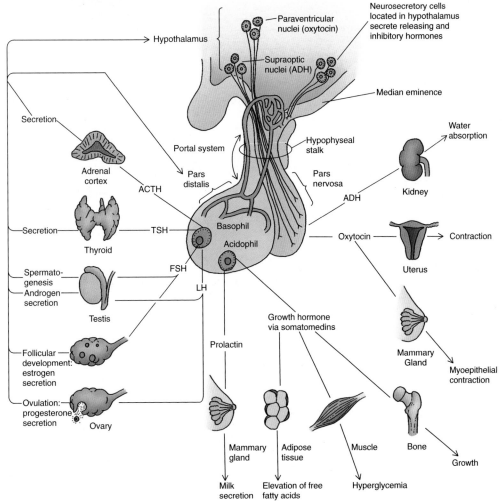

Hypothalamus

Paraventricular nuclei (oxytocin)

Neurosecretory cells located in hypothalamus secrete releasing and inhibitory hormones

Supraoptic nuclei (ADH)

Median eminence

Secretion

Adrenal cortex

ACTH

Portal system

Pars distalis

Hypophyseal stalk

Pars nervosa

ADH

Water absorption

Kidney

Secretion

Thyroid

TSH

Basophil

Acidophil

Oxytocin

Contraction

Uterus

Spermato-genesis

Androgen secretion

FSH

LH

Testis

Growth hormone via somatomedins

Prolactin

Mammary Gland

Myoepithelial contraction

Follicular development: estrogen secretion

Ovulation: progesterone secretion

Ovary

Mammary gland

Adipose tissue

Muscle

Bone

Growth

Milk secretion

Elevation of free fatty acids

Hyperglycemia

Figure 13.4 The pituitary gland and its target organs. *(From Gartner LP, Hiatt JL: Color Textbook of Histology, 3rd ed. Philadelphia, Saunders, 2007, p 305.)*

Table 13.3 PHYSIOLOGIC EFFECTS OF PITUITARY HORMONES

Hormone	Releasing/Inhibiting	Function
Pars Distalis		
Somatotropin (growth hormone)	*Releasing*—SRH/*Inhibiting*—somatostatin	Generalized effect on most cells is to increase metabolic rates; stimulate liver cells to release somatomedins (insulin-like growth factors I and II), which increases proliferation of cartilage and assists in growth in long bones
Prolactin	*Releasing*—PRH/*Inhibiting*—PIF	Promotes development of mammary glands during pregnancy; stimulates milk production after parturition (prolactin secretion is stimulated by suckling)
Adrenocorticotropic hormone (ACTH, corticotropin)	*Releasing*—CRH	Stimulates synthesis and release of hormones (cortisol and corticosterone) from suprarenal cortex
FSH	*Releasing*—LHRH/*Inhibiting*—inhibin (in males)	Stimulates secondary ovarian follicle growth and estrogen secretion; stimulates Sertoli cells in seminiferous tubules to produce androgen-binding protein
LH	*Releasing*—LHRH	Assists FSH in promoting ovulation, formation of corpus luteum, and secretion of progesterone and estrogen, forming a negative feedback to the hypothalamus to inhibit LHRH in women
Interstitial cell–stimulating hormone (ICSH) in men		Stimulates Leydig cells to secrete and release testosterone, which forms a negative feedback to the hypothalamus to inhibit LHRH in men
TSH (thyrotropin)	*Releasing*—TRH/*Inhibiting*—negative feedback suppresses via CNS	Stimulates synthesis and release of thyroid hormone, which increases metabolic rate
Pars Nervosa		
Oxytocin		Stimulates smooth muscle contractions of uterus during orgasm; causes contractions of pregnant uterus at parturition (stimulation of cervix sends signal to hypothalamus to secrete more oxytocin); suckling sends signals to hypothalamus, resulting in more oxytocin, causing contractions of myoepithelial cells of the mammary glands, assisting in milk ejection
Vasopressin (antidiuretic hormone [ADH])		Conserves body water by increasing resorption of water by kidneys; thought to be regulated by osmotic pressure; causes contraction of smooth muscles in arteries, increasing blood pressure; may restore normal blood pressure after severe hemorrhage

CNS, central nervous system.
From Gartner LP, Hiatt JL: Color Textbook of Histology, 3rd ed. Philadelphia, Saunders, 2007, p 307.

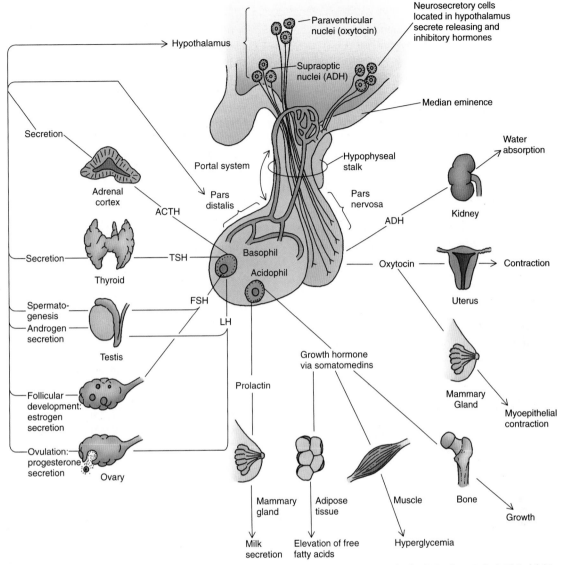

Figure 13.5 The pituitary gland and its target organs. *(From Gartner LP, Hiatt JL: Color Textbook of Histology, 3rd ed. Philadelphia, Saunders, 2007, p 305.)*

CLINICAL CONSIDERATIONS

Nontoxic goiter refers to enlargement of the thyroid gland that is not associated with overproduction of thyroid hormone or malignancy. Numerous factors may cause the thyroid to become enlarged. A diet deficient in iodine can cause goiter, but this is rarely the case because of the iodine available in the diet. A more common cause of goiter is an increase in thyroid-stimulating hormone (TSH) in response to a defect in normal hormone synthesis within the thyroid gland. In this situation, TSH causes the thyroid to enlarge over several years. Most small to moderate-sized goiters can be treated with thyroid hormone in the form of a pill. This treatment reduces TSH production from the pituitary gland, which should result in stabilization in size of the gland. This treatment often does not cause the size of the goiter to decrease, but usually keeps it from growing any larger. Patients who do not respond to thyroid hormone therapy are often referred for surgery if it continues to grow.

Thyroid Gland

The thyroid gland is a bilobed gland located in the neck, anteroinferior to the larynx (Fig. 13.6). The right and left lobes are connected across the midline by the isthmus. Occasionally, ascending from the isthmus, there is a pyramidal lobe, a remnant of the thyroglossal duct from which the thyroid develops in the posterior region of the embryonic tongue. A thin **capsule** surrounds the gland, and embedded in its posterior aspect are the **parathyroid glands**. The capsule sends septa into the substance of the gland, subdividing it into lobes, and conveys the gland's vascular, neural, and lymphatic supply to its parenchyma, which is arranged in cystlike **follicles** (≤1 mm in diameter) whose lumen contains a colloid that is surrounded by simple cuboidal follicular cells and occasional parafollicular cells.

Each follicle is surrounded by the basal lamina, manufactured by the **follicular cells** (Fig. 13.7).

- Binding of **TSH**, produced by the anterior pituitary, to TSH receptors on the basal cell membranes of follicular cells and the presence of **iodide**, which enters the cells via iodide pumps of the basal plasmalemmae of follicular cells, stimulate these cells to synthesize the hormones **tetraiodothyronine (thyroxine, T_4)** and **triiodothyronine (T_3)**.
  - Iodination of the hormones is preceded by the **oxidation** of **iodide** at the follicular cell–colloid interface by the enzyme **thyroid peroxidase**.
  - Tyrosine residues, bound to the secretory glycoprotein, **thyroglobulin**, are iodinated by the attachment of one or two oxidated iodides, forming **monoiodinated tyrosine (MIT)** or **diiodinated tyrosine (DIT)**.
  - The active hormones T_3 and T_4 are produced by combining one MIT and one DIT or two DITs.
  - When formed, T_3 and T_4, bound to the secretory glycoprotein thyroglobulin, are released into the colloid for storage.
- Release of T_3 and T_4 occurs in response to TSH, occupying TSH receptor sites on the follicular cell basal plasmalemma. Follicular cells:

- Form **filopodia** that extend into the colloid capturing and endocytosing a small amount of it in endocytic vesicles.
- Have colloid-filled endocytic vesicles that deliver their content into the endosomal compartment where MIT, DIT, T_3, and T_4 are stripped from the thyroglobulin and are released into the cytosol.
- Secrete T_3, but predominantly T_4, and are exocytosed into the capillary beds of the richly vascularized connective tissue stroma of the thyroid gland.
- Within the bloodstream are bound to **plasma proteins** and are delivered to their target cells throughout the body.
- T_3 binds less avidly to the plasma proteins than T_4, and T_3 is more likely to be endocytosed by its target cell than is T_4.
  - When in the cytosol, T_3 complexes much more readily than does T_4 to **nuclear thyroid receptor protein**, but both complexes enter the nucleus to initiate transcription (Table 13.4); T_3 is more physiologically active than is T_4.
  - T_3 and T_4 boost the metabolic rates of their target cells, promote the rate of growth in growing individuals, enhance mental acuity, stimulate carbohydrate and lipid metabolism, and increase heart rate, respiration, and muscle action.
  - T_3 and T_4 decrease the production of fatty acids, cholesterol, and triglycerides, and facilitate weight loss.

Parafollicular cells (C cells, clear cells) stain lightly and are located at the periphery of follicles but share the basal lamina of the follicle. These cells produce the peptide hormone **calcitonin**, which is released directly into the capillary beds of the thyroid connective tissue stroma, attaches to calcitonin receptors of osteoclasts, and inhibits them from resorbing bone (see Table 13.4). Calcitonin is released by parafollicular cells if the plasma calcium levels are greater than normal.

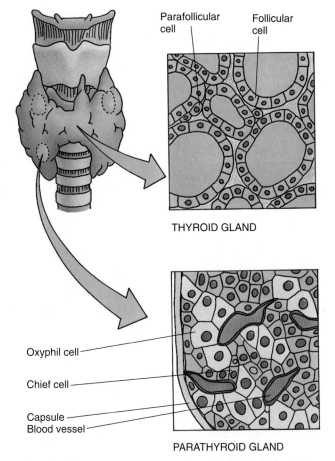

Figure 13.6 The thyroid and parathyroid glands. *(From Gartner LP, Hiatt JL: Color Textbook of Histology, 3rd ed. Philadelphia, Saunders, 2007, p 313.)*

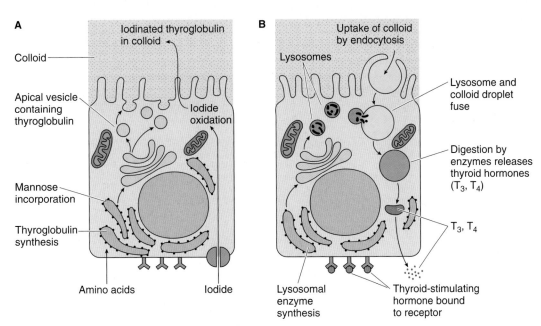

Figure 13.7 The synthesis and iodination of thyroglobulin (**A**) and release of thyroid hormone (**B**). *(From Gartner LP, Hiatt JL: Color Textbook of Histology, 3rd ed. Philadelphia, Saunders, 2007, p 315.)*

Parathyroid Glands

The **parathyroid glands** (Fig. 13.8) are represented as four small (5 × 4 × 2 mm) individual glands located on the posterosuperior and posteroinferior poles of the thyroid gland. Each parathyroid gland is enveloped in its own connective tissue **capsule**, which may become infiltrated by adipose cells in an adult. Connective tissue **septa** entering the substance of the glands convey nerves, blood vessels, and lymph vessels, and support the cords of parenchymal cells and the rich capillary network. The parathyroid glands produce **parathyroid hormone (PTH)**, which (see Table 13.4):

- Increases blood calcium levels and, in concert with **calcitonin**, produced by the parafollicular cells of the thyroid, maintains optimal concentrations of calcium within the bloodstream and the interstitial fluid.
- Binds to PTH receptors of osteoblasts, prompting them to release **osteoclast-stimulating factor** to increase the number and activity of osteoclasts.
- Acts on the kidneys to conserve calcium and to increase the production of **vitamin D**, which enhances the ability of the alimentary canal to increase the amount of calcium absorption.

The parenchyma of the parathyroid gland is composed of two cell populations, chief cells and oxyphil cells.

- **Chief cells**, small, round, eosinophilic cells that form clusters of cells throughout the richly vascularized substance of the parathyroid glands, manufacture **preproparathyroid hormone** on their rough endoplasmic reticulum. This prohormone is cleaved within the rough endoplasmic reticulum to form **proparathyroid hormone**, which is transported to the Golgi complex where it is cleaved to form **PTH**. The packaged hormone is stored in secretory granules until its release via exocytosis.
- **Oxyphil cells** are larger, stain darker, and are much fewer in number than chief cells. They appear in small clusters, and their function is unknown, although some investigators suggest that they are inactive chief cells.

CLINICAL CONSIDERATIONS

Primary hyperparathyroidism, a condition most prevalent in women, is an overproduction of PTH. The word *primary* in this case indicates that overproduction is due to a nonmalignant hyperplasia of one or more of the parathyroid glands. Excess plasma levels of PTH cause an overabundance of calcium and decreased phosphate levels in the blood and interstitial fluid. This condition results in bone mineral loss; bone pain and fractures; muscle weakness; paresthesia; fatigue; development of kidney stones, nausea, vomiting, confusion, and depression.

Hypoparathyroidism results from a deficiency in secreting PTH. A common cause is injury to one or more of the parathyroid glands during thyroid surgery. Hypoparathyroidism is characterized by low blood calcium levels, retention of bone calcium, and increased phosphate resorption in the kidneys. Symptoms include muscle spasms, paresthesia, numbness, tingling, muscle tetany in facial and laryngeal muscles, cataract formation, mental confusion, and loss of memory. Intravenous doses of calcium gluconate, vitamin D, and oral calcium are the only treatment for survival.

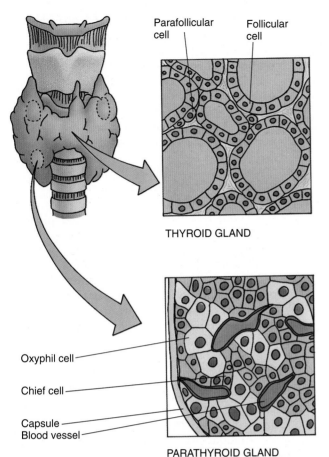

Parafollicular cell

Follicular cell

THYROID GLAND

Oxyphil cell

Chief cell

Capsule
Blood vessel

PARATHYROID GLAND

Figure 13.8 The thyroid and parathyroid glands. *(From Gartner LP, Hiatt JL: Color Textbook of Histology, 3rd ed. Philadelphia, Saunders, 2007, p 313.)*

CLINICAL CONSIDERATIONS

Graves' disease is the most common form of hyperthyroidism, resulting from the immune system attacking the thyroid gland, causing an overproduction of the hormone thyroxine. When severe, it attacks the tissues behind the eyes, producing exophthalmos and skin lesions around the shins and tops of the feet. Additionally, Graves' disease can increase the body's metabolic rate, leading to a number of health problems, including increased heart rate. It is most common in women older than 20 years. Treatments do not stop the immune attacks, but they can ease symptoms and decrease thyroxine production.

Simple goiter is an enlargement of the thyroid gland resulting from an insufficient intake of iodine. Simple goiter is associated with neither hyperthyroidism nor hypothyroidism and can be treated with supplemental intake of iodine in the diet.

Hypothyroidism, or underactive thyroid, is a condition in which the thyroid gland does not produce enough hormones. It is most common in women older than 50 years. When left untreated, it upsets the normal balance in the body and can cause many health problems, including fatigue, obesity, joint pain, heart disease, mental sluggishness, loss of hair, and failure of body functions. Synthetic thyroid hormone is the effective treatment of choice.

Myxedema is an extreme form of hypothyroidism resulting in several health problems, including depression, mental slowness, weakness, bradycardia, and fatigue. Additional symptoms include a swollen face, bagginess under the eyes, and nonpitting edema of the skin as a result of excesses of glycosaminoglycans and proteoglycans infiltrating the extracellular matrix. Patients with myxedema need immediate medical attention.

Cretinism is a severe form of hypothyroidism occurring in fetal life through childhood as a result of the congenital absence of a thyroid gland. Patients with cretinism display severely stunted physical and mental growth.

Suprarenal Glands (Adrenal Glands)

The paired **suprarenal glands** are surrounded by an abundance of adipose tissue in their position on the superior pole of each kidney. Each of these small glands weighs less than 10 g and is invested by its **capsule** that provides slender connective tissue elements that convey neural elements and a profuse blood supply into the substance of the gland. The glands are subdivided into an outer **cortex** and a small, inner **medulla** (Fig. 13.9), each with a different embryonic origin; the cortex is derived from mesoderm, whereas the medulla arises from neural crest. Each suprarenal gland has three arteries supplying it: the superior, middle, and inferior suprarenal arteries. These vessels perforate the capsule and form the **subcapsular plexus** from which short and long cortical arteries arise.

- Short cortical arteries give rise to:
  - Fenestrated **sinusoidal capillaries**, whose fenestrae increase in diameter as the capillaries penetrate deeper into the cortex.
  - Sinusoidal capillaries, which are drained by small **venules** that pass through the medulla and deliver their blood into the **suprarenal vein**
- **Long cortical arteries** have no branches in the cortex; they enter the medulla and form a capillary plexus, which is drained by small venules that deliver their blood into the suprarenal vein.

The **suprarenal cortex** is composed of three overlapping concentric zones: the outermost zona glomerulosa; the middle and widest region, the zona fasciculata; and the innermost zone, the zona reticularis (see Fig. 13.9). These regions secrete the cholesterol-based hormones, mineralocorticoids, glucocorticoids, and androgens, in response to the binding of ACTH to their ACTH receptors (see Table 13.4).

- The parenchymal cells of the **zona glomerulosa**, the outermost of the three concentric regions of the suprarenal cortex, display occasional lipid droplets and a wealth of smooth endoplasmic reticulum. These cells manufacture, in response to ACTH and angiotensin II, **aldosterone** and a limited quantity of **deoxycorticosterone**. Mineralocorticoids help regulate electrolyte and water balance by acting on distal convoluted tubules of the kidneys.
- The widest region of the cortex is the **zona fasciculata**, whose large cells, arranged in longitudinal columns, are so well-endowed by lipid droplets that in histologic sections they resemble sponges—hence they are called **spongiocytes**. In response to the presence of ACTH, these cells secrete the glucocorticoids **cortisol** and **corticosterone**, hormones that control the metabolism of lipids, proteins, and carbohydrates. They enhance gluconeogenesis and glycogen synthesis in the liver, and lipolysis and proteolysis in adipocytes and muscle cells. In excess levels, they suppress the immune system and have anti-inflammatory properties.
- The thinnest and innermost region of the cortex is the **zona reticularis**, whose cells resemble the spongiocytes of the zona fasciculata but with smaller lipid droplets. The parenchymal cells of this zone are arranged in networks of anastomosing cords and manufacture **androgens**, predominantly **dehydroepiandrosterone** and **androstenedione**; neither dehydroepiandrosterone nor androstenedione exerts any significant effects in a healthy individual.

The **suprarenal medulla** (see Fig. 13-9 and Table 13.4) is quite small, constituting approximately 10% of the suprarenal gland in weight. The richly vascularized medulla has an ample neural supply and is composed of two types of parenchymal cells, the more populous **chromaffin cells** and the large, **sympathetic ganglion cells**.

- **Chromaffin cells** received their name because they have a great affinity to chromaffin salts, indicating that their cytoplasm is well endowed with **catecholamines**, specifically **epinephrine** and **norepinephrine**. These cells are ubiquitous throughout the suprarenal medulla and are arranged in cordlike clusters. Chromaffin cells are innervated by preganglionic sympathetic neurons. When these neurons release their neurotransmitter, **acetylcholine**, it binds to the acetylcholine receptors of chromaffin cells, depolarizing their plasmalemma and resulting in the release of epinephrine (if the stimulus is physiologic) or norepinephrine (if the stimulus is emotional) into the capillary beds.
  - **Epinephrine** increases blood pressure and heart rate and depresses gastrointestinal smooth muscle motility.
  - **Norepinephrine** increases blood pressure by causing vascular smooth muscle contraction.
- **Sympathetic ganglion cells** are scattered throughout the suprarenal medulla and modified so that they are without dendrites and axons.

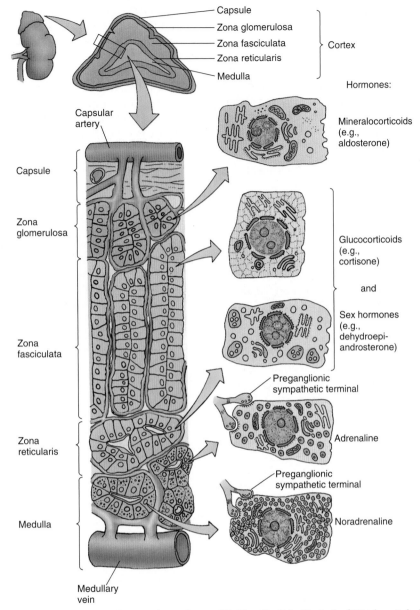

Capsule
Zona glomerulosa
Zona fasciculata
Zona reticularis
Medulla
Cortex

Hormones:

Capsular artery

Capsule

Zona glomerulosa

Mineralocorticoids (e.g., aldosterone)

Zona fasciculata

Glucocorticoids (e.g., cortisone)

and

Sex hormones (e.g., dehydroepi-androsterone)

Zona reticularis

Preganglionic sympathetic terminal

Adrenaline

Medulla

Preganglionic sympathetic terminal

Noradrenaline

Medullary vein

Figure 13.9 The suprarenal gland and its cell types. *(From Gartner LP, Hiatt JL: Color Textbook of Histology, 3rd ed. Philadelphia, Saunders, 2007, p 319.)*

CLINICAL CONSIDERATIONS

Cushing's syndrome (hyperadrenocorticism) results from adenomas located in the anterior pituitary gland leading to an increase in ACTH production. Excess ACTH causes the adrenal glands to be enlarged, the suprarenal cortex to be hypertrophied, and the overproduction of cortisol. Patients are obese, especially in the face, neck, and trunk. They exhibit muscle wasting and osteoporosis. Men become sterile, and women have amenorrhea.

Addison's disease is an adrenocortical insufficiency resulting from destruction of the adrenal cortex from some diseases. It is most often caused by an autoimmune process. It can be caused by tuberculosis and some other infectious diseases. Symptoms develop over several months and include fatigue, muscle weakness, low blood pressure, nausea, vomiting, joint pains, decreased blood glucose, weight loss, and depression. Treatment is by replacement hormones.

Pineal Gland (Pineal Body)

The **pineal gland**, an evagination of the roof of the diencephalon (see Table 13.4), is a small endocrine gland weighing less than 150 mg. It is covered by **pia mater**, which, acting as a capsule, sends blood vessel–bearing septa into the substance of the gland, subdividing it into partial lobules. Two cell types compose the parenchyma of this gland—pinealocytes and interstitial cells.

- **Pinealocytes**, the principal cells of the pineal gland, possess one or two long tortuous processes whose terminals are flattened and dilated as they approach the capillaries. These cells possess a well-developed cytoskeleton and specialized tubular structures of unknown function, called **synaptic ribbons**, whose numbers increase during the dark segment of the diurnal cycle. Postganglionic sympathetic fibers form synapses with pinealocytes, stimulating them to release **melatonin** at night but not during the day, establishing the body's diurnal rhythm. By inhibiting the release of growth hormone and gonadotropin, they regulate certain bodily functions. Levels of melatonin in the blood are highest before bedtime.

- The glia-like **interstitial cells** are more prominent in the pineal stalk than in the bulk of the gland. They stain deeply and possess long cellular processes containing intermediate filaments, microfilaments, and microtubules. These cells, along with connective tissue, provide support to the pinealocytes.

- The pineal gland contains calcified structures known as **corpora arenacea (brain sand)** of unknown function or origin. Calcification begins early in childhood and increases throughout life.

CLINICAL CONSIDERATIONS

The central nervous system may be protected to some degree by the action of melatonin in scavenging and eliminating free radicals resulting from oxidative stress. Some individuals use melatonin as a supplement to combat mood and sleep disorders and depression. It has been reported that exposure to bright artificial light may inhibit the production of melatonin, easing depression. Additionally, many individuals suggest that doses of melatonin taken at the *proper* time may reduce jet lag.

Table 13.4 HORMONES AND FUNCTIONS OF THE THYROID, PARATHYROID, ADRENAL, AND PINEAL GLANDS

Hormone	Cell Source	Regulating Hormone	Function
Thyroid Gland			
Thyroxine (T_4) and triiodothyronine (T_3)	Follicular cells	TSH	Facilitate nuclear transcription of genes responsible for protein synthesis; increase cellular metabolism, growth rates; facilitate mental processes; increase endocrine gland activity; stimulate carbohydrate and fat metabolism; decrease cholesterol, phospholipids, and triglycerides; increase fatty acids; decrease body weight; increase heart rate, respiration, muscle action
Calcitonin (thyrocalcitonin)	Parafollicular cells	Feedback mechanism with parathyroid hormone	Decreases plasma calcium concentration by suppressing bone resorption
Parathyroid Gland			
Parathyroid hormone (PTH)	Chief cells	Feedback mechanism with calcitonin	Increases calcium concentration in body fluids
Suprarenal (Adrenal) Glands and Suprarenal Cortex			
Mineralocorticoids: aldosterone and deoxycorticosterone	Cells of zona glomerulosa	Angiotensin II and ACTH	Control body fluid volume and electrolyte concentrations by acting on distal tubules of the kidney, causing excretion of potassium and resorption of sodium
Glucocorticoids: cortisol and corticosterone	Cells of zona fasciculata (spongiocytes)	ACTH	Regulate metabolism of carbohydrates, fats, and proteins; decrease protein synthesis, increasing amino acids in blood; stimulate gluconeogenesis by activating liver to convert amino acids to glucose; release fatty acid and glycerol; act as anti-inflammatory agents; reduce capillary permeability; suppress immune response
Androgens: dehydroepiandrosterone and androstenedione	Cells of zona reticularis	ACTH	Provides weak masculinizing characteristics
Suprarenal Medulla			
Catecholamines: epinephrine and norepinephrine	Chromaffin cells	Preganglionic, sympathetic, and splanchnic nerves	*Epinephrine*—operates "fight or flight" mechanism preparing the body for severe fear or stress; increases cardiac heart rate and output, augmenting blood flow to organs and release of glucose from liver for energy *Norepinephrine*—Causes elevation in blood pressure by vasoconstriction
Pineal Gland			
Melatonin	Pinealocytes	Norepinephrine	May influence cyclic gonadal activity

From Gartner LP, Hiatt JL: Color Textbook of Histology, 3rd ed. Philadelphia, Saunders, 2007, p 312.

14 INTEGUMENT

The **integument**, the largest and heaviest organ in the body (weighing approximately 15% of total body weight and having an average surface area of about 2 m²), comprises the skin, hair, sebaceous glands, nails, and sweat glands. It covers the entire surface of the body and becomes continuous with the mucous membranes of the digestive, respiratory, and urogenital systems at their external orifices. Skin lines the outer ear canal, covers the eardrums, and is continuous with the conjunctiva of the eye at the eyelid.

Skin

Skin is composed of two layers: the outer stratified squamous keratinized epithelium, known as the **epidermis**, which overlies the connective tissue layer, called the **dermis** (Fig. 14.1). The epidermis is separated from the dermis by a **basement membrane**. The junction is not a flat plane; instead, the dermis forms conelike and ridge-like elevations—**dermal ridges (dermal papillae)**. The dermal ridges are precisely matched by the contours of the epidermis—the **epidermal ridges (epidermal papillae)**. The epidermal ridges and dermal ridges together are known as the **rete apparatus**. Deep to the dermis is a fascial layer, the **hypodermis (superficial fascia)**, which may contain a considerable amount of adipose tissue in overweight individuals, but the hypodermis is not considered to be a component of skin.

Skin has a plethora of functions. The most prevalent are:

- Forming a supple cover for the body
- Protecting against impact and abrasion injury, bacterial assault, and dehydration
- Absorbing ultraviolet (UV) radiation for vitamin D production
- Receiving information from the external milieu (e.g., touch, pain, temperature)
- Regulating temperature
- Excreting sweat
- Producing melanin (protecting the deeper layers from excessive UV radiation)

The presence of raised ridges with intervening grooves in the forms of loops, whorls, and arches—**dermatoglyphs (fingerprints)**—on the pads of the fingertips and toes provides for a less slippery surface so that smaller objects may be held more securely and provides sensory input for the identification of the object being handled.

> **KEY WORDS**
> - **Skin**
> - **Keratinocytes**
> - **Nonkeratinocytes of the epidermis**
> - **Dermis**
> - **Glands of skin**
> - **Hair**
> - **Nails**

EPIDERMIS

The **epidermis**, the outer layer of skin, is avascular and receives its nutrients via diffusion from the capillary networks of the dermis. The epidermis is composed of a stratified squamous keratinized epithelium whose average thickness is less than 0.1 mm, although on the palm of the hand it may be almost 1 mm in thickness, and on the sole of the foot it may be 1.4 mm thick. There are two types of skin (Table 14.1; see Fig. 14.1):

- **Thick skin**, present on the palm of the hand and the sole of the foot, is hairless, has no arrector pili muscles, and has no sebaceous glands, although it does have sweat glands.
- **Thin skin**, present on the remainder of the body, possesses hair follicles, arrector pili muscles, sebaceous glands, and sweat glands.

Four different cell types compose the epidermis—**keratinocytes**, **Langerhans cells**, **melanocytes**, and **Merkel cells**—of which keratinocytes are the most populous and are the ones that are derived from ectoderm. The other three cell types are distributed among the keratinocytes.

Because the cells on the epithelial surface are desquamated, the lost cells are replaced by mitotic activity of keratinocytes occupying the deeper layers of the epidermis. It is believed that **epidermal growth factor** and **interleukin-1α** induce mitotic activity of keratinocytes, and **transforming growth factor** is believed to inhibit such activity. Cell division occurs only at night, and the newly formed cells push the cells above them toward the surface, eventually to be sloughed off. It takes approximately 1 month for a newly formed cell to reach the free surface and be desquamated. As keratinocytes move toward the free surface, they undergo **cytomorphosis**, which permits the epidermis to be divided into five layers. Only three of the five layers are evident in thin skin, whereas all five layers are observable in thick skin.

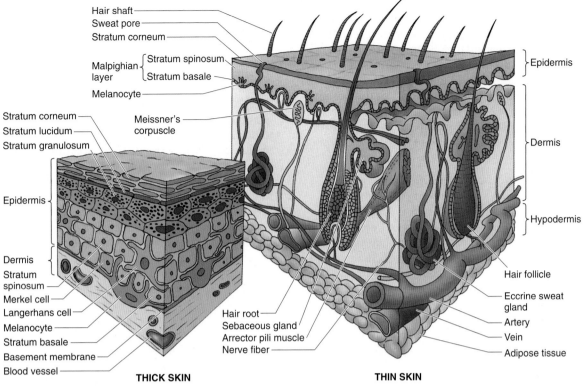

Figure 14.1 Comparison of thick skin and thin skin. *(From Gartner LP, Hiatt JL: Color Textbook of Histology, 3rd ed. Philadelphia, Saunders, 2007, p 328.)*

Table 14.1 CHARACTERISTICS OF THICK AND THIN SKIN

Skin Type	Examples	Thickness (μm)	Strata	Appendages
Thick skin	Palms, soles	400–600	All five strata	Without hair follicles, arrector pili muscles, and sebaceous glands
Thin skin	Remainder of the body	75–150	Without distinct stratum lucidum and granulosum	With hair follicles, arrector pili muscles, and sebaceous and sweat glands

Layers of the Epidermis

The five layers of the epidermis of **thick skin** are stratum basale (stratum germinativum), sitting directly on the basement membrane; stratum spinosum; stratum granulosum; stratum lucidum; and stratum corneum (Fig. 14.2 and Table 14.2). Keratinocytes of the five layers adhere to adjacent cells via desmosomal contacts. Isolated cells of the strata granulosum and lucidum are present in **thin skin**, but their cells do not form distinct layers as they do in thick skin. Thin skin has only three of the five strata.

- The **stratum basale (stratum germinativum)**, composed of a single layer of cuboidal to low columnar-shaped cells, sits on the basement membrane. These cells undergo cell division, and the newly formed cells push the older cells lying above them toward the free surface. Stratum basale cells form hemidesmosomes with the underlying basal lamina and desmosomes with their adjacent cells. The desmosomal and hemidesmosomal plaques have bundles of intermediate filaments (**tonofilaments**) associated with them. Their cytoplasm has a limited organelle content but is rich in ribosomes.

- The **stratum spinosum** is a substantial region composed of several layers of cells that are polyhedral in shape in the vicinity of the stratum basale but become flatter as the cells migrate away from the basement membrane. The polyhedral cells display mitotic activity, but cells in the more superficial layers of the stratum spinosum no longer divide. The organelles of these cells resemble those of the stratum basale; however, their tonofilaments are better developed, especially in the more superficially located flattened cells, forming thicker bundles known as **tonofibrils**. In the same region, the flattened cells house secretory granules called membrane-coating granules (**lamellar granules**), which are less than 0.5 μm in diameter and contain lamellar deposits of lipid. Cytoplasmic extensions of these cells resemble spines—hence the name of this layer. The spines of adjacent cells interdigitate with each other, and by forming desmosomes these cells adhere to each other and to cells of the strata basale and granulosum.

- Cells of the **stratum granulosum** house membrane-coating granules and non–membrane-bound deposits of **keratohyalin** in which bundles of tonofilaments are embedded. The contents of the membrane-coating granules are exocytosed into the extracellular space superficial to the stratum spinosum so that there is a pool of **lipid barrier** that accumulates between the stratum granulosum and the stratum lucidum that prevents aqueous fluid from penetrating in either direction. The presence of this lipid makes the epidermis impermeable to water, preventing fluid loss from the underlying dermis and the entry of water into the dermis from outside the body.

- The **stratum lucidum** is a transparent layer of cells whose organelles, including its nucleus, have been eliminated by lysosomal action. These are dead cells, but they are packed with a significant amount of tonofilaments enveloped by **eleidin**, a derivative of keratohyalin. The cell membranes of these cells are coated on their cytoplasmic aspect by the protein **involucrin**, whose function is not understood.

- The **stratum corneum**, the most superficial layer, is usually the thickest layer of the epidermis of thick skin. The plasma membranes of these dead cells, known as **squames**, are thickened, and they are filled with **keratin filaments**. Cells of the most superficial layers of the stratum corneum cannot maintain desmosomal contact with their neighbors and are sloughed off.

Table 14.2 STRATA AND HISTOLOGIC FEATURES OF THICK SKIN

Layer	Histologic Features
Epidermis	Derived from ectoderm; composed of stratified squamous keratinized epithelium (keratinocytes)
Stratum corneum	Numerous layers of dead flattened keratinized cells, keratinocytes, without nuclei and organelles (squames, or horny cells) that are sloughed off
Stratum lucidum*	Lightly stained thin layer of keratinocytes without nuclei and organelles; cells contain densely packed keratin filaments and eleidin
Stratum granulosum*	Three to five cell layers thick. These keratinocytes still retain nuclei; cells contain large, coarse keratohyalin granules and membrane-coating granules
Stratum spinosum	Thickest layer of epidermis, whose keratinocytes, known as prickle cells, interdigitate with one another by forming intercellular bridges and numerous desmosomes; prickle cells have numerous tonofilaments and membrane-coating granules and are mitotically active; this layer also houses Langerhans cells.
Stratum basale (germinativum)	Single layer of cuboidal to low columnar, mitotically active cells, separated from the papillary layer of the dermis by a well-developed basement membrane; Merkel cells and melanocytes are also present in this layer.
Dermis	Derived from mesoderm; composed mostly of type I collagen and elastic fibers, subdivided into two regions—papillary layer and reticular layer, a dense, irregular collagenous connective tissue
Papillary layer	Interdigitates with epidermis, forming the dermal papilla component of the rete apparatus; type III collagen and elastic fibers in loose arrangement and anchoring fibrils (type VII collagen); abundant capillary beds, connective tissue cells, and mechanoreceptors are located in this layer; occasionally, melanocytes are also present in the papillary layer.
Reticular layer	Deepest layer of skin; type I collagen, thick elastic fibers, and connective tissue cells; contains sweat glands and their ducts, hair follicles and arrector pili muscles, and sebaceous glands and mechanoreceptors (e.g., pacinian corpuscles)

*Present only in thick skin. All layers are usually thinner in thin skin.
From Gartner LP, Hiatt JL: Color Textbook of Histology, 3rd ed. Philadelphia, Saunders, 2007, p 329.

CLINICAL CONSIDERATIONS

Psoriasis is a chronic, noncontagious autoimmune disease that affects the skin and joints. It is characterized by patchy lesions especially around the joints called **psoriatic plaques**, which are brought about by an increase in the number of proliferating cells of the stratum basale, resulting in an accumulation of cells of the stratum corneum. Plaques frequently occur on the skin of the elbows and knees but can affect any area, including the scalp and genitals; even the fingernails and toenails may be affected. Psoriasis can also cause inflammation of the joints, which is known as **psoriatic arthritis**. Of individuals with psoriasis, 10% to 15% have psoriatic arthritis.

Epidermolysis bullosa, one of a group of hereditary diseases, is characterized by blistering of the skin after minor trauma. It is caused by defects in the intermediate filaments of the keratinocytes that prevent stability in these cells and defects in anchoring fibrils between the dermis and epidermis.

Nonkeratinocytes in the Epidermis

There are three types of **nonkeratinocytes** in the epidermis (see Fig. 14.2):

- **Langerhans cells**, antigen-presenting cells derived from the bone marrow, are scattered throughout the stratum spinosum; there may be 800 Langerhans cells per square millimeter. The nuclei and cytoplasm are not unusual except for the presence of cytoplasmic **Birbeck granules** (**vermiform granules**), which resemble table tennis paddles in section and whose function is unknown. These cells appear clear with the light microscope and may be differentiated from surrounding keratinocytes by the absence of tonofilaments. Similar to other antigen-presenting cells, Langerhans cells possess Fc and C3 receptors, phagocytose antigens, form epitope–major histocompatibility complexes, and migrate to nearby lymph nodes, where they present their epitope–major histocompatibility complexes to T cells.
- **Merkel cells**, derived from neural crest, are clear cells located in the stratum basale, especially in the oral mucosa, hair follicles, and tips of the fingers. The nuclei of these cells have deep grooves, their cytoskeleton is rich in cytokeratins, and they are closely linked with myelinated sensory fibers, forming **Merkel cell–neurite** associations. Merkel cells function as **mechanoreceptors** responsible for light touch.

- **Melanocytes** also are neural crest derivatives and are located in the stratum basale, but they have long, slender, finger-like processes that extend into the stratum spinosum, where their tips are surrounded by cytoplasmic extensions of keratinocytes. Melanocytes possess oval-shaped granules (except in individuals with red hair these granules are spherical) containing the enzyme tyrosinase, known as **melanosomes**. In these melanosomes, the tyrosinase converts tyrosine into the dark pigment **melanin**. Melanosomes migrate into the tip of the melanocyte processes accumulating more and more melanin along the way, a process stimulated by UV radiation. The tips of these melanocyte processes are nipped off by keratinocytes, a process known as **cytocrine secretion**, and the melanosomes located within the keratinocytes of the stratum spinosum are attacked by lysosomal enzymes, to be degraded within a few days. Meanwhile, the melanin acts to protect the keratinocytes from UV irradiation. Although the population density of melanocytes varies with regions of the body of a single individual, the numbers are essentially the same across the races. The differences in skin color are due not to a greater number of melanocytes but to the greater production and slower degradation of melanin.

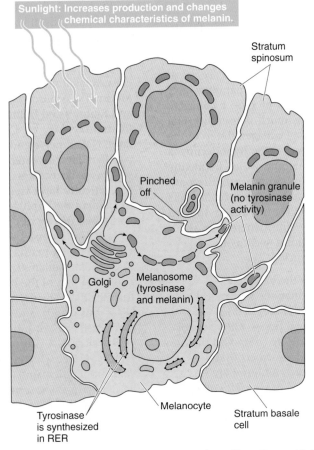

Sunlight: Increases production and changes chemical characteristics of melanin.

Stratum spinosum

Pinched off

Melanin granule (no tyrosinase activity)

Golgi

Melanosome (tyrosinase and melanin)

Tyrosinase is synthesized in RER

Melanocyte

Stratum basale cell

Figure 14.2 Melanocytes and their function. RER, rough endoplasmic reticulum. *(From Gartner LP, Hiatt JL: Color Textbook of Histology, 3rd ed. Philadelphia, Saunders, 2007, p 334.)*

CLINICAL CONSIDERATIONS

In the presence of UV light, tyrosinase activity is increased, resulting in acceleration of melanin production. Also, melanin is darkened by the presence of UV light. Pigmentation is also influenced by adrenocorticotropic hormone of the pituitary gland. In certain instances, such as in patients with **Addison's disease**, the production of cortisol is insufficient, causing an excess of adrenocorticotropic hormone that results in hyperpigmentation.

Vitiligo is a disease in which certain areas of the skin (often the face and hands) are devoid of pigmentation. This autoimmune disease destroys the melanocytes, resulting in an area devoid of pigmentation, although keratinocytes are unaffected. Vitiligo is usually associated with other autoimmune disorders.

Albinism is a genetic defect resulting in the complete lack of melanin production. Individuals with albinism possess melanosomes but fail to produce tyrosinase, and so they are devoid of melanin.

Moles (nevi) are benign accumulations of melanocytes in the epidermis. They vary in size from small dots to more than 1 inch in diameter. They may be flat or raised, may be smooth or rough (wartlike), and may have hairs growing from them. Although they are usually brown or dark brown, some moles are flesh-colored.

UV rays are of two types. UVB rays are responsible for sunburn, whereas UVA rays tan the skin. It has been shown that UV radiation may be an important factor in photoaging and in the development of basal cell carcinoma and melanoma later in life.

DERMIS

The connective tissue layer deep to the epidermis, known as the **dermis**, is composed of two regions: the superficial **papillary layer** and the deeper **reticular layer**. Both layers are composed of a dense, irregular fibroelastic connective tissue. The papillary layer is loose, with slender bundles of type I collagen, whereas the reticular layer is much denser, housing thick, coarse bundles of type I collagen. Deep to the dermis, but not a part of skin, is the **hypodermis**, a superficial fascia of gross anatomy, which frequently houses a variable layer of adipose tissue, the **panniculus adiposus**, which can be several centimeters thick in obese individuals. The dermis is thin in certain regions, as in the eyelids, where it is about 0.6 mm thick. In other regions, such as the sole of the foot, it may be 3 mm thick.

- The **papillary layer** abuts the basement membrane, forming evaginations known as **dermal ridges (dermal papillae)** that interdigitate with epidermal ridges. The fibers of this loose connective tissue are composed of type III collagen and slender elastic fibers that intertwine with one another. Additionally, anchoring fibrils, composed of type VII collagen fibers, attach to the reticular fibers to assist in securing the basement membrane to the papillary layer and, in this fashion, affixing the epidermis to the dermis. The cells of the papillary layer are the normal cells of connective tissue proper, but this region also houses capillary loops to provide nutrients for the avascular epidermis and aid in regulating body temperature. Additionally, encapsulated neural nerve endings, such as Meissner's corpuscles for mechanoreception and Krause's end bulbs, which may be thermoreceptors, are located in the papillary layer. Naked nerve endings penetrate the papillary layer to enter the epidermis, where they serve as pain receptors.

- The **reticular layer** is a much denser connective tissue than the papillary layer, and its fibers are composed mostly of coarse bundles of type I collagen interspersed with thick elastic fibers embedded in a matrix of ground substance rich in dermatan sulfate. The cellular composition is similar to that of the papillary layer but not quite as rich. The deep aspects of sweat glands, sebaceous glands, and hair follicles, with their associated arrector pili muscles, are located in the dermis. A rich plexus of blood and lymph vessels, which give rise to smaller vessels that supply the papillary layer, also is located in the dermis. Encapsulated neural elements such as **pacinian corpuscles** and **Ruffini's corpuscles** respond to deep pressure and tensile forces.

The three types of malignant tumors of the skin are basal cell carcinoma, squamous cell carcinoma, and malignant melanoma. **Basal cell carcinoma**, the most common malignancy in humans, affects approximately 1 million Americans each year. Almost all basal cell carcinomas occur on parts of the body excessively exposed to the sun, especially the face, ears, neck, scalp, shoulders, and back. Individuals at highest risk have fair skin and light-colored hair. It most often affects older individuals, but younger individuals have become more affected in recent years. Individuals who work or spend their leisure time in the sun are particularly susceptible. Basal cell carcinoma arises in the cells of the stratum basale. A lesion forms at the affected site, which may appear as psoriasis or eczema or as a small sore (e.g., on the face) that bleeds and does not heal. Only a trained physician can diagnose basal cell carcinoma, and it must be confirmed by biopsy. Surgical removal is the usual treatment. Although basal cell carcinomas normally do not metastasize, individuals who have experienced one episode are at risk for recurrence.

Squamous cell carcinoma is the second most common skin cancer. More than 250,000 new cases are diagnosed each year in the United States. Middle-aged and older individuals with fair complexions who have been exposed to the sun for a prolonged period are most likely to be affected. The keratinocytes of the skin are affected, and the lesions appear as crusted or scaly patches on the skin with a red, inflamed base or a nonhealing ulcer. They are generally found in sun-exposed areas, but they may occur on the lips, inside the mouth, on the genitalia, or anywhere on the body. Any lesion, especially lesions that enlarge, bleed, change in appearance, or do not heal, should be evaluated by a dermatologist. Early diagnosis and treatment are important because lesions can increase in size and metastasize. Surgical intervention is the usual treatment.

Malignant melanoma is a very serious malignant tumor of melanocytes. These transformed cells multiply, invade the dermis, enter the lymphatic and circulatory systems, and metastasize to many organs. Melanoma affects fair-skinned individuals more frequently, especially when these individuals are exposed to excessive UV rays. Evidence suggests that UV radiation used in indoor tanning equipment may cause melanoma. The risk may also be inherited. Malignant melanoma is curable when detected early, but can be fatal if allowed to progress and spread. The usual treatment after early detection is surgical excision.

Glands of the Skin

Although skin has four different types of **glands** (Fig. 14.3), only three of them are described in this chapter: eccrine sweat glands, apocrine sweat glands, and sebaceous glands. The fourth type of skin gland, the mammary gland, which is a highly modified sweat gland, is described with the female reproductive system in Chapter 20.

- Almost 4 million **eccrine sweat glands** are distributed throughout most of the skin covering the body. Each of these **simple coiled tubular glands** is an ectodermal derivative (invested by a basement membrane) that grows down through the epidermis and dermis and frequently enters the hypodermis. There it forms the highly coiled, **merocrine secretory portion** of the gland. Arising from the secretory portion is the narrower, corkscrew-shaped **duct** that pierces the tip or crest of a dermal ridge and enters the epidermis to end at its free surface as a sweat pore.
- The simple cuboidal to low columnar epithelium of the secretory portion is composed of dark cells and clear cells. **Myoepithelial** cells, rich in actin and myosin filaments, surround the cells of the secretory portion, assisting in the expression of sweat from its lumen.
  - **Dark cells** (**mucoid cells**) viewed with the electron microscope are seen to be pyramidal in shape, where the base is at the lumen and the apex of the cell may or may not reach the basal lamina. These cells manufacture and release a mucous type of secretion.
  - **Clear cells** are similar in shape to dark cells, with their bases abutting the basal lamina and their apex barely reaching the lumen. These cells exhibit a rich glycogen content and an intricately folded basal plasmalemma on electron micrographs, indicative of participating in epithelial transport. These cells manufacture and release into the lumen a serous secretory product.

The stratified cuboidal epithelium of the eccrine sweat gland duct is composed of a **basal layer** housing numerous mitochondria and a **luminal layer** with a scant amount of cytoplasm and an irregularly shaped nucleus.

Sweat produced by the secretory portion is more or less iso-osmotic with plasma, but the cells of the duct portion conserve sodium, chloride, and potassium, and excrete lactic acid, urea, and some ingested material, such as certain drugs and the essence of garlic.

- **Apocrine sweat glands** are similar to, but are much larger than, eccrine sweat glands and are located in the armpit (axilla), areola of the nipple, and circumanal area. Despite their name, they most probably secrete via the merocrine mode. They begin secretion only after puberty, are associated with and deliver their secretory product into the canals of hair follicles, and, in some women, undergo periodic alteration associated with the menstrual cycle. Although their secretion is odorless, bacterial metabolism converts it into an odoriferous substance, 3-methyl-1,2-hexanic acid, which may have pheromonal properties. There are certain modified apocrine sweat glands in the external ear canal, wax-producing ceruminous glands, and the glands of Moll in the eyelids.
- **Sebaceous glands** are **holocrine** glands that are associated with hair follicles. The ducts of these glands empty their secretory product, the oily **sebum**, into the canals of hair follicles; they are located only in glabrous (hairy) skin. The most peripheral cells of these globular glands are flat; they sit on a basement membrane and undergo cell division to produce more flat cells and larger, round cells. The larger cells are centrally located, and they accumulate lipid droplets that eventually displace the organelles of the cells, causing their degeneration, necrosis, and transformation into sebum that coats the hair shaft and skin surface. Sebum makes the hair less brittle and the skin more supple. Sebaceous glands, similar to apocrine sweat glands, are under hormonal control and become more active after puberty.

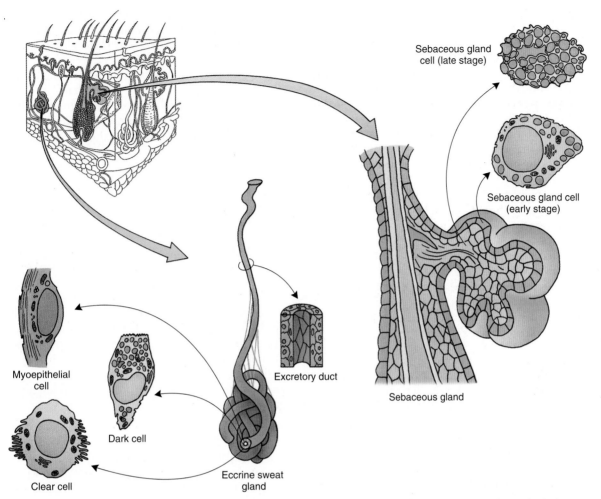

Sebaceous gland cell (late stage)

Sebaceous gland cell (early stage)

Sebaceous gland

Myoepithelial cell

Dark cell

Clear cell

Excretory duct

Eccrine sweat gland

Figure 14.3 An eccrine gland and a sebaceous gland and their constituent cells. *(From Gartner LP, Hiatt JL: Color Textbook of Histology, 3rd ed. Philadelphia, Saunders, 2007, p 337.)*

Hair

The surface of thin skin is covered with **hair** (Fig. 14.4), a keratinous filament whose amino acid composition determines whether it is soft and supple or coarse and wiry. Humans have three types of hair: **lanugo**, present only on fetuses and newborns; **vellus**, a soft, short, very fine hair, such as that present on the eyelids; and **terminal hairs**, the coarse, hard, dark hair that is located on the scalp and eyebrows and face in men. Humans appear to be much less hairy than other primates; however, that is because most human hair is vellus, whereas most primate hair is terminal hair. The number of hairs per square centimeter is the same in humans as in other primates.

Hair develops from **hair follicles**, epidermal invaginations that frequently extend into the hypodermis. They are enveloped in a basement membrane, known as the **glassy membrane**, which is surrounded by dermally derived connective tissue membrane. There are several components of a hair follicle:

- The **hair root** is an enlarged, hollow terminus whose concavity is occupied by vascular connective tissue elements known as the **dermal papilla**; the two together are known as the **hair bulb**.
- The core of the hair root consists of cells known as the **matrix**; the mitotic activity of these cells is responsible for hair growth.
- Immediately deep to the glassy membrane is a single layer of cells at the hair bulb that increase in number in the vicinity of the stratum corneum; this layer of cells is known as the **external root sheath**.
- The **internal root sheath**, surrounded by the external root sheath, is composed of three layers of cells: **Henley's layer**; **Huxley's layer**; and the deepest layer, the **cuticle of the internal root sheath**. The internal root sheath develops from the most peripheral cells of the matrix; it extends from the matrix to where the duct of the sebaceous gland enters the hair canal. The absence of the internal root sheath from that point leaves a space known as the **canal of the hair follicle**.
- The **hair shaft**, the part of the hair follicle that extends through the epidermis, has three layers:
  - Most peripheral is the **cuticle of the hair**, which arises from peripheral cells of the matrix.
  - Slightly peripheral, the **cortex** arises from the cells of the matrix peripheral to the center. During their migration away from their site of origin, the cells of the cortex manufacture and accumulate **keratin filaments** that become embedded in a matrix of **trichohyalin**, a substance similar to keratohyalin of the stratum granulosum, and form the hard keratin characteristic of the hair shaft.
- The central core of the hair shaft, the **medulla**, arises from the most central cells of the matrix. The medulla is displaced by the cells of the cortex as the hair shaft extends above the skin surface.

HAIR COLOR

Hair color is due to the production of melanin by melanocytes that occupy a position in the matrix along the basal lamina adjacent to the dermal papilla. The tips of the dendritic processes of the melanocytes become engulfed and are pinched off by cells of the cortex; depending on the quantity of melanin that the cells of the cortex carry with them, hair color ranges from light blond to dark black. As mentioned earlier, individuals with red hair have spherical rather than oval melanosomes. Gray hair of older individuals is due to the reduced activity of tyrosinase that prevents melanocytes from producing an adequate quantity of melanin pigment.

ARRECTOR PILI

Arrector pili are smooth muscle bundles that insert into the papillary layer of the dermis and, at an oblique angle, into the connective tissue sheet surrounding the external root sheet of the hair follicle. When these smooth muscle cells contract, they raise the hair shaft and depress the skin at the site of muscle attachment. The nondepressed regions of the epidermis seem to be elevated, giving the appearance of *goose bumps*.

HAIR GROWTH

The **growth of hair**, about 2 to 3 mm per week, occurs in three phases: the **anagen phase**, when the growth period may be 6 years for hair on the scalp but only a few months for hair in the underarm; the **catagen phase**, when the hair bulb involutes for a short time; and the **telogen phase**, when the hair follicle is at rest until the hair shaft falls out and a new hair shaft is formed in its place. Hair follicles in specific regions of the body alter from vellum hair to terminal hair in response to the presence of hormones. At puberty, pubic hairs and underarm hairs develop in boys and girls, and facial hair becomes coarse in boys.

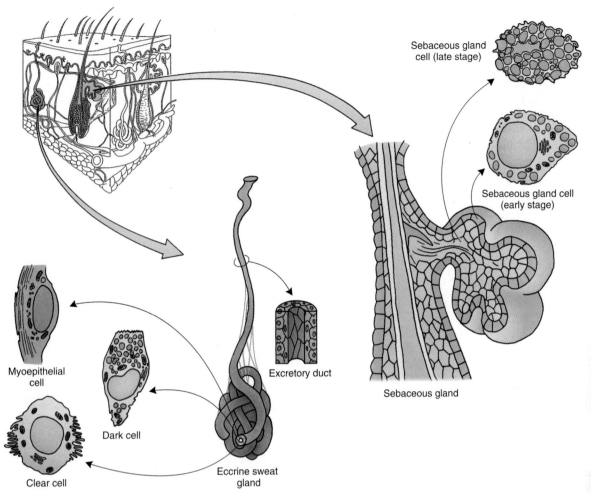

Sebaceous gland cell (late stage)

Sebaceous gland cell (early stage)

Sebaceous gland

Myoepithelial cell

Dark cell

Clear cell

Excretory duct

Eccrine sweat gland

Figure 14.4 An eccrine gland and a sebaceous gland and their constituent cells. *(From Gartner LP, Hiatt JL: Color Textbook of Histology, 3rd ed. Philadelphia, Saunders, 2007, p 337.)*

CLINICAL CONSIDERATIONS

Acne, a disease of the skin, is the most common disease seen by dermatologists. Acne is the term for plugged pores (blackheads and whiteheads), pimples, and deeper lumps (cysts or nodules) that occur on the face, neck, chest, back, shoulders, and upper arms. It affects nearly 100% of teenagers to some extent. Acne is not restricted to any age group, however; adults in their 40s can get acne. When severe, acne can lead to serious and permanent scarring. Several factors contribute to the development of acne. Acne is a result of obstructions causing an impacting of sebum within the hair follicle. The bacteria *Propionibacterium acnes* produce substances that cause redness and inflammation, and they produce enzymes, which dissolve the sebum into irritating substances that exacerbate the inflammation. Androgens, male hormones that are present in both sexes, enlarge the sebaceous glands and increase sebum production (during puberty), which may lead to plug formation progressing to acne. **Estrogens**, female hormones, improve acne in girls. The monthly menstrual cycle is due to changes in the estrogen levels, which is why acne in a girl may get better and then get worse as she goes through her monthly cycle. It is also believed that there is a genetic factor in acne, but the factor has not been identified.

Nails

Nails (**nail plates**) (Fig. 14.5), composed of thick plates of horny keratin, are located on the distal phalanx of each of the 20 digits. Each nail plate lies on the epidermal **nail bed** and grows from the **nail matrix** that is located in that part of the **nail root** that is directly deep to the **proximal nail fold**, a doubling over of the epidermis. The stratum corneum of the nail fold, known as the **eponych-ium** (**cuticle**), overlies the **lunula**, the white region of the nail plate. On the lateral aspects of the nail plate, the epidermis folds down to form the **lateral nail walls**, where each nail wall borders a longitudinal depression, the **nail groove**. Under the free end of the nail plate, the epidermis folds down, and its stratum corneum forms the cuticle-like **hyponychium**. Fingernails grow very slowly, about 2 mm per month, and toenails grow even more slowly.

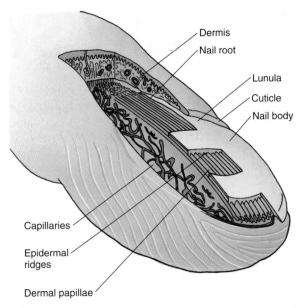

Dermis
Nail root
Lunula
Cuticle
Nail body
Capillaries
Epidermal ridges
Dermal papillae

Figure 14.5 Structure of the thumbnail. *(From Gartner LP, Hiatt JL: Color Textbook of Histology, 3rd ed. Philadelphia, Saunders, 2007, p 343.)*

CLINICAL CONSIDERATIONS

Onychomycosis is a common fungal disease, affecting mostly adults and particularly elderly adults, that attacks fingernails or toenails, causing them to thicken, discolor, disfigure, or split. The toenails are more likely to be affected. Without treatment, the nails can become so thickened that they may rub against the shoe, causing pain and inflammation.

15 RESPIRATORY SYSTEM

The respiratory system—the lungs and the airways leading to and from the lungs—distributes oxygen (O_2) to and removes carbon dioxide (CO_2) from the cells of the body. The ability of the respiratory system to accomplish these essential responsibilities depends on:

- **Ventilation (breathing)** that propels air to and from the lungs
- **External respiration**—transferring, in the bloodstream, the inhaled O_2 for the CO_2 released by cells
- O_2 and CO_2 **delivery**
- **Internal respiration**—exchange of O_2 for CO_2 in the cellular environment.

Ventilation and external respiration are the domains of the respiratory system, the delivery of O_2 and CO_2 is the function of the circulatory system, and internal respiration is a cellular event that occurs in the vicinity of all living cells. Proper function of the respiratory system requires that the inspired air be delivered by the **conducting portion** to the **respiratory portion**, where exchange of gases (external respiration) can occur.

Conducting Portion of the Respiratory System

The **conducting portion of the respiratory system** consists of the nasal cavity, mouth, nasopharynx, pharynx, larynx, trachea, primary bronchi, secondary bronchi, bronchioles, and terminal bronchioles. This system of conduits is kept patent by bone, cartilage, and fibroelastic connective tissue. As the passageways branch and get closer to the respiratory portion, they decrease in diameter but increase in number; the total cross-sectional areas *increase* at deeper levels, causing a *decrease* in the velocity of airflow as the inspired air approaches its final destination, the alveolus. Concomitantly, the velocity of the expired air increases as it approaches the nares and the lips.

The **nasal cavity** begins at the **nostrils (nares)**, ends at the **choanae**, and is divided into two halves by the bony and cartilaginous **nasal septum**.

- The **anterior aspect** is lined by thin skin (Table 15.1) with vibrissae, which filter larger particulate matter present in the inspired air.

- The pseudostratified columnar epithelium of the **posterior aspect** of the nasal cavity is rich in goblet cells (see Table 15.1). The underlying connective tissue has an abundant vascular supply with large venous sinusoids, seromucous glands, a rich supply of lymphoid cells and antibodies.
- The **olfactory region**, located in the posterosuperior aspect of the nasal cavity, is yellowish and houses the olfactory epithelium that perceives odors (Fig. 15.1). Cells of the olfactory epithelium include basal, sustentacular, and olfactory cells.
- **Basal cells** are small regenerative cells of two types: **horizontal**, which give rise to the second type, **globose**, which divide to form sustentacular and olfactory cells.
- **Sustentacular cells** make the yellow pigment that gives the olfactory epithelium its color. These cells establish junctional complexes with the sustentacular and olfactory cells that adjoin them, and provide support and electrical insulation to olfactory cell. Sustentacular cells live for 12 months.
- **Olfactory cells**, bipolar neurons of cranial nerve I (the olfactory nerve), are responsible for perception of odors. The dendrites of these cells extend to form a slight bulge, the olfactory vesicle, from which nonmotile olfactory cilia extend into the mucous layer of the nasal cavity. The axoneme of the cilia have the nine doublets surrounding the two singlets configuration, but distally the nine doublets degenerate into nine singlets that surround the pair of singlets in the middle. The opposite end of the olfactory cell body is its axon, which joins axons of other olfactory cells to form olfactory nerve fiber bundles, which pass through foramina in the cribriform plate and synapse with cells in the olfactory bulb.

The vascularized **lamina propria** possesses lymphatic elements and **Bowman's glands** that secrete a watery fluid containing odorant binding protein, IgA, and antimicrobial agents.

Table 15.1 CHARACTERISTIC FEATURES OF THE RESPIRATORY SYSTEM

Division	Region	Support	Glands	Epithelium	Cell Types	Additional Features
Extrapulmonary conducting	Nasal vestibule	Hyaline cartilage	Sebaceous and sweat glands	Stratified squamous keratinized	Epidermis	Vibrissae
	Nasal cavity: respiratory	Hyaline cartilage and bone	Seromucous glands	Respiratory	Basal, goblet, ciliated, brush, serous, DNES	Erectile-like tissue
	Nasal cavity: olfactory	Bone	Bowman's glands	Olfactory	Olfactory, sustentacular, and basal	Olfactory vesicle
Extrapulmonary conducting	Nasopharynx	Skeletal muscle	Seromucous glands	Respiratory	Basal, goblet, ciliated, brush, serous, DNES	Pharyngeal tonsils and eustachian tubes
	Larynx	Hyaline and elastic cartilages	Mucous and seromucous glands	Respiratory and stratified squamous nonkeratinized	Basal, goblet, ciliated, brush, serous, DNES	Epiglottis, vocal folds, and vestibular folds
Intrapulmonary conducting	Trachea and primary bronchi	Hyaline cartilage and dense, irregular collagenous CT	Mucous and seromucous glands	Respiratory	Basal, goblet, ciliated, brush, serous, DNES	C-rings and trachealis muscle (smooth muscle) in adventitia
	Secondary (intrapulmonary) bronchi	Hyaline cartilage and smooth muscle	Seromucous glands	Respiratory	Basal, goblet, ciliated, brush, serous, DNES	Plates of hyaline cartilage and two ribbons of helically oriented smooth muscle
	(Primary) bronchioles	Smooth muscle	No glands	Simple columnar to simple cuboidal	Ciliated cells and Clara cells (and occasional goblet cells in larger bronchioles)	<1 mm in diameter; supply air to lobules; two ribbons of helically oriented smooth muscle
	Terminal bronchioles	Smooth muscle	No glands	Simple cuboidal	Some ciliated cells and many Clara cells (no goblet cells)	<0.5 mm in diameter; supply air to lung acini; some smooth muscle
Respiratory	Respiratory bronchioles	Some smooth muscle and collagen fibers	No glands	Simple cuboidal and highly attenuated simple squamous	Some ciliated cuboidal cells, Clara cells, and types I and II pneumocytes	Alveoli in their walls; alveoli have smooth muscle sphincters in their opening
	Alveolar ducts	Type III collagen (reticular) fibers and smooth muscle sphincters of alveoli	No glands	Highly attenuated simple squamous	Types I and II pneumocytes of alveoli	No walls of their own, only a linear sequence of alveoli
	Alveolar sacs	Type III collagen and elastic fibers	No glands	Highly attenuated simple squamous	Types I and II pneumocytes	Clusters of alveoli
	Alveoli	Type III collagen and elastic fibers	No glands	Highly attenuated simple squamous	Types I and II pneumocytes	200 μm in diameter; have alveolar macrophages

CT, connective tissue; DNES, diffuse neuroendocrine system.
From Gartner LP, Hiatt JL: Color Textbook of Histology, 3rd ed. Philadelphia, Saunders, 2007, pp 346–347.

HISTOPHYSIOLOGY OF THE NASAL CAVITY

The richly vascularized nasal mucosa has an abundance of glands that produce mucus and watery fluid that keep the surface of the epithelium moist.

- The mucous layer traps particulate matter suspended in the inspired air.
- The cilia of the columnar cells of the pseudostratified epithelium sweep the mucus, with its entrapped particulate matter, toward the back of the throat to be eliminated.
- The rich vascular supply is arranged in such a fashion that a countercurrent mechanism is established that humidifies and warms the inspired air.
- The lymphoid elements present in the lamina propria capture allergens and antigens to ensure that foreign antigens are eliminated, although frequently symptoms associated with hay fever and colds are induced.

The olfactory epithelium (see Fig. 15.1), by sensing various odors, provides most of the information that is recognized as taste. Although the system of olfaction is not well understood, it is believed to be similar to the immune system, in that **odorants**—molecules that dissolve in the mucus—bind to **odor receptor molecules** on the surface of the olfactory cilia.

- When odorants have bound to the required number of odor receptor molecules, the olfactory cell membrane depolarizes, and the **action potential** travels along its axon to stimulate collections of **mitral cells**, located in small regions known as **glomeruli** within the **olfactory bulb**.
- The 1000 or so glomeruli located in the olfactory bulb receive input from about 2000 olfactory neurons.
- The particular permutations and combinations of possible inputs permit humans to recognize approximately 10,000 different odors, which requires each glomerulus to participate in the recognition of numerous different scents.
- The odorants are quickly washed away from the olfactory cilia by the copious fluid flow from Bowman's glands, preventing multiple responses from a single odorant.

LARYNX

The **larynx** is a short musculocartilaginous segment of the conducting portion of the respiratory system interposed between the pharynx and the trachea. It permits phonation and averts the entry of food or drink material into the respiratory system during the process of deglutition.

- The larynx comprises several cartilages that are connected to one another by ligaments and by extrinsic and intrinsic skeletal muscles.
- The **aditus**, the superior opening of the larynx, is guarded by the **epiglottis**, a cartilaginous flap that stays open during phonation and breathing but closes over the aditus during swallowing.

The laryngeal lumen displays two pairs of folds:

- The superior **vestibular folds**, which do not move
- The inferior **vocal folds**, which contain a dense regular elastic connective tissue, the **vocal ligament**, and its adhering **vocalis muscle**; these assist intrinsic muscles in tensing the vocal ligaments and moving them in a medial direction, narrowing the **rima glottidis**, the space between the right and left vocal folds.

As the exhaled air rushes past the vocal folds, it vibrates them and produces a **sound** that, by being modulated by the tongue and lips, creates **speech**. The length of the vocal fold and the degree of tension placed on it modulates the pitch of the sound that is being produced; the shorter the fold and the greater the tension on the vocal cord, the higher the pitch of the sound that is being produced.

The superior aspects of the vocal folds and of the epiglottis are covered by **stratified squamous non-keratinized epithelium**, and the remainder of the laryngeal lumen is lined by **pseudostratified ciliated columnar epithelium**. The cilia of the columnar cells of this epithelium transport mucus toward the pharynx to be eliminated.

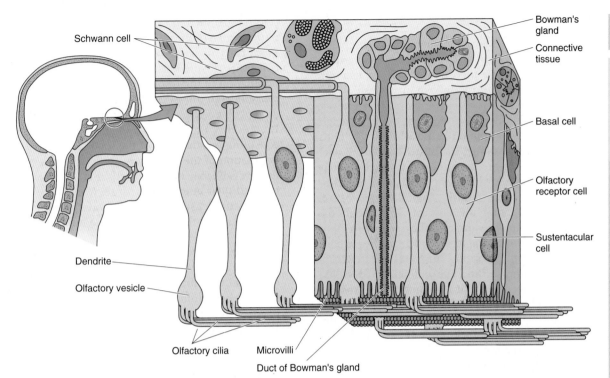

Figure 15.1 The olfactory epithelium and its various cell types—basal, sustentacular, and olfactory cells. *(From Gartner LP, Hiatt JL: Color Textbook of Histology, 3rd ed. Philadelphia, Saunders, 2007, p 348.)*

CLINICAL CONSIDERATIONS

A common problem with many individuals is a nosebleed (**epistaxis**). In children, nosebleeds are usually the result of nasal drying, whereas in adults, they may be a warning sign of high blood pressure. Nosebleed usually occurs in the anteroinferior region of the nasal septum (**Kiesselbach's area**) an area rich in blood vessels. Bleeding may be stopped by applying pressure or packing the nasal cavity with cotton. Any nasal bleeding that persists, recurs, or is severe needs to be evaluated by a physician.

Within the lamina propria of the respiratory epithelium covering the conchae are large venous plexuses known as **swell bodies**. Every 20 to 30 minutes, the swell bodies on one side of the nasal fossa become engorged with blood that distends the mucosa slightly, impeding airflow. At this time, most of the airflow passes through the opposite nasal fossa. This cycling assists the respiratory mucosa in maintaining a hydrated state.

Acute or chronic **laryngitis** is an inflammation of the larynx resulting from overuse, irritation, or infection of the vocal folds (the mucous membrane covering of the vocal cords). Normally, the vocal folds open and close smoothly, forming sounds as air passes by them, causing them to vibrate. During laryngitis, the vocal folds become inflamed or irritated and they swell, resulting in the creation of hoarse sounds. Most cases of laryngitis are triggered by temporary viral infections or vocal strain and are not serious. Persistent hoarseness can sometimes signal a more serious underlying medical condition, however.

Cough reflex is initiated by particulate matter or irritants in the upper passageways of the respiratory system, including the trachea and the bronchi. The reflex begins with a large volume of air being inhaled. This inhalation is followed by closing the glottis and epiglottis, followed by a powerful contraction of the muscles of expiration (abdominal and intercostal muscles) and then an immediate opening of the glottis and epiglottis. This last event permits a powerful rush of air (velocity of which may reach 100 mph) forcing the irritant out of the upper respiratory passages.

TRACHEA

The **trachea**, a 12-cm-long tube, is always patent because of the 10 to 12 C-shaped hyaline cartilage rings, called **C-rings**, that support it along its entire length. Each C-ring, positioned in such a fashion that its closed portion faces in an anterior direction, has its own perichondrium. The perichondria of neighboring C-rings are connected to each other by fibroelastic connective tissue. The posteriorly facing open ends of the C-rings are connected to each other by slips of smooth muscle—the **trachealis muscle**—whose contraction reduces the diameter of the trachea, accelerating the flow of air through this tubular structure. The lumen of the trachea resembles the shape of the capital letter *D*. The trachea is composed of three layers: the innermost mucosa, the middle submucosa, and the outermost adventitia. The **mucosa** of the trachea is composed of **respiratory epithelium**, subepithelial connective tissue (lamina propria), and a thick sheet of elastic fibers that separates the mucosa from the submucosa. The **respiratory epithelium**, pseudostratified ciliated columnar epithelium (Fig. 15.2), is composed of goblet cells, ciliated columnar cells, basal cells, brush cells, serous cells, and diffuse neuroendocrine system (DNES) cells. All cells of this epithelium sit on the basement membrane, but not all of them reach the lumen.

- Almost one third of the cells of this epithelium are **goblet cells** (Fig. 15.3), unicellular glands that manufacture the slippery secretion known as **mucinogen**, which they store in secretory vesicles in the expanded apical region of their cytoplasm, known as the **theca**. Most of the organelles, including the nucleus of goblet cells, are located in the thin, basal part of the cell known as the **stem**. When the mucinogen is released into the lumen of the trachea, it becomes hydrated and is known as **mucin**. When mucin is mixed with particulate matter in the lumen, it becomes known as **mucus**.
- There are approximately as many **ciliated columnar cells** as there are goblet cells. These tall cells have numerous cilia that propel the mucus in the lumen of the trachea toward the larynx.
- **Basal cells** are short, regenerative cells; they constitute slightly less than one third of the cell population of the respiratory epithelium. These cells undergo mitosis and replace the dead and dying goblet cells, ciliated cells, and brush cells.
- **Brush cells**, also known as small granule cells, constitute less than 3% of the total cell population of the respiratory epithelium. These narrow cells may be goblet cells that have released their **mucinogens**, or they may have some **neurosensory** function because they have long microvilli that extend into the lumen of the trachea.
- There are approximately as many **serous cells** as there are brush cells. Serous cells are also tall columnar cells that display apical secretory granules containing a serous secretion whose function is not understood.
- **DNES cells** compose about 3% of the total cell population. These cells manufacture and release paracrine or endocrine hormones in response to stimuli such as hypoxia. DNES cells are frequently innervated, and the nerve fiber DNES cell complex is known as **pulmonary neuroepithelial bodies**, which, under hypoxic conditions, may be able to activate neurons in the respiratory center of the hypothalamus.

The **lamina propria** of the trachea is a fibroelastic connective tissue housing lymphoid elements and serous and mucous glands that deliver their secretion into the lumen. A thick **elastic sheet**, the outermost layer of the lamina propria, separates the mucosa from the submucosa.

A richly vascularized dense irregular fibroelastic connective tissue forms the **submucosa** of the trachea. It houses numerous seromucous glands and an abundance of lymphoid elements. The C-rings of the trachea are located in the fibroelastic connective tissue of the **adventitia**. This outermost layer binds the trachea to the surrounding structures, such as the esophagus.

CLINICAL CONSIDERATIONS

Individuals who are chronically exposed to irritants such as tobacco smoke or coal dust may display alteration of their respiratory epithelium, known as **metaplasia**, so that instead of the normal pseudostratified ciliated columnar morphology, their ciliated cells are greatly reduced in height, goblet cells become abundant, and a thicker layer of mucus is produced attempting to remove the irritants. The decrease in the number of ciliated cells hinders the clearance of mucus, however, increasing congestion. Additionally, seromucous glands of the lamina propria and the submucosa become enlarged and produce more secretory products. If the environmental conditions are changed and the irritants are eliminated, the respiratory epithelium returns to its previously normal, healthy state.

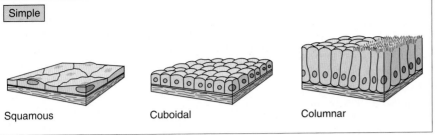

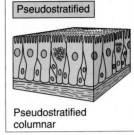

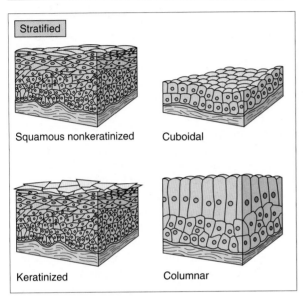

Figure 15.2 Types of epithelia. *(From Gartner LP, Hiatt JL: Color Textbook of Histology, 3rd ed. Philadelphia, Saunders, 2007, p 87.)*

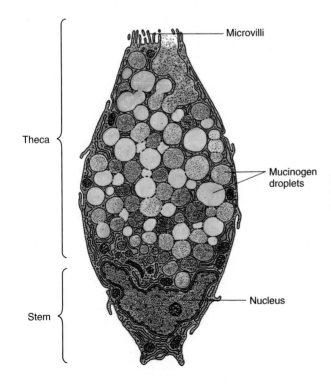

Figure 15.3 Ultrastructure of a goblet cell. *(From Lentz TL: Cell Fine Structure: An Atlas of Drawings of Whole-Cell Structure. Philadelphia, Saunders, 1971.)*

BRONCHIAL TREE

The bifurcation of the trachea signals the beginning of the **bronchial tree**, the conducting portion of the respiratory system, which extends all the way into the lungs down to the level of the terminal bronchioles. As the branches of the bronchial tree bifurcate, their diameter decreases, and their numbers increase, and, as stated earlier, the total cross-sectional area of the bronchial tree increases in size, slowing the velocity of the inspired airflow and increasing the velocity of the expired airflow. The bronchial tree comprises primary bronchi, secondary and tertiary bronchi, bronchioles, and terminal bronchioles (Fig. 15.4). General comments concerning the histology of the bronchial tree as it progresses from primary bronchi to terminal bronchioles are that:

- The size of cartilage and glands decreases.
- The percent of goblet cells and the epithelial thickness decrease.
- The amount of elastic tissue and smooth muscle, relative to the thickness of its wall, increases.

The trachea bifurcates to form the left and right **primary (extrapulmonary) bronchi**, which resemble the trachea except that they are smaller in diameter and their walls are thinner. The left primary bronchus is not as straight as the right bronchus, and it bifurcates. The right one trifurcates before entering the lung tissue to become intrapulmonary (secondary) bronchi. Each branch of the left and right primary bronchi serves one of the five lobes of the lung.

Secondary bronchi (intrapulmonary bronchi, lobar bronchi) resemble primary bronchi, but the supporting hyaline cartilage is no longer in the shape of a C-ring. Instead, it is composed of small cartilage pieces that surround the circumference of the lumen, giving the cross-sectional circumference of the lumen a round shape.

- Because the cartilage no longer has open arms facing in a posterior direction, the smooth muscle migrates toward the lumen, occupying a position between the lamina propria and the submucosa, and is arranged in two helically disposed layers.
- The fibroelastic adventitia has elastic fibers radiating from it in such a fashion that the fibers are positioned more or less perpendicularly to a tangent placed at their contact with the wall of the secondary bronchus.
- These elastic fibers contact other elastic fibers that ramify throughout the substance of the lungs.

Secondary bronchi, when in the lung, arborize to form **tertiary (segmental) bronchi**, each of which serves 1 of the 10 relatively large, **bronchopulmonary segments** of each lung. As these tertiary bronchioles arborize, they form smaller and smaller cylindrical conduits that eventually have no hyaline cartilage in their wall, and possess, relative to the thickness of their walls, more smooth muscle cells disposed in two helically oriented bundles. The smallest of these segmental bronchi serve two or more **pulmonary lobules**, small subdivisions of a bronchopulmonary segment, and arborize to form bronchioles.

A convenient, but not universally accepted, working definition of a **bronchiole** is that it is less than 1 mm in diameter and serves a single pulmonary lobule. Bronchioles possess:

- No cartilage in their walls
- A relatively thick smooth muscle coat compared with the thickness of their wall
- Elastic fibers that emanate from the connective tissue, enveloping the smooth muscle bundles in:
  - Such a fashion that they are positioned more or less perpendicular to a tangent placed at their contact with the wall of the bronchiole
  - Contact with other elastic fibers arising from various sources, placing tension on the entire circumference of the bronchiole and maintaining its patency
- No glands in their lamina propria
- A simple columnar ciliated to a simple cuboidal ciliated epithelial lining
- No goblet cells in the epithelial lining of smaller bronchioles
- Columnar **Clara cells** in bronchioles of all sizes that:
  - Secrete a surfactant-like substance that assists in maintaining bronchiolar patency
  - Destroy inhaled toxins and act as regenerative cells to maintain the epithelial lining

Bronchioles arborize to give rise to **terminal bronchioles** (see Fig. 15.4), the smallest segments of the conducting portion of the respiratory system (<0.5 mm in diameter), each of which serves a small segment of a lung lobule, the **lung acinus**. Terminal bronchioles resemble bronchioles but are much more slender and are lined by a simple epithelium composed of cuboidal cells (some with cilia) and Clara cells. Their narrow lamina propria is surrounded by some smooth muscle cells and kept patent by elastic fibers radiating from the fibroelastic connective tissue wall. Terminal bronchioles give rise to respiratory bronchioles.

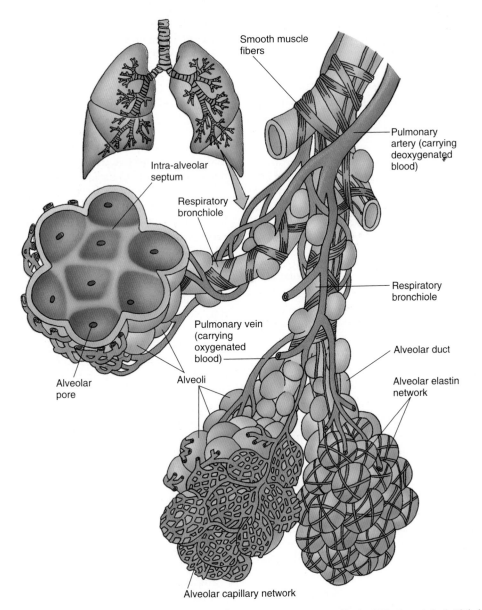

Figure 15.4 The conduits of the respiratory system. *(From Gartner LP, Hiatt JL: Color Textbook of Histology, 3rd ed. Philadelphia, Saunders, 2007, p 355.)*

Respiratory Portion of the Respiratory System

The **respiratory portion of the respiratory system** consists of respiratory bronchioles, alveolar ducts, alveolar sacs, and alveoli. **Respiratory bronchioles** (Fig. 15.5) resemble terminal bronchioles with the exception of the occasional alveoli that balloon out of their walls permitting the exchange of gases to occur, which does not happen in terminal bronchioles. Respiratory bronchioles undergo branching and eventually give rise to **alveolar ducts** (see Fig. 15.5), which are simply a linear sequence of alveoli that branch to form many additional alveolar ducts.

- Each of these alveolar ducts ends as a cul-de-sac formed by two or three groups of alveoli.
- Each alveolar group is referred to as an **alveolar sac**.
- The common airspace from which these groups of alveolar sacs originate is known as the **atrium**.
- Alveolar ducts, alveolar sacs, and alveoli possess their own basal lamina, and they maintain their patency by the presence of slender elastic fibers that attach to the slight connective tissue elements of these structures and to other elastic fibers in their vicinity.

Alveoli (see Fig. 15.5) are small airspaces lined by two types of cells: highly attenuated **type I pneumocytes (type I alveolar cells)** and **type II pneumocytes (septal cells)**. The very thin wall of the alveolus permits the exchange of O_2 for CO_2. A smooth muscle cell and its surrounding reticular fibers encircle the opening of each alveolus controlling the size of its aperture. It has been estimated that there are 300 million alveoli in the two lungs, where each alveolus is approximately 0.002 mm^3 providing a total surface area of 140 m^2 devoted to the exchange of O_2 for CO_2.

- **Type I pneumocytes** are highly attenuated cells that form greater than 95% of the alveolar surface. Most of the organelles of this cell are crowded around the region of the nucleus, whereas the remaining regions of the cell are approximately 80 nm wide and house mostly the fluid cytosol. Adjacent type I pneumocytes form occluding junctions with each other to avoid the entry of extracellular fluid from the interalveolar connective tissue compartment into the alveolus.
- **Type II pneumocytes** (Fig. 15.6) are cuboidal-shaped cells that form only 5% of the alveolar surface even though they outnumber the type I pneumocytes. These cells house **lamellar bodies** that they discharge into the lumen of the alveolus as **pulmonary surfactant**, a substance composed of dipalmitoyl phosphatidylcholine and surfactant apoproteins SP-A, SP-B, SP-C, and SP-D that coats the wall of the alveolar airspace

and, by reducing surface tension, assists in maintaining alveolar patency. These cells not only manufacture and resorb surfactant in a continuous manner, but they also have the ability to enter the cell cycle and form more type II and type I pneumocytes.

The region between two neighboring alveoli is known as an **interalveolar septum**, which is a slender, **continuous, capillary-rich** (see Figs. 15.5 and 15-6) connective tissue element that provides a degree of stability to these delicate structures. **Monocytes**, derived from bone marrow, populate interalveolar septa and enter the lumina of alveoli, becoming known as **alveolar macrophages (dust cells)**, which phagocytose not only particulate matter and microorganisms that gain access to the alveoli with the inhaled air but also surfactant to ensure a constant exchange of old for newly formed surfactant. Dust cells, engorged with phagocytosed material, either reenter the interalveolar septum to leave the lung via lymph vessels or migrate up the bronchial tree to enter the pharynx to be eliminated with the mucus by being swallowed or expectorated.

Interalveolar septa may be very narrow, housing only a continuous capillary whose basal lamina is fused with the basal lamina of the type I pneumocyte; or a capillary and connective tissue elements, including lymphoid cells, fibroblasts, and macrophages surrounded by reticular fibers, elastic fibers, ground substance, and extracellular fluid. The exchange of CO_2 in the capillaries for oxygen in the alveolus occurs best in the region of the narrowest possible interalveolar septum, known as the **blood-gas barrier**, a structure composed of:

- Capillary endothelium
- Fused basal laminae of the capillary endothelium and type I pneumocytes
- Attenuated type I pneumocyte
- Surfactant

CLINICAL CONSIDERATIONS

Chronic obstructive pulmonary disease (COPD) is a combination of lung diseases that includes emphysema and bronchitis. Emphysema is a chronic disease in which the alveoli become damaged, resulting in difficulty breathing; chronic bronchitis is a disease in which a bronchial obstruction impedes breathing. It becomes chronic, resulting in swelling, inflammation, wheezing, coughing, and increased difficulty in breathing. It can begin as a mild condition, and over time it can lead to a greatly reduced quality of life and respiratory failure resulting in death of the individual.

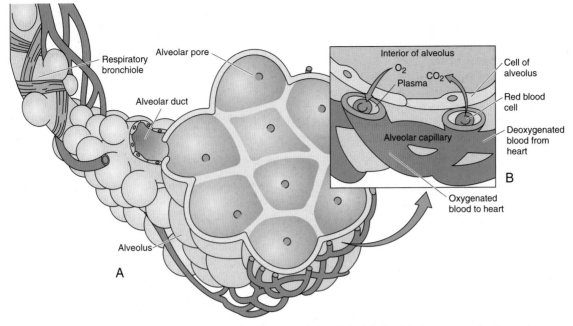

Figure 15.5 **A,** Respiratory bronchiole, alveolar duct, alveolar sac, and alveoli. **B,** Relationship between an alveolus and continuous capillaries. *(From Gartner LP, Hiatt JL: Color Textbook of Histology, 3rd ed. Philadelphia, Saunders, 2007, p 358.)*

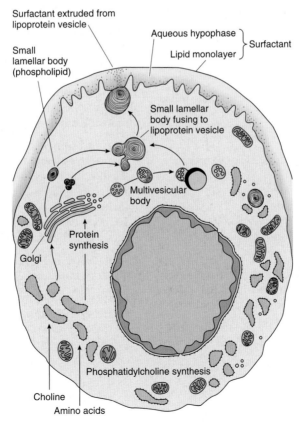

Figure 15.6 Type II pneumocyte. *(From Gartner LP, Hiatt JL: Color Textbook of Histology, 3rd ed. Philadelphia, Saunders, 2007, p 361.)*

EXCHANGE OF GASES BETWEEN THE TISSUES AND THE LUNGS

Cellular respiration in the entire body results in the formation of approximately 200 mL of CO_2 per minute that enters the capillaries to be transported to the lungs (Fig. 15.7A and B), where it is exchanged for O_2. Because the partial pressure of CO_2 is greater in the tissues than in blood, the gas enters the capillaries via simple diffusion. The 200 mL of CO_2 that enters the capillaries every minute is distributed in the following manner:

- 20 mL becomes dissolved gas in the plasma.
- 40 mL binds to globin component of hemoglobin.
- 140 mL enters the erythrocyte where **carbonic anhydrase** catalyzes its reaction with water to form H_2CO_3, which dissociates to form H^+ and HCO_3^-. The bicarbonate ion diffuses out of the red blood cell (RBC) cytosol into the plasma; to compensate for the change in ionic balance, Cl^- enters the RBC cytosol from the plasma, a process known as the **chloride shift** (Fig. 15.7C).

In the alveoli of the lungs, the partial pressure of oxygen is greater than that of the oxygen entering blood. The two gases are again exchanged by simple diffusion, a process that does not require the expenditure of energy. The release of CO_2 and the uptake of O_2 occur in the following manner (Fig. 15.7D):

- Bicarbonate ions of the plasma enter the RBC cytosol necessitating the exit of Cl^- ions from the cytosol, a reversal of what happened before (constituting another chloride shift).
- Carbonic acid forms by binding bicarbonate ions with H^+ ions.
- Oxygen enters the RBC and binds to the heme portion of hemoglobin.
- The enzyme carbonic anhydrase cleaves carbonic acid to form water and CO_2.
- The 200 mL of CO_2 that enters the bloodstream in the tissues per minute is released from the bloodstream, diffuses across the blood-gas barrier, enters the alveolar airspaces, and is exhaled.

Because of its ability to bind to two separate sites on the hemoglobin molecule, **nitric oxide (NO)** plays an important role in the process of gas exchange.

- In the tissues, NO is released by endothelial cells in the lung and binds to one site on the hemoglobin molecule; when it reaches the tissues, it is released, causing relaxation of the vascular smooth muscles with a resultant dilation of the vessel, facilitating the release of oxygen.
- NO occupies the second binding site on hemoglobin by binding to the site of the released oxygen; in this fashion, NO is conveyed to the lungs, where it is released and enters the alveolar airspaces to be exhaled with carbon dioxide.

MECHANISM OF VENTILATION

The processes of **inhalation** and **exhalation** depend on the anatomic relationship of the lungs, the pleural membranes, the pleural cavities, and the elastic fiber components of lung tissue. Each lung is covered by visceral pleura, which is continuous, at the root of each lung, with the parietal pleura.

- The **parietal pleura** adheres to the walls of the thoracic cage and to the connective tissue components of the mediastinum.
- The **visceral pleura** adheres to the surface the lung.
- The space between the parietal pleura and the visceral pleura is a serous cavity known as the **pleural cavity**, an empty space lubricated by a thin, serous fluid whose function is to reduce friction caused by the movements of the lung.

Inhalation is facilitated by the contraction of the muscles of chest wall and the diaphragm (respiratory muscles). As these muscles contract, an energy-requiring process, the thoracic cage enlarges and pulls on the adhering parietal pleura, enlarging the pleural cavities and consequently reducing the pressure inside the pleural cavities.

- The atmospheric pressure is now greater than that of the pleural cavities, causing the influx of air into the lungs.
- The entry of air into the lungs stretches the lung, including its elastic fibers, and reduces the formerly enlarged volume of the pleural cavities, increasing the pressure inside these cavities.

Exhalation is facilitated by the relaxation of the respiratory muscles, permitting:

- Elastic fibers that were stretched to begin to return to their normal length
- Increased pressure within the pleural cavities to drive air out of the lungs

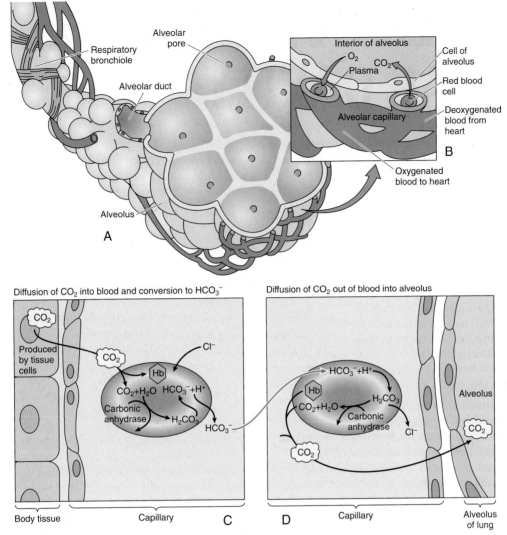

Figure 15.7 A, Respiratory bronchiole, alveolar duct, alveolar sac, and alveoli. **B,** Relationship between an alveolus and continuous capillaries. **C,** CO_2 uptake from body tissues by erythrocytes and plasma. **D,** CO_2 release by erythrocytes and plasma in the lung. (Compare **A** with the alveolar duct shown in Fig. 15.4.) *(From Gartner LP, Hiatt JL: Color Textbook of Histology, 3rd ed. Philadelphia, Saunders, 2007, p 358.)*

CLINICAL CONSIDERATIONS

Patients with pulmonary congestion and congestive heart failure have lungs that are congested with extravasated blood. RBCs gain entrance into the alveoli, where they are phagocytosed by alveolar macrophages. In these instances, these macrophages are called **heart failure cells** when they are present in the lung and sputum.

Lung cancer is the most common cause of cancer-related death among men and women in the United States. It claims more lives each year than colon, prostate, and breast cancers combined. Lung cancer is a disease of uncontrolled cell growth in lung tissue that may lead to metastasis with invasion of adjacent tissue and other organ systems. Most lung cancers are **carcinomas of the lung**, derived from epithelial cells. Almost 90% of lung cancer is caused by long-term exposure to tobacco smoke. The most common symptoms are shortness of breath, coughing, coughing up blood, and weight loss. There are two main types of lung cancer: small cell lung carcinoma, which responds to chemotherapy, and non–small cell lung carcinoma, which responds better to surgery. Radical radiation is often used in the treatment of small cell lung carcinoma.

16 DIGESTIVE SYSTEM: ORAL CAVITY

The digestive system is a complex, continuous tube that includes the functions of modified ingestion, swallowing (deglutition), digestion, absorption of nutrients and fluids, and elimination of indigestible residues and gases. The glandular portion of the digestive system may be intramural or extramural.

Oral Cavity

The **oral cavity (mouth)**, lined by a wet **stratified squamous epithelium**, is subdivided into two spaces—the **vestibule** and the **oral cavity proper**. The **subepithelial connective tissue** and the epithelium together are known as the **oral mucosa**.

- When epithelium is **keratinized** or **parakeratinized** because of friction, the mucosa is referred to as **masticatory mucosa**, located on the gingiva, hard palate, and dorsal tongue.
- Most of the oral cavity has a **lining mucosa**.
- The dorsum of the tongue and areas of the soft palate and pharynx possess taste buds, and those regions are referred to as **specialized mucosa**.

The paired major salivary glands produce **saliva**, which possesses **salivary amylase**, the antimicrobial agents **lactoferrin** and **lysozyme**, and **IgA** and maintains a moist environment. During eating, flow of saliva allows macerated food to be formed into **bolus** that can be swallowed.

Lips

Each lip (Fig. 16.1A) has three surfaces: the hairy external **skin aspect**, the red **vermilion zone**, and the wet **mucosal (internal) aspect**. The tall rete apparatus of the vermilion zone brings capillaries near the surface imparting a pink color to it. The mucosal aspect is always wet and has a lining mucosa whose richly vascularized connective tissue possesses mucous (but some serous) **minor salivary glands**.

Teeth

Humans have 20 **deciduous teeth** that are replaced and supplanted by the **permanent dentition**.

Each tooth (Fig. 16.1B) is hollow and has an enamel-covered **crown** and cementum-covered **root**, which meet at the **cervix**. The hollow **pulp cavity** is divided into the **root canal** and the **pulp chamber** housing the **pulp**, and is surrounded by a mineralized **dentin**. The root is suspended in the bony **alveolus** by a dense collagenous **periodontal ligament (PDL)**.

The pulp has a neurovascular **core** surrounded by three concentric layers:

- The **cell-rich zone**, which is surrounded by
- The **cell-poor zone** and
- The outermost zone, the **odontoblastic** layer

A plexus of sensory nerve fibers, **Raschkow's plexus**, located at the interface of the pulp core and the cell-rich zone, conveys pain sensation to the brain. Nerve fibers and vascular supply enter the pulp through the **apical foramen** of the root tip.

Enamel, the hardest tissue in the body, is translucent and covers the crown. It is composed of 4% organic matrix and water and 96% calcium hydroxyapatite, large crystals coated by an organic matrix (**enamelins** and **tuftelins**), formed into **enamel rods** (**enamel prisms**). Each enamel prism is manufactured by specialized cells, **ameloblasts**, which die after tooth eruption; enamel cannot repair itself.

Dentin, yellowish in color, is located in the crown and in the root. It is composed of a type I collagen–based organic matrix and 65% to 70% calcium hydroxyapatite. Its elastic property protects the overlying enamel from being fractured easily. Dentin is manufactured by cells called **odontoblasts**, whose long **processes** occupy the tunnel-like spaces, **dentinal tubules**, in the substance of dentin.

Cementum, composed of 50% to 55% of type I collagen–based organic matrix and bound water and 45% to 50% calcium hydroxyapatite, is located only on the root. Cementum of the apical aspect of the root possesses **lacunae** occupied by **cementocytes** (**cellular cementum**); cementum of the coronal aspect lacks cementocytes (**acellular cementum**). Both types of cementum are covered by a single layer of **cementoblasts**, which manufacture cementum. **Cementoclasts (odontoclasts)** resorb cementum.

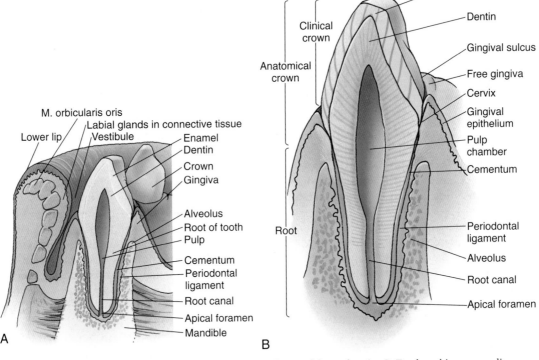

Figure 16.1 **A**, A tooth in situ, presenting the lower lip, vestibule, and part of the oral cavity. **B**, Tooth and its surrounding tissues. The enamel of the crown meets the cementum of the root at the cervix of the tooth. Dentin is located in the crown and in the root. *(A and B, From Gartner LP, Hiatt JL: Color Textbook of Histology, 3rd ed. Philadelphia, Saunders, 2007, pp 368 and 369.)*

CLINICAL CONSIDERATIONS

LIP

Angular cheilitis is a painful condition in which the corners of the **lips** become dry and cracked; it is frequently due to dietary deficiency of vitamin B_2, zinc deficiency, or iron deficiency anemia. The lesions are most common in elderly individuals who have poorly fitting dentures, and the area becomes infected with pathogens such as *Candida albicans*.

ORAL CAVITY

The lining mucosa of the lips and cheeks may become ulcerated, small areas that are characterized by small, red-rimmed, white, painful spots known as **canker sores** (or **aphthous ulcers**). These lesions are usually stress-related and resolve within 7 to 10 days. The pain can be relieved by the application of a local anesthetic ointment.

Squamous cell carcinoma is the most common oral cancer. It is initially painless and appears as a smooth or rough-surfaced red or white lesion that may be in the form of a hard lump or an ulcerated depression that bleeds occasionally. In almost half of affected individuals, these carcinomas occur on the lining mucosa of the lip, whereas in the remaining individuals the affected area is the tongue or the floor of the mouth. Frequently, squamous cell carcinoma is caused by smoking, alcohol use, or the use of smokeless tobacco, but individuals who neither drink alcohol nor use tobacco products may have the disease. The treatment is usually a combination of surgery and radiation therapy.

AGE-RELATED CHANGES IN TEETH

Because **enamel** is nonvital, and the cells manufacturing enamel are no longer present after completion of tooth eruption, enamel cannot be regenerated. The frictional and attritional forces of mastication continuously remove enamel from the occlusal and incisal surfaces, reducing the total amount of enamel. To compensate for the reduction in the size of the crown, cementum is added onto the apical surface, causing the tooth to continue to erupt. This posteruptive movement of the tooth insures that it remains in contact with the tooth opposing it in the other arch.

ODONTOGENESIS BEFORE THE BELL STAGE

Odontogenesis, or tooth development, begins between the sixth and seventh weeks of development when the ectodermal oral epithelium proliferates to form a horseshoe-shaped **dental lamina**, one on the maxillary arch and one on the mandibular arch (Fig. 16.2). The dental lamina is separated from the neural crest–derived ectomesenchyme by a basement membrane.

- In 10 different regions of each dental lamina, a bud forms, beginning the **bud stage** of odontogenesis. Each of the 20 buds presages a specific deciduous tooth. The ectomesenchyme at the tip of each bud condenses to form **dental papilla**.

- Each bud enlarges by mitotic activity and forms a three-layered **enamel organ**—the **cap stage** of odontogenesis. The simple squamous epithelium, the **outer enamel epithelium (OEE)**, is continuous at the rimlike **cervical loop** with the concave simple squamous-cuboidal **inner enamel epithelium (IEE)**. The stellate-shaped cells of the **stellate reticulum** are located between the IEE and OEE. The basement membrane completely surrounds the enamel organ whose concavity is filled with the **dental papilla**, a well-vascularized ectomesenchyme. The enamel organ and dental papilla together are known as the **tooth germ**. The later stage of the enamel organ alters its morphology to form a template that is incisiform, caniniform, or molariform. This ability of the enamel organ depends on the **enamel knot**, a cluster of cells located among the cells of the stellate reticulum. It is the principal signaling center of tooth formation. The dental papilla manufactures **fibroblast growth factor 4 (FGF-4)** and **epidermal growth factor (EGF)**, both necessary for the survival of the enamel knot, which synthesizes FGF-4, **Sonic Hedgehog**, and various **bone morphogenetic proteins** that direct the transformation of the enamel organ into a molariform template. When the transformation is complete, the dental papilla ceases to express EGF and FGF-4, and the enamel knot undergoes apoptosis. The dental papillae of incisiform and caniniform enamel organs never express FGF-4 or EGF, and their enamel knots undergo apoptosis during the cap stage. The absence of the enamel knot results in the formation of a default noncusped tooth. The dental papilla forms the **dentin** and the **pulp** of the tooth. The ectomesenchyme surrounding the tooth germ forms a thin, dense connective tissue layer, the **dental sac**, which forms the **alveolus**, **PDL**, and

cementum of the tooth. **Enamel** is synthesized by ameloblasts, cells that are differentiated from the IEE. The permanent teeth arise from the **succedaneous laminae** of the 20 tooth buds. The 12 permanent molars arise from the extensions of the two dental laminae that begin to elongate.

- As the cap grows in size, a fourth layer, the **stratum intermedium**, appears that is characteristic of the **bell stage (stage of histodifferentiation and morphodifferentiation)**. As development continues, the cells of the IEE at the region farthest from the cervical loop become elongated cells known as **preameloblasts** as they begin to manufacture enamel matrix; these cells mature into **ameloblasts** (Fig. 16.3). In response to the initial formation of enamel, the layer of dental papilla cells that abut the basal lamina differentiate into **preodontoblasts**, and when they begin to manufacture dentin matrix, they mature into **odontoblasts** (see Fig. 16.3).

- The **dentinoenamel junction** is established, and the **appositional stage** of tooth development begins. Initially, the dentinoenamel junction is just a microscopic region that continues to spread along the concavity of the enamel organ and eventually reaches the cervical loop. While that is taking place, ameloblasts and odontoblasts continue to manufacture enamel and dentin, respectively. Both hard tissues become thicker, and the two cell types are displaced farther and farther from each other.

- When enamel formation is completed, the cervical loop elongates, forming a cylindrical sheet, **Hertwig's epithelial root sheath (HERS)**, composed only of OEE and IEE that encloses, and is surrounded by, ectomesenchymal cells. The enclosed ectomesenchymal cells are continuous with the dental papilla and form **radicular pulp** and **radicular dentin**. The older regions of HERS begin to disintegrate, and some ectomesenchymal cells surrounding HERS migrate onto the radicular dentin surface, differentiate into **cementoblasts**, and manufacture **cementum**. As HERS continues to lengthen, more and more of the root is formed, and finally the last region of the root housing the **apical foramen** is produced. As the root becomes longer, the tooth is erupting into the oral cavity. The eruptive motion is independent of root elongation even though the two processes occur concurrently. Eruption is effected by the activity of specialized **myofibroblasts** of the dental sac that, by tugging on the type I collagen fibers of the dental sac (future PDL) attached to the cementum, drag the developing tooth into occlusion.

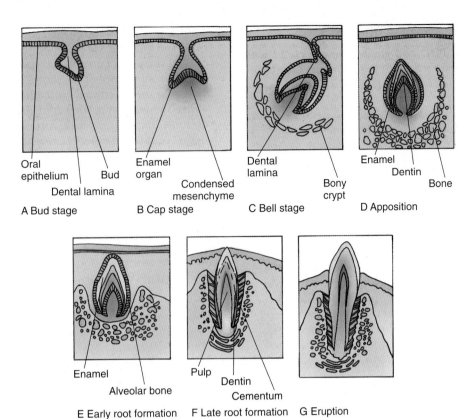

Oral
epithelium — Bud
Dental lamina

A Bud stage

Enamel
organ
Condensed
mesenchyme

B Cap stage

Dental
lamina
Bony
crypt

C Bell stage

Enamel
Dentin
Bone

D Apposition

Enamel
Alveolar bone

E Early root formation

Pulp
Dentin
Cementum

F Late root formation

G Eruption

Figure 16.2 A–G, Odontogenesis. *(From Gartner LP, Hiatt JL: Color Textbook of Histology, 3rd ed. Philadelphia, Saunders, 2007, p 372.)*

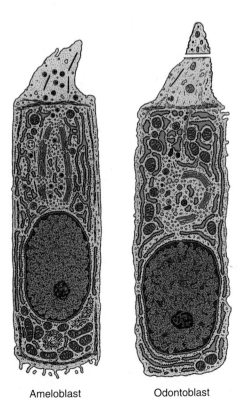

Ameloblast   Odontoblast

Figure 16.3 Ameloblast and odontoblast. The long odontoblastic process of the odontoblast was shortened by cutting out a long portion of it (*white space*). *(From Lentz TL: Cell Fine Structure: An Atlas of Drawings of Whole-Cell Structure. Philadelphia, Saunders, 1971.)*

STRUCTURES ASSOCIATED WITH TEETH

The alveolus, PDL, and gingiva are associated with teeth and assist each tooth in maintaining its proper position in the oral cavity (Fig. 16.4).

- The **PDL**, composed of a cellular, neurovascular, dense, irregular collagenous connective tissue, occupies the narrow PDL space (width ≤0.5 mm in a healthy mouth) between the cementum of the root and the alveolus (see Fig. 16.4). The type I collagen fibers of the PDL are arranged in **principal fiber groups**, which resist and accommodate the forces of mastication. They suspend the tooth in its alveolus via **Sharpey's fibers** embedded in the cementum and in the alveolar bone. The most numerous cells of the PDL are fibroblasts, which not only synthesize the extracellular matrix but also degrade its collagen, accounting for its exceptionally high turnover rate in this tissue. The PDL possesses autonomic, sensory, and proprioceptive nerve fibers, the last of which provide information about spatial orientation.

- The bony housing of the root of each tooth, known as the **alveolus** (see Fig. 16.4), is composed of three regions: the cone-shaped thin compact bone that has numerous perforations and is in contact with the PDL, known as the **alveolar bone proper**; surrounded by cancellous bone, the **spongiosa**; and the outermost thick compact bone—the **cortical plate**—which is disposed lingually and labially. Neurovascular supply of the alveolus resides in tunnel-shaped **nutrient canals**. The blood vessels and nerve fibers of the alveolus pass through the perforations in the alveolar bone proper, serving not only the alveolus but also the PDL.

- The stratified squamous orthokeratinized or parakeratinized epithelium of the **gingiva (gum)** attests to the harsh frictional forces to which it is exposed (see Fig. 16.4). Similar to the PDL, the type I collagen fiber bundles of its dense irregular collagenous connective tissue are arranged in **principal fiber groups**. As the gingival epithelium reaches the enamel, it makes a sharp bend and attaches, via hemidesmosomes, to the enamel surface as an epithelial band around the entire circumference of the tooth, which is known as the **junctional epithelium**. This thin, wedge-shaped, 1-mm-long epithelial collar that is no more than 50 cells wide coronally and less than 7 cells broad apically prevents the abundant population of microorganisms of the oral cavity from invading the sterile connective tissue of the gingiva.

Palate

The **palate**, composed of the anterior, immovable hard palate and posterior, movable, muscular soft palate, separates the nasal and oral cavities from each other.

- On the oral surface, the **hard palate** is lined by a masticatory mucosa whose connective tissue has adipose tissue anteriorly and **minor mucous salivary glands** posteriorly. The connective tissue of the hard palate adheres to the **bony shelf** in its core. The nasal side of the hard palate possesses a dense, irregular collagenous connective tissue covered by a pseudostratified ciliated columnar epithelium with an abundance of goblet cells.

- The oral surface of the **soft palate** is covered by a **lining mucosa**. The connective tissue is rich in **minor mucous salivary glands** that are continuous with the glands of the hard palate. The core of the soft palate is composed of **skeletal muscles**, some of which originate from the anterior edge of the bony shelf of the hard palate. The nasal aspect of the soft palate is identical to the nasal aspect of the hard palate.

- The soft palate ends in the conical **uvula**, which is covered by a lining mucosa on all of its surfaces with some minor mucous salivary glands interspersed among the connective tissue elements. The core of the uvula contains skeletal muscle fibers that function in elevating the uvula during swallowing.

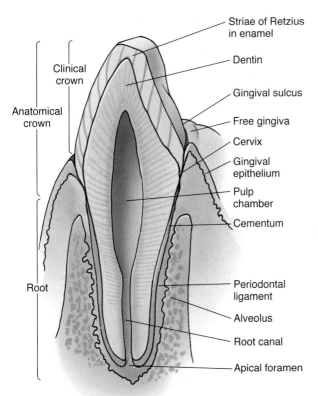

Striae of Retzius in enamel
Dentin
Gingival sulcus
Free gingiva
Cervix
Gingival epithelium
Pulp chamber
Cementum
Periodontal ligament
Alveolus
Root canal
Apical foramen

Clinical crown
Anatomical crown
Root

Figure 16.4 Tooth and its surrounding tissues. The enamel of the crown meets the cementum of the root at the cervix of the tooth. Dentin is located in the crown and in the root. *(From Gartner LP, Hiatt JL: Color Textbook of Histology, 3rd ed. Philadelphia, Saunders, 2007, p 369.)*

CLINICAL CONSIDERATIONS

The **jaw-jerk reflex** is responsible for the opening of the mouth when one unexpectedly encounters a hard object while chewing one's food. This reflex is initiated when the sudden force encountered by the PDL causes the proprioceptive fibers to inhibit the muscles of mastication from continuing to contract, protecting the teeth from being fractured.

Occlusal trauma from atypical activities such as bruxing (grinding the teeth at night) or excessive clenching of the teeth may result in thrombosis or, in the worst case, ischemic necrosis of the PDL. Such lesions are responsible for the widening of the PDL space (i.e., the space between the cementum of the tooth and the bony alveolus) with a concomitant increase in the mobility of the tooth and, if untreated, the loss of that tooth.

Alveolar damage may occur because of excessively rapid orthodontic forces placed on the tooth. The forces placed on the tooth become transferred to the PDL causing it to become inflamed, and in response osteoclasts are recruited to the PDL, where they resorb the alveolus to a greater extent than intended by the dental practitioner. The greater than anticipated widening of the PDL space may result in a possible loss of the tooth owing to irreversible motility.

Halitosis, or bad breath, is usually caused by food particles that have not been removed from between the teeth, from the crevices of the tongue, or from the pits of the palatine tonsils where this debris begins to decompose and emit an unpleasant odor. Additionally, individuals with poor oral hygiene or endodontics problems that have resulted in abscess formation usually have halitosis. The ingestion of certain foods, such as raw garlic or onion, gives the breath an unpleasant odor that disappears when the volatile oils present in these substances clears the bloodstream. Infections with certain bacteria, such as *Haemophilus influenzae,* produce characteristic sweet, mousy odors that a physician well trained in microbiology should be able to recognize. Less frequently, organic problems may also impart a specific odor to the breath; the breath has an acetone odor in diabetes, smells like urine in kidney failure, and smells mousy in liver disease. Certain esophageal and gastric tumors can impart a foul odor to the breath as well.

Tongue

The **tongue** (Figs. 16.5 and 16.6) is a large, exceptionally mobile, muscular organ that not only assists in mastication by positioning food on the occlusal plane but also functions in the formation and swallowing of the bolus. The tongue also possesses four types of **lingual papillae**, most of which jut above the surface and have a masticatory mucosa whose highly keratinized stratified squamous epithelium allows the papillae to scrape food off a surface. Other lingual papillae are covered by a nonkeratinized stratified squamous epithelium that houses taste buds to determine the taste of food.

The muscles of the tongue are voluntary and divided into two categories:

- **Extrinsic muscles** originate outside, but insert into, the tongue and move it.
- **Intrinsic muscles** are contained wholly within the tongue and alter its shape.

The tongue has three surfaces: dorsal, ventral, and lateral. The **dorsal surface** is separated into an anterior two thirds and a posterior one third by the V-shaped **sulcus terminalis**, whose posteriorly positioned apex is marked by the pitlike **foramen cecum**. The posterior one third is characterized by a lining mucosa whose surface is irregular because its subepithelial connective tissue is rich in lymph nodes, collectively termed the **lingual tonsil**. The **root of the tongue** attaches this muscular organ to the floor of the mouth and to the pharynx.

LINGUAL PAPILLAE

Three of the four types of **lingual papillae** are located on the dorsum of the anterior two thirds of the tongue.

- The most numerous of these, the long, fingerlike, highly keratinized **filiform papillae**, have no taste buds. They project above the surface of the tongue and function in scraping food off a surface.
- **Fungiform papillae** are much fewer in number, resemble a mushroom, project above the surface, and are dispersed in an apparent random fashion among the filiform papillae. Because fungiform papillae are covered by a nonkeratinized stratified squamous epithelium, they appear as red dots on the surface of the tongue. The epithelium of their dorsal surface houses three or four taste buds.

- The 12 or so **circumvallate papillae** are located in front of the sulcus terminalis. They are depressed into the surface and are surrounded by a furrow whose epithelial lining possesses taste buds. The floor of this furrow accepts small ducts from the **glands of von Ebner**.
- The lateral surface of the posterior aspect of the anterior two thirds of the tongue has longitudinally disposed groove-like regions, the **foliate papillae**, that resemble leaves of a book. The taste buds of these papillae degenerate by the third year of age. The depth of the furrows receives small ducts of the minor serous salivary **glands of Ebner**.

TASTE BUDS

Taste buds (see Figs. 16.5 and 16.6) are an intraepithelial collection of neural crest–derived cells that form a barrel-shaped structure whose opening, the **taste pore**, has microvilli—known as **taste hairs**—protruding from it. The taste bud is composed of approximately 60 to 80 spindle-shaped cells that are constantly being shed and replaced by new cells. The 3000 or so taste buds function in the sensation of the five (or perhaps six) primary taste sensations: bitter, sweet, salty, sour, umami (delicious), and, for some people, fat. Each taste bud is completely intraepithelial and is composed of four types of cells, three of which have a life span of 10 days. The fourth cell type, the **basal cell (type IV cell)**, is a regenerative cell whose mitotic activity is responsible for generating new cells. The other three cell types are:

- **Type I cell** (dark cell)
- **Type II cell** (light cell)
- **Type III cell** (intermediate cell)

It is believed that basal cells give rise to type I cells that differentiate into type II cells that begin to degenerate and become type III cells and then die. Types I, II, and III all possess microvilli (taste hairs), structures that have the ability to respond to **tastants**, chemicals present in food that become dissolved in saliva. Some of these tastants activate ion channels (salt and sour), others activate G protein–linked receptors (umami, sweet, and bitter), and still others activate fatty acid transporters (lipids). Most of the taste that people associate with food depends on the odor of food rather than on the taste that is perceived by taste buds.

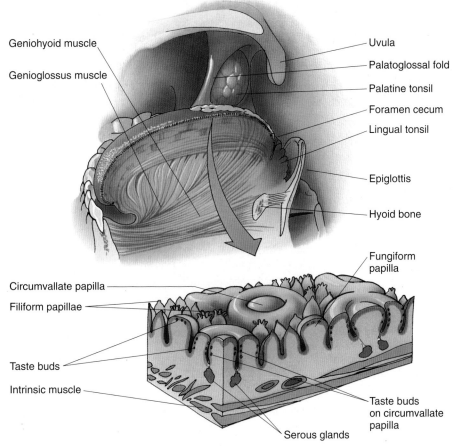

Geniohyoid muscle

Genioglossus muscle

Uvula

Palatoglossal fold

Palatine tonsil

Foramen cecum

Lingual tonsil

Epiglottis

Hyoid bone

Fungiform papilla

Circumvallate papilla

Filiform papillae

Taste buds

Intrinsic muscle

Taste buds on circumvallate papilla

Serous glands

Figure 16.5 Tongue in the oral cavity and a section from the posterior aspect of its anterior two thirds showing the various types of lingual papillae. *(From Gartner LP, Hiatt JL: Color Textbook of Histology, 3rd ed. Philadelphia, Saunders, 2007, p 377.)*

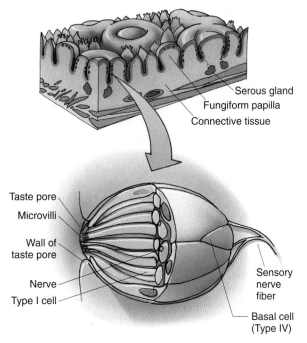

Serous gland

Fungiform papilla

Connective tissue

Taste pore

Microvilli

Wall of taste pore

Nerve

Type I cell

Sensory nerve fiber

Basal cell (Type IV)

Figure 16.6 Section of the tongue showing the various types of lingual papillae and a diagram of a taste bud. *(From Gartner LP, Hiatt JL: Color Textbook of Histology, 3rd ed. Philadelphia, Saunders, 2007, p 378.)*

17 DIGESTIVE SYSTEM: ALIMENTARY CANAL

The 9-meter-long alimentary canal is a tubular structure composed of the esophagus, stomach, small and large intestines, and anal canal. It digests food, absorbs nutrients and water, and compacts and eliminates the indigestible components of the ingested food.

General Organization of the Alimentary Canal

The digestive tract is composed of concentric cylinders around a **lumen**. These layers are modified along the canal, but before discussing the modifications, the general pattern is described (Fig. 17.1):

- The lumen is lined by an **epithelial layer** and a subepithelial connective tissue, the **lamina propria**, which houses glands and lymphatic nodules that constitute the **mucosa-associated lymphoid tissue**. The lamina propria is surrounded by the **muscularis mucosae**, two smooth muscle layers arranged in a helical fashion: an inner circular and an outer longitudinal layer. The epithelium, lamina propria, and muscularis mucosae together are the **mucosa**.
- Surrounding the mucosa is a dense, collagenous connective tissue, the **submucosa**, which is a vascularized region that houses glands but only in the esophagus and duodenum. **Meissner's submucosal plexus**, a component of the **enteric nervous system**, occupies the most peripheral layer of the submucosa, serving intramural glands, vascular supply, and muscularis mucosae, and acts locally.
- The **muscularis externa** is composed of smooth muscle in two helically disposed layers—an **inner circular** and an **outer longitudinal layer**. **Auerbach's (myenteric) plexus** lies between these two smooth muscle layers and controls **peristalsis**. Auerbach's plexus acts locally and also over long stretches of the alimentary canal.
- The alimentary canal is covered by either connective tissue (**adventitia**), which affixes

regions of the gut to the body wall, or by a moist simple squamous epithelium (**serosa**), which reduces friction as the gut moves during peristalsis.

The enteric nervous system can act completely on its own; however, it is modulated by the **sympathetic** and **parasympathetic nervous systems**.

Esophagus

The **esophagus**, a 25-cm-long muscular tube whose wall is collapsed unless it is transmitting a bolus into the stomach, closely follows this general plan.

- The esophageal **mucosa** is composed of a stratified squamous nonkeratinized epithelium, a lamina propria whose **esophageal cardiac glands** produce mucus that aids in swallowing the bolus. These glands are located in the regions near the pharynx and near the stomach. The muscularis mucosa is composed of a longitudinally disposed smooth muscle layer.
- The vascular **submucosa** has the **esophageal glands proper**, which produce mucous and serous secretions. The serous component of this gland manufactures **pepsinogen** (a proenzyme) and **lysozyme**, an antibacterial agent. The mucous component lubricates the epithelium. The esophagus has glands in its submucosa.
- The **muscularis externa**, composed of an inner circular and an outer longitudinal layer, is unusual because in the upper one third of the esophagus, near the pharynx, both layers are composed of skeletal muscle; in the middle third, they are composed of skeletal and smooth muscles; and in the lower third, near the stomach, they are composed solely of smooth muscle.
- The outermost layer of the esophagus is the **adventitia** in the thorax and a **serosa** once it enters the abdominal cavity.

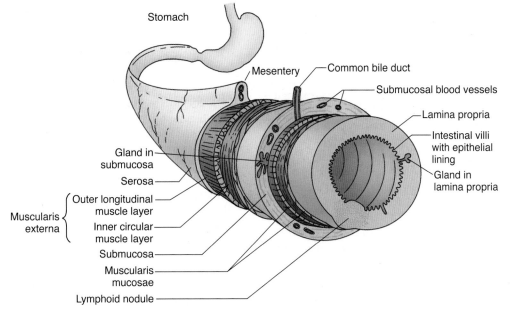

Stomach

Mesentery

Common bile duct

Submucosal blood vessels

Lamina propria

Intestinal villi
with epithelial
lining

Gland in
lamina propria

Gland in
submucosa

Serosa

Outer longitudinal
muscle layer

Muscularis
externa

Inner circular
muscle layer

Submucosa

Muscularis
mucosae

Lymphoid nodule

Figure 17.1 General plan of the alimentary canal. *(From Gartner LP, Hiatt JL: Color Textbook of Histology, 3rd ed. Philadelphia, Saunders, 2007, p 382.)*

CLINICAL CONSIDERATIONS

The most common symptoms that are indicative of disorders of the digestive system include dysphagia (problems with swallowing), regurgitation, constipation, diarrhea, and bleeding from the digestive tract. **Dysphagia** may have numerous causes, including physical obstructions in the pharynx or esophagus, muscular or neural problems, and psychogenic problems. **Regurgitation** is not accompanied by nausea or by violent constriction of the abdominal musculature that occurs during vomiting. The process of regurgitation may be due to neural or muscular problems associated with the esophageal sphincter or due to stenosis of the esophagus as a result of a malignancy or untreated acid reflux. Regurgitation in the absence of a physical cause is known as **rumination**; in this condition, the swallowed food returns to the mouth, where it may be chewed and swallowed again. Rumination is common in infants; it may occur in adults also and is usually stress-related.

Constipation is a condition in which bowel movements occur less than three times per week. It is more common in women than in men, in adults older than 65 years, and in women who are pregnant. Individuals who are constipated usually produce small, dark, dry, hard stools that are difficult to eliminate. The causes of constipation may be dietary (e.g., low fiber consumption, eating too much dairy, not drinking enough fluids);

sedentary lifestyle; certain medications, including overuse of laxatives; disruption of the daily routine as in traveling; and ill health, such as stroke and intestinal disorders. **Diarrhea** refers to the production of loose, watery stool at least three times in one day. There are two types of diarrhea—acute and chronic. **Acute diarrhea** is quite common, lasts for 1 or 2 days, and resolves itself; if it lasts for more than 2 days, it is considered to be **chronic diarrhea**, and a physician should be consulted to prevent dehydration and rule out organic disease. Most cases of acute diarrhea are due to bacterial, viral, or parasitic infections, whereas chronic diarrhea is usually due to problems with the alimentary canal, such as irritable bowel syndrome.

Bleeding from the digestive tract may occur from the mouth as bloody vomiting or from the anus as bloody discharge or bloody stool. The blood may be fresh or coagulated. Usually, if the blood is fresh, it is red in color and originates near the oral cavity or the anus. If the blood is coagulated, it appears as black particulate matter that resembles coffee grounds in the vomit or it stains the stool black (melena). Bleeding from the alimentary canal may be caused by peptic ulcers, varices that leak blood, use of certain anti-inflammatory agents, inflammatory bowel disease, and cancer.

Stomach

The **stomach** has an inlet, where the esophagus joins it, and an outflow, where it is joined by the duodenum. It can expand from a 50-mL volume when empty to approximately 1500 mL when distended. As the stomach receives a bolus from the esophagus, it secretes gastric juices to liquefy the bolus into an acidic fluid known as **chyme** and to begin to digest it via hydrochloric acid and its enzymes, **rennin**, **pepsin**, and **gastric lipase**. The hormone **ghrelin** maintains a constant intraluminal pressure by allowing the muscularis externa to adapt to the expanding volume and sustains the feeling of hunger as the stomach is being distended. The acidic chyme is released in 1- to 2-mL aliquots into the duodenum through the **pyloric sphincter**, the modified inner circular layer of the muscularis externa. The stomach has:

- A **cardiac region** at the concave lesser curvature
- A **pyloric region** at the greater curvature
- Two additional anatomic regions, the **fundus** and the **body**, which are identical histologically and are referred to as the **fundic region** (Fig. 17.2)

The lumen of the empty stomach presents **rugae**, folds of the mucosa and submucosa, which disappear when the stomach is distended. The stomach lining displays numerous epithelially lined depressions, **gastric pits (foveolae)**, whose floor is perforated by many tubular gastric glands populating the highly vascular **lamina propria**. The **muscularis mucosae** has three layers of smooth muscle—inner circular, outer longitudinal, and a poorly defined outermost oblique layer. The **submucosa** is unremarkable. The **muscularis externa** has inner circular, outer longitudinal, and innermost oblique layers.

- The simple columnar **epithelium** of the fundic stomach is composed of tightly packed **surface lining cells** and **regenerative cells**; the lateral cell membranes of these cells form tight junctions with each other. Surface lining cells produce the thick, visible mucus that guards the epithelium from the acidic chyme, and regenerative cells proliferate to replace the stomach's epithelial lining.
- The gastric pits of the fundic and cardiac regions extend one third of the way into the **lamina propria**, which is crowded with **gastric glands**.
- Each gland possesses six cell types, distributed disproportionately, in its three regions: the **isthmus**, which pierces the gastric pit; the **neck**; and the **base**, which abuts the muscularis mucosae. The gastric pits of the pyloric region extend halfway into the lamina propria.

CELLULAR COMPOSITION OF FUNDIC GLANDS

See Figure 17.2.

- **Mucous neck cells** manufacture **soluble mucus** that becomes part of the chyme and lubricates the alimentary canal. The plasmalemmae of these cells form tight junctions with their neighbors.
- The **regenerative cells'** rapid mitotic rate replaces the entire epithelial lining every 5 to 7 days.
- **Parietal (oxyntic) cells** are usually not present in the base of the gland. They have deep **intracellular canaliculi** that are lined by microvilli. An intracellular vesicular network, the **tubulovesicular system** whose membrane component is rich in the proton pump H^+,K^+-**ATPase**, parallels the intracellular canaliculi. Parietal cells produce **hydrochloric acid** and **gastric intrinsic factor**. During HCl production, the tubulovesicular system is reduced in size with a concomitant increase in the number of microvilli, suggesting that the vesicular network is used to store membranes destined for microvillus production, enabling the cell to increase its surface area during its secretory activity. With the cessation of HCl production, the microvillus membranes are returned to the tubulovesicular system. This energy-requiring process is fueled by the abundant mitochondrial content of parietal cells. The glycoprotein gastric intrinsic factor is released into the lumen of the stomach where it complexes with **vitamin B_{12}**, to be absorbed by cells of the ileum.
- **Chief (zymogenic) cells**, located mostly in the base of fundic glands and not at all in cardiac or pyloric glands, manufacture pepsinogen, rennin, and gastric lipase. The proenzyme **pepsinogen** is converted to the proteolytic enzyme **pepsin** in the acidic milieu of the stomach; rennin (chymosin) is a proteolytic enzyme that curdles milk, and the enzyme gastric lipase degrades lipids. These enzymes are present within vesicles in the apical cytoplasm of chief cells and are released because of the interaction of **acetylcholine** and **secretin** as they bind to their respective receptors on the basal plasma membrane of chief cells to activate their **second messenger systems**.
- **Diffuse neuroendocrine system (DNES) cells** are of two types—open and closed—where the former reach the lumen, and the latter do not. Each DNES cell produces a particular hormone that it releases into the lamina propria. These hormones are **autocrine** if destined for the releasing cell, **paracrine** if destined for a cell nearby, and **endocrine** if they have to travel via the bloodstream.

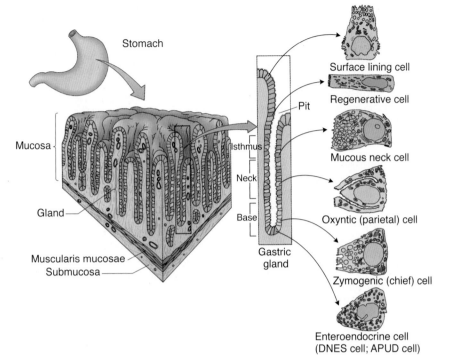

Figure 17.2 Graphic representation of the mucosa of the fundic region of the stomach displaying the fundic glands of the lamina propria. The various cell types composing the epithelium of the stomach and fundic glands are displayed. *(From Gartner LP, Hiatt JL: Color Textbook of Histology, 3rd ed. Philadelphia, Saunders, 2007, p 386.)*

CLINICAL CONSIDERATIONS

Too much HCl production in the stomach may be due to many causes, one of which is a malignancy involving G cells, the DNES cells that produce the paracrine hormone gastrin. Individuals with this type of cancer have **Zollinger-Ellison syndrome**, and the tumor may be located in various areas of the digestive system, such as the bile duct, duodenum, or pancreas. These patients have recurring ulcers that do not respond to normal ulcer treatments, such as antibiotics against *Helicobacter pylori* or histamine$_2$ blockers. Proton pump inhibitors are effective, but cure involves surgical excision of the tumor.

The normal position of the stomach and the gastroesophageal junction is below the diaphragm in the abdominal cavity. In some cases, however, the stomach may protrude into the thoracic cavity, a condition known as **hiatal hernia**. This is a very common condition, and the incidence increases with the age of the individual. There are two types of hiatal hernia. In **sliding hiatal hernia**, which is more common, the gastroesophageal junction and part of the stomach slide up and down through weakness in the esophageal hiatus of the diaphragm. The second type, **paraesophageal**

hiatal hernia, is less common but may be more serious. In this condition, the gastroesophageal junction remains in the abdominal cavity, but a part of the stomach protrudes into the thoracic cavity through the esophageal hiatus and lies alongside the esophagus; if it becomes trapped in that location, possible strangulation of that portion of the stomach may result. If the stomach does not retract on its own, surgical intervention becomes necessary.

Sliding hiatal hernia is usually asymptomatic, although it may manifest with gastric reflux, heartburn, and indigestion, especially in individuals who lie down after eating. The same symptoms accompany paraesophageal hiatal hernia; however, if strangulation occurs, the patient experiences substernal pain. Because this symptom resembles a possible heart attack, an individual with substernal pain should seek immediate medical attention. In most cases, surgery is not required. Treatment of hiatal hernias involve changes in dietary habits; the patient should eat more frequently and smaller quantities at each meal. Also, antacids and elevating the head of the bed usually relieve the symptoms.

GASTRIC HISTOPHYSIOLOGY

On a daily basis, the glands of the stomach produce about 2 to 3 L of secretions whose main constituents are water, HCl, enzymes, intrinsic factor, and soluble and visible mucus. By coating the lining of the stomach, the neutral pH of the visible mucus protects the stomach lining from the acidic gastric juices. The visible mucus also affords a beneficial environment for *H. pylori*, the bacterium that resides within it.

- The **muscularis externa** of the stomach functions in churning and liquefying ingested food, forming a thick chyme that resembles split pea soup.
- The **muscularis mucosae** ensure that the entire epithelial surface of the stomach comes into contact with the chyme. When the chyme is of proper consistency, and depending on its acidity, osmolality, and lipid and caloric content, **DNES cells** of the duodenum release the hormone **gastrin**, which induces the pyloric sphincter to open and the longitudinal muscles of the pylorus to contract, injecting 1 to 2 mL of chyme into the duodenum. If the chyme is not ready to be discharged, DNES cells release the hormones **cholecystokinin** and **gastric inhibitory peptide**, which inhibit the pyloric sphincter from opening, and the chyme remains in the stomach.

HCl production in the stomach has three phases: **cephalic**, referring to the thought, smell, or sight of food; **gastric**, the presence of food in the lumen of the stomach; and **intestinal**, the presence of food in the duodenum. The mechanism of HCl production by parietal cells is the same, however, regardless of the phase that induced it. The basal aspect of the cell membrane of parietal cells possesses receptors for the neurotransmitter **acetylcholine** and for the paracrine hormones **gastrin** and **histamine$_2$**. When all three sites have bound their respective signaling molecules, HCl production and its secretion into the intracellular canaliculi occurs in the following manner (Fig. 17.3):

1. **Carbonic anhydrase**, present in the cytosol, catalyzes the production of H_2CO_3, which dissociates into H^+ and HCO_3^-.
2. **Active transport** exchanges intracellular H^+ for extracellular K^+ located in the intracellular canaliculi. Although K^+ is also actively transported into the parietal cell at its basal cell membrane, it also leaves the parietal cell via K^+ channels located in the basal plasmalemma.
3. K^+ and Cl^- are actively transported out of the cell and into the intracellular canaliculi, where H^+ and Cl^- combine to form **HCl**.

4. The circulation of ions between the parietal cell and the extracellular fluid of the lamina propria alters **osmotic pressures**, causing the flow of H_2O into the parietal cell.
5. The **movement of ions** between the parietal cell and the intracellular canaliculi alters the osmotic pressure within the parietal cell, causing the movement of H_2O into the intracellular canaliculi.
6. HCl and water, the main components of the gastric juice, are released into the intracellular canaliculi, spaces that are continuous with the lumen of the stomach.

The presence of tight junctions formed by the epithelial lining of the gastric mucosa prevents the entry of HCl from the gastric lumen into the lamina propria. Additionally, the HCO_3^- that is produced by the parietal cell is released into the lamina propria and, by its buffering action, protects the lamina propria from the accidental leakage of HCl from the gastric lumen. Another possible protection is afforded by the release of **prostaglandins** in areas whose epithelial barrier is accidentally breached. Prostaglandins in the lamina propria amplify blood flow to the area, facilitating the elimination of H^+ from the affected region.

The **inhibition** of HCl production and secretion is controlled by four hormones:

- **Prostaglandin**, **gastric inhibitory peptide**, and **urogastrone** act directly on parietal cells, inhibiting their secretory activity.
- The fourth hormone, **somatostatin**, inhibits the release of gastrin by G cells and histamine by enterochromaffin-like cells, eliminating the signaling molecules necessary for inducing parietal cells to make and secrete HCl.

Small Intestine

The small intestine (Fig. 17.4) is approximately 7 m in length and is said to have three regions. The first portion is the very short **duodenum**, about 25 cm long; the middle portion is the **jejunum**, whose wall is relatively thick and is a little less than 3 m long; and the third portion is the ileum, which is the narrowest, has the thinnest walls, and is about 4 m in length. The small intestine receives digestive enzymes from the pancreas and bile from the gallbladder, which assist it in digesting the food in its lumen and absorbing water and the nutrients generated. Histologically, the three regions are quite similar to each other. After a general description of their common features, the differences among the three regions are described in detail.

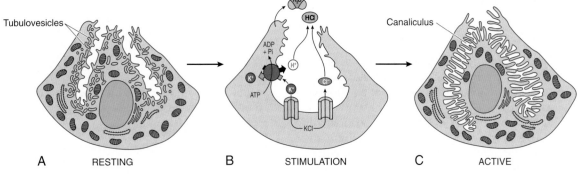

Figure 17.3 Graphic representation of hydrochloric acid production by parietal cells. **A,** Resting cell. **B,** Mechanism of HCl release. **C,** Numerous microvilli in an active cell. *(From Gartner LP, Hiatt JL: Color Textbook of Histology, 3rd ed. Philadelphia, Saunders, 2007, p 397.)*

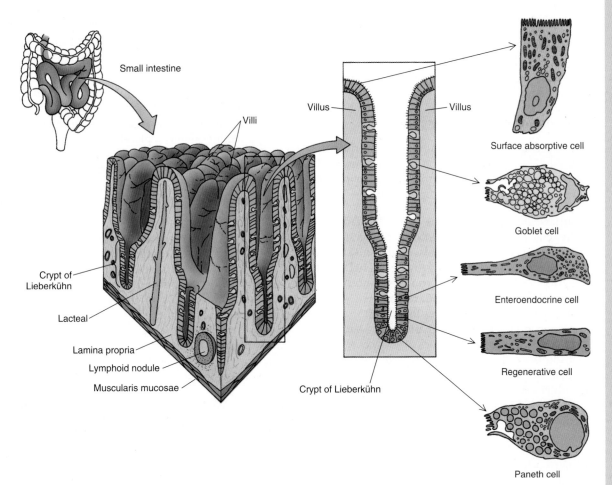

Figure 17.4 Graphic representation of the small intestine and the cell types composing its epithelial lining. *(From Gartner LP, Hiatt JL: Color Textbook of Histology, 3rd ed. Philadelphia, Saunders, 2007, p 399.)*

COMMON HISTOLOGIC FEATURES

To increase the luminal surface area of the small intestine, its submucosa and mucosa have:

- Transverse folds, **plicae circulares (valves of Kerckring)**, begin in the duodenum and extend into the ileum, retard the velocity of chyme, and augment the surface area two- to threefold.
- Finger-like extensions of the lamina propria, **villi**, are covered by a simple cuboidal epithelium and enlarge the luminal surface 10-fold; these **villi** are 1.5 mm tall in the duodenum, 1 mm tall in the jejunum, and 0.5 mm tall in the ileum; each villus possesses a vascular, loose connective tissue core with a blindly ending lymph capillary, the **lacteal**.
- Simple columnar epithelial cells covering each villus possess abundant **microvilli** that augment the luminal surface area 20-fold.
- Intervillous spaces of the small intestine display openings of the **crypts of Lieberkühn**, which increase the luminal surface area by a factor of 3 to 4.

HISTOLOGY OF THE SMALL INTESTINE

The **mucosa** of the small intestine comprises the epithelial lining, lamina propria, and muscularis mucosae (Fig. 17.5). The simple columnar epithelium covering the villus is composed of:

- **Surface absorptive cells**, the most abundant of the cells, function in the end stage of digestion and in absorbing amino acids, lipids, and sugars. These cells possess 3000 microvilli covered with a glycocalyx; the glycocalyx comprises mostly **enterokinases**, **aminopeptidases**, and **oligosaccharidases**, enzymes that digest oligopeptides and oligosaccharides. The lateral aspects of the cell membranes of surface absorptive cells adhere to the membranes of adjacent cells by forming junctional complexes.
- **Goblet cells** manufacture **mucinogen**, a complex protein polysaccharide that, when in contact with water, becomes **mucin**. When released into the lumen, it mixes with the luminal content and becomes a slippery substance known as **mucus**.
- **DNES** cells constitute about 1% of the villous epithelial cells, each producing a specific paracrine/endocrine hormone.
- **Microfold cells (M cells)**, located where lymphoid nodules of the lamina propria contact the epithelium, have deep folds—**intercellular pockets**. M cells phagocytose intraluminal antigens and transfer them to lymphocytes present in their intercellular pockets, which then transfer the antigens to APCs of the lamina

propria to initiate an immune response. Some of the IgA manufactured by plasma cells is endocytosed by epithelial cells that couple secretory component to it and release the complex into the lumen. Most of the IgA travels to the liver; hepatocytes complex it with secretory component and release it into the bile to be transported to the gallbladder (Fig. 17.6).

The **lamina propria** of the mucosa is a loose connective tissue that is rich in lymphoid and capillary elements, and, in the core of the villus, possesses **lacteals** (see Fig. 17.5). The deeper aspect of the lamina propria, between the base of the villi and the muscularis mucosae, is quite vascular, although it is mostly displaced by the abundance of intestinal intramural glands, the **crypts of Lieberkühn**. These glands extend from the intervillous spaces to the muscularis mucosae, and their epithelium consists of the same cell types as those covering the villus, and:

- **Regenerative cells** proliferate to form new cells of the epithelial lining. The new cell migrates along the basal lamina to the tip of the villus, where it is sloughed off into the lumen 5 to 7 days after its formation; the epithelial lining of the small intestine is replaced once every week.
- **Paneth cells** live longer (20 days), are located at the base of the crypts of Lieberkühn, and house large eosinophilic granules that contain **lysozyme** and **defensins**, antimicrobial agents, and **tumor necrosis factor-α**.

The **muscularis mucosa** is composed of an **inner circular** and an **outer longitudinal layer** of smooth muscle. Occasional smooth muscle cells enter the core of the villus extending to its tip. The **submucosa** of the small intestine is unremarkable, and its **muscularis externa** is composed of an inner circular and an outer longitudinal layer. **Meissner's** and **Auerbach's plexuses** occupy their normal positions. The outermost layer is a **serosa** except in parts of the duodenum where it is an **adventitia**.

CLINICAL CONSIDERATIONS

Defensins are produced by Paneth cells, in response to tumor necrosis factor-α and because of the presence of metabolic by-products released by microorganisms. Defensins insert into the phospholipid membranes of microorganisms, where they form ion channels that permit the leakage of ions from the invading organism, killing it. **Lysozyme**, a proteolytic enzyme also manufactured by Paneth cells, breaks down the bacterial membrane component—peptidoglycan—killing the organism.

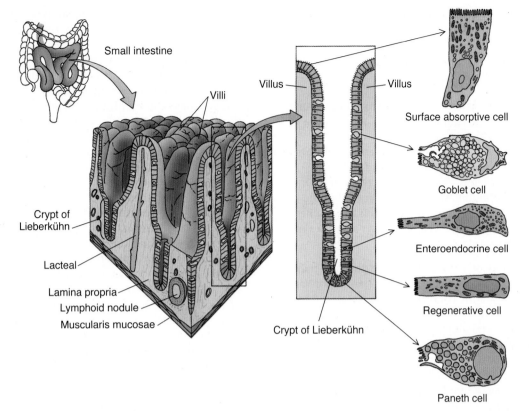

Figure 17.5 Graphic representation of the small intestine and the cell types composing its epithelial lining. *(From Gartner LP, Hiatt JL: Color Textbook of Histology, 3rd ed. Philadelphia, Saunders, 2007, p 399.)*

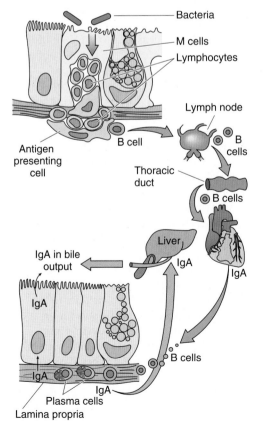

Figure 17.6 Graphic representation of the role of M cells and the circulation of IgA in the small intestine. *(From Gartner LP, Hiatt JL: Color Textbook of Histology, 3rd ed. Philadelphia, Saunders, 2007, p 405.)*

Regional Differences in the Histology of the Small Intestine

The three regions of the small intestine may be differentiated from one another by minor variations in their histologic appearance.

- The villi are tallest in the duodenum (1.5 mm), shorter in the jejunum (1 mm), and shortest in the ileum (0.5 mm).
- The major difference is the presence of Brunner's glands in the submucosa of the duodenum.
- Peyer's patches, which are collections of lymphoid nodules, are present in the lamina propria of the ileum. The jejunum has neither glands in its submucosa nor Peyer's patches in its lamina propria.

The duodenum receives the **bile duct** and **pancreatic duct** at the **duodenal papilla** (papilla of Vater). **Brunner's glands (duodenal glands)** are tubuloalveolar, branched glands that open into the base of the crypts of Lieberkühn. Brunner's glands manufacture a seromucous fluid rich in bicarbonates that acts to buffer the acidic chyme delivered from the stomach. These glands also manufacture the hormone **urogastrone (human epidermal growth factor)**, which inhibits parietal cells from manufacturing HCl and stimulates the mitotic activities of epithelial cells.

HISTOPHYSIOLOGY OF THE SMALL INTESTINE

The **motility** of the small intestine has two phases—**mixing contractions**, which are localized events that function in exposing the luminal contents to the epithelial lining of the gut, and **propulsive contractions (peristaltic waves)**, which move the luminal contents along the length of the small intestine. This movement is slow, about 1 to 2 cm/min, and chyme entering the duodenum from the stomach spends 6 to 12 hours in the small intestine. The propulsive contractions are controlled by **Auerbach's plexus** and by the DNES-derived hormones cholecystokinin, gastrin, motilin, substance P, and serotonin, which increase motility, and secretin and glucagon, which retard motility (see Table 17.1).

- **Glands of the small intestine secrete** 2 L of a seromucous secretion on a daily basis. The secretory process is mostly under the control of Meissner's submucosal plexus, but also is influenced by the DNES-derived hormones secretin and cholecystokinin.
- **Digestion** of the food material present in the lumen of the small intestine is due to the presence of enzymes, mostly derived from the pancreas and bile from the liver and concentrated in and delivered from the gallbladder. The process of digestion begins in the oral cavity and stomach and continues in the duodenum, where pancreatic enzymes degrade the various components of the chyme into oligopeptides and dipeptides and oligosaccharides and disaccharides. **Enterokinases** and **aminopeptidases**, located in the glycocalyx of the microvilli, complete protein digestion into amino acids and dipeptides and tripeptides that are absorbed into the surface absorptive cells to be converted into amino acids by **cytoplasmic peptidases**. The glycocalyx also contains **oligosaccharidases (lactase, maltase, sucrase, and α-dextrinase)** that complete the digestion of dietary carbohydrates by degrading oligosaccharides into monosaccharides that are absorbed by the surface absorptive cells. Lipids present in the chyme are emulsified by the bile salts into **micelles**, and the pancreatic lipase breaks down the lipids into fatty acids and monoglycerides, which diffuse through the plasmalemma of the microvilli.
- **Absorption** (Fig. 17.7) of the end products of digestion and electrolytes and water occurs mostly in the small and large intestines, although certain substances, such as alcohol, are also absorbed in the stomach. Enormous quantities enter the surface absorptive cells of the small intestine, including 1 kg of fat, 0.5 kg of proteins and carbohydrates, about 35 g of sodium, and 7 L of fluid per day. **Amino acids** and **monoglycerides** are released into the core of the villus, enter the tributaries of the hepatic portal vein, and go to the liver for further action. Monoglycerides and **long-chain fatty acids** bind to intracellular fatty acid–binding proteins, and enter the smooth endoplasmic reticulum to be esterified by **acyl CoA synthetase** and **acyltransferases** into triglycerides. These triglycerides, coupled to proteins, are transported to the basolateral membrane to be released into the core of the villus as **chylomicrons** that enter the lacteals, which become filled with the lipid-rich fluid, **chyle**. The lacteal is emptied because of the rhythmic contractions of the slips of smooth muscle derived from the inner circular layer of the muscularis mucosae, discharging the chyle into the submucosal lymphatic plexus. The chyle is transported to the thoracic duct to be delivered into the junction of the subclavian vein with the left internal jugular vein. Fatty acids that are less than 12 carbons long avoid the re-esterification process; instead, they pass to the basolateral cell membrane to be released into the core of the villus to travel to the hepatic portal vein and from there to the liver.

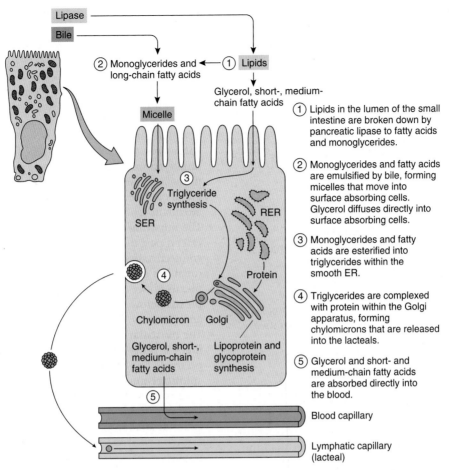

① Lipids in the lumen of the small intestine are broken down by pancreatic lipase to fatty acids and monoglycerides.

② Monoglycerides and fatty acids are emulsified by bile, forming micelles that move into surface absorbing cells. Glycerol diffuses directly into surface absorbing cells.

③ Monoglycerides and fatty acids are esterified into triglycerides within the smooth ER.

④ Triglycerides are complexed with protein within the Golgi apparatus, forming chylomicrons that are released into the lacteals.

⑤ Glycerol and short- and medium-chain fatty acids are absorbed directly into the blood.

Figure 17.7 Graphic representation of fat absorption by the surface absorptive cells in the small intestine. *(From Gartner LP, Hiatt JL: Color Textbook of Histology, 3rd ed. Philadelphia, Saunders, 2007, p 407.)*

Table 17.1 DIFFUSE NEUROENDOCRINE SYSTEM CELLS OF THE GASTROINTESTINAL TRACT

Cell	Location	Hormone Produced	Function
A	Stomach, small intestine	Glucagon	Elevates blood glucose
D	Stomach, intestines	Somatostatin	Inhibits hormone release by DNES cells
EC	Stomach, intestines	Serotonin, substance P	Increases peristaltic movement
ECL	Stomach	Histamine	Stimulates HCl secretion
G	Stomach, small intestine	Gastrin	Stimulates HCl secretion; gastric motility
GL	Stomach, intestines	Glicentin	Elevates blood glucose levels
I	Small intestine	Cholecystokinin	Stimulates release of pancreatic enzymes and contraction of gallbladder
K	Small intestine	Gastric inhibitory peptide	Inhibits HCl secretion
Mo	Small intestine	Motilin	Increases intestinal peristalsis
N	Small intestine	Neurotensin	Decreases intestinal peristalsis
PP	Stomach, large intestine	Pancreatic polypeptide	Stimulates enzyme release by chief cells; inhibits release of pancreatic enzymes
S	Small intestine	Secretin	Stimulates release of pancreatic buffer
VIP	Stomach, intestines	Vasoactive intestinal peptide	Increases peristalsis of intestines; stimulates elimination of water and ions

EC, enterochromaffin cell; ECL, enterochromaffin-like cell; G, gastrin-producing cell; GI, gastrointestinal; GL, glicentin-producing cell; HCl, hydrochloric acid; MO, motilin-producing cell; N, neurotensin-producing cell; PP, pancreatic polypeptide–producing cell; VIP, vasoactive intestinal peptide–producing cell.

From Gartner LP, Hiatt JL: Color Textbook of Histology, 3rd ed. Philadelphia, Saunders, 2007, p 392.

Large Intestine

The **large intestine**, approximately 1.5 m long, comprises the cecum, appendix, colon, rectum, and anus. Histologically, except for the appendix and the anus, these regions are very similar and are referred to as the **colon**. The colon functions in the absorption of water, electrolytes, and gases and in the compaction of chyme it receives from the ileum into feces.

The colon resembles the small intestine except that it has a greater diameter and possesses no villi.

- The **crypts of Lieberkühn** resemble their counterparts in the small intestine, but they lack Paneth cells, possess few DNES cells, and have a greater number of goblet cells (Fig. 17.8). Although it would appear at first glance that most of the epithelial cells are goblet cells, actually more than half of them are surface absorptive cells. As in other regions of the alimentary canal, the entire epithelial lining is replaced via mitotic activity of the regenerative cells at least once per week.
- The lamina propria, muscularis mucosae, and submucosa are unremarkable.
- The **muscularis externa** is modified in that many of the smooth muscle fibers of the outer longitudinal layer are collected into three slim bands of muscle, the **taeniae coli**, that are almost in constant tonus, making them shorter than the colon.
- The colon forms a linear sequence of pouches, called **haustra coli**, along its length.
- The entire colon is invested by a **serosa** except at the anus, where it is attached to the body wall by a connective tissue adventitia. Along the length of the colon, the serosa forms fat-filled pouches known as **appendices epiploicae**.

The **function** of the **colon** is the secretion of bicarbonate-rich mucus; it also **absorbs** more fluid and electrolytes from the intestinal contents, accomplishing the **compaction** of the feces. Every day, the colon reclaims about 1.4 L of electrolyte-containing fluids and reduces the daily feces volume to approximately 100 mL. The colon absorbs approximately 6 to 9 L of gases a day, releasing only about 0.5 to 1 L of gas as flatus. The crypts of Lieberkühn of the **rectum** are sparsely distributed and deeper than those of the colon; otherwise, the rectum greatly resembles the colon.

- The 3- to 4-cm-long **anal canal** is narrower than the rectum, and in its lower half it does not possess even the shallow crypts of Lieberkühn present in its upper half.
- The anal mucosa presents longitudinal folds, **anal columns** (of Morgagni), that converge at the **pectinate line** to form the **anal valves** that house the pocket-like **anal sinuses**.
- The anal canal is lined by a simple cuboidal epithelium that becomes stratified squamous nonkeratinized below the pectinate line. The fibroelastic **lamina propria** houses **circumanal glands** at the anus; hair follicles and their attendant sebaceous glands are present here.
- The **muscularis mucosae** is present but does not extend past the pectinate line. The fibroelastic connective tissue of the **submucosa** of the anal canal has an **internal hemorrhoidal venous plexus** above and **external hemorrhoidal venous plexus** below the pectinate line, just above the anal orifice.
- The **muscularis externa** is unremarkable except that the inner **circular layer** is thickened at the pectinate line to form the **internal anal sphincter muscle**, and the external longitudinal layer is replaced by a fibroelastic membrane that surrounds the internal anal sphincter. The **external anal sphincter muscle** is formed by thickenings of the skeletal muscle of the floor of the pelvis and surrounds the internal anal sphincter and the fibroelastic sheath. This skeletal muscle sphincter muscle permits voluntary control over the anus.
- The outermost layer of the colon is a **serosa**.

The **appendix** is a narrow 5- to 6-cm-long outpocketing of the cecum whose stellate lumen is lined by simple columnar epithelium composed of surface absorptive cells, goblet cells, and M cells that adjoins the lymphoid nodules present in the lamina propria. The crypts of Lieberkühn are sparse and shallow and are composed of surface absorptive cells, goblet cells, regenerative cells, numerous DNES cells, and occasional Paneth cells. The lamina propria is a loose connective tissue richly endowed with lymphoid cells and lymphoid nodules. The **muscularis mucosae**, **submucosa**, and **muscularis externa** follow the common organization of the digestive tract. The outermost layer of the appendix is a **serosa**.

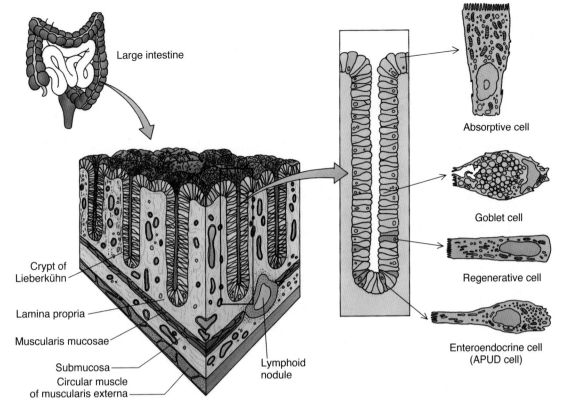

Figure 17.8 Graphic representation of the colon and the cell types composing its epithelial lining. *(From Gartner LP, Hiatt JL: Color Textbook of Histology, 3rd ed. Philadelphia, Saunders, 2007, p 408.)*

CLINICAL CONSIDERATIONS

Crohn's disease is a chronic inflammation of the wall of the alimentary canal that occurs most frequently in the ileum and the colon. It is believed to be an immune-related disorder that may have genetic and environmental components. It occurs in equal distribution among men and women, making its first appearance usually between ages 15 and 25 years, but almost always before age 35. The usual symptoms are fever, chronic diarrhea that may or may not be accompanied by bleeding, abdominal cramps of varied severity, weight loss, and lack of appetite. The symptoms may last several weeks and then resolve by themselves, only to recur at various indeterminate intervals with variable degrees of severity. The location of the inflammation may be the same as before, or it may spread to other regions of the alimentary canal. Common complications are the formation of fistulas and obstruction of the digestive canal, and in the colon it may lead to colorectal cancer. Although Crohn's disease is incurable, palliative treatments include the use of antidiarrheal and anti-inflammatory agents, antibiotics, immunomodulators, dietary modifications, and, if necessary, surgical resection of the affected areas.

Individuals with **cholera** have ingested water or food infected with *Vibrio cholerae,* an organism that produces cholera toxin. Although cholera is a very easily treated disease, it is widespread in the tropical and subtropical regions in developing countries, where it is responsible for a high degree of fatality. Cholera is prevented successfully by employing proper sanitary conditions and is treated by antibiotics and the rapid administration of electrolyte-balanced fluids to replace fluid and electrolyte losses, which may be 10 L/day owing to uncontrolled diarrhea.

Intestinal gas is a by-product of bacterial metabolism and some swallowed air. The odoriferous components of feces are mercaptans, indole, and hydrogen sulfide, and the odoriferous component of flatus is methane. Because the methane gas is mixed with O_2, CO_2, and H_2, it is quite flammable, and occasionally during cauterization as part of sigmoidoscopy, small, localized explosions may occur.

18 DIGESTIVE SYSTEM: GLANDS

The **glands** of the digestive system are located within the wall of the alimentary canal—the **intramural glands** and outside the wall the **extramural glands**, including the major salivary glands (parotid, submandibular, and sublingual glands), pancreas, and liver (and gallbladder), whose secretions gain access to the lumen of the alimentary canal by a system of ducts.

Major Salivary Glands

The **major salivary glands** (Fig. 18.1)—parotid, submandibular, and sublingual—are compound tubuloalveolar glands that secrete saliva.

- Each major salivary gland is surrounded by a connective tissue **capsule** that sends connective tissue **septa** into the substance of the gland dividing it into lobes and lobules.
- The neurovascular elements travel in these connective tissue septa to supply the **parenchyma** of the gland. The parenchyma is the secretory portion, consisting of acini or tubules or both, and a duct portion that culminates in the principal duct of the gland.
- The functional unit of a salivary gland, the **salivon**, is composed of an acinus and its intercalated and striated ducts.

Three types of cells form the secretory portion of a salivary gland: serous, mucous, and myoepithelial.

- **Serous cells** resemble a truncated pyramid, and they produce a watery fluid composed mostly of water, electrolytes, and enzymes (**salivary amylase** and **lipase**) that begin digestion in the oral cavity. Other secretions include kallikrein and the antibacterial agents lysozyme and lactoferrin. The secretions are stored in apically located **zymogen granules** (secretory granules) until their release is prompted.
- **Mucous cells** resemble serous cells, but their apical cytoplasm houses secretory granules filled with **mucinogen**, a proteoglycan that, when released, becomes hydrated to form **mucin**. When mucin mixes with the secretion, it becomes **mucus**.

- **Acini** are composed of serous cells only, mucous cells only, or mucous cells only but capped by a few serous cells as **serous demilunes**. Each acinus is surrounded by a basal lamina, and **myoepithelial cells** whose contraction assists in delivering the secretory product of the acinus into the lumen to enter the ducts.

The **ducts** of salivary glands begin as very slender conduits lined by simple cuboidal epithelium known as **intercalated ducts**.

- The secretion entering these ducts and isotonic with blood is known as the **primary saliva**. Larger, **striated ducts**, lined with low columnar epithelial cells, receive the primary saliva.
- The basal cell membranes of these cells display numerous mitochondria-rich folds that actively transport Na^+ out of the lumen and K^+ and HCO_3^- into the lumen of the duct, modifying the primary saliva into hypotonic **secondary saliva**. Several striated ducts unite to form intralobular ducts, which unite to form larger excretory ducts.
- The principal excretory duct that delivers the saliva into the oral cavity is usually lined by a stratified cuboidal to pseudostratified epithelium.

Plasma cells of the connective tissue **stroma** make **IgA dimers** that are held to each other by a **J chain**. These dimers are taken up by the acinar cells and by striated duct cells where the secretory component is added, forming secretory IgA that is transferred into the lumen of the acinus and striated duct.

In contrast to the minor salivary glands, the major salivary glands secrete on demand, and their secretion is controlled by the process of smelling food, chewing, and vomiting. Saliva output is about 1 L/day and is reduced with fear and fatigue and while sleeping. Parasympathetic innervation induces flow mainly of watery saliva, whereas sympathetic innervation induces the release of more viscous saliva.

Of the major salivary glands, the **parotid gland** produces a serous secretion, about 30% of the saliva, whereas the **submandibular gland** produces 60%, and the **sublingual gland** produces only 5% of saliva. The latter two glands release a **mixed saliva**.

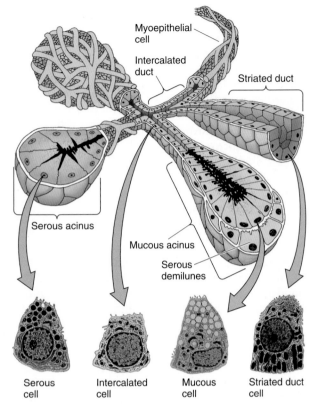

Figure 18.1 Generalized depiction of a major salivary gland. *(From Gartner LP, Hiatt JL: Color Textbook of Histology, 3rd ed. Philadelphia, Saunders, 2007, p 414.)*

CLINICAL CONSIDERATIONS

The **flow of saliva** is essential for the maintenance of a healthy mouth because saliva cleanses the teeth, keeps the oral mucosa moist, and offers the first line of defense against invading microorganisms. Also, by moistening the food, it allows the formation of a compact, but pliable and slippery bolus that can be swallowed easily. Salivary flow is normal when one is relaxed; however, when an individual is scared or nervous, the mouth becomes dry. This condition was well known during the time of the Inquisition and was used by the court in trying the individual. The accused was given flour to swallow with the assumption that if the individual was not guilty, he or she would not be nervous or scared and could produce enough saliva to swallow the flour. Naturally, the accused was always nervous and scared, and because of the limited salivary flow could not swallow the flour; this was taken as undeniable evidence that the accused was guilty as charged.

Mumps is a viral disease that most commonly occurs in children 5 to 15 years old. It is spread by droplets of virus-containing saliva that become airborne after an infected individual coughs near an uninfected individual or if an uninfected individual has contact with an object on which saliva from an infected individual has landed. The incubation period for mumps is 2 to 3 weeks, after which the patient becomes lethargic, has a headache, and experiences a lack of appetite. The most frequent symptom is painful swelling of the parotid glands that is accompanied by a high fever of 103°F to 104°F. Most children in the United States are immunized against mumps, so incidence of this disease is very low. Mumps is much more serious in men because it may spread to one or both testes, where it may cause sterility, or to the meninges and pancreas, but usually the infection resolves itself.

Pancreas

The **pancreas** is a 25-cm-long gland that weighs about 150 g and has an exocrine and an endocrine component. Its insubstantial connective tissue capsule sends septa into the substance of the gland, which not only subdivide it into lobes and lobules but also convey a system of ducts and neurovascular elements to serve the gland. The **exocrine portion** occupies most of the gland, and the **endocrine component**, the islets of Langerhans, is distributed as richly vascularized spherical clusters of endocrine cells among the secretory acini (Fig. 18.2).

The **exocrine pancreas**, composed of tubuloacinar units with its associated system of ducts, manufactures and releases:

- Approximately 1.2 L of a buffered fluid that is designed to neutralize the acidic chyme released by the stomach into the duodenum
- **Proenzymes** that are activated when in the lumen of the duodenum to break down the nutrient-rich chyme

Each **acinus** is composed of 40 to 50 **acinar cells**. The lumen of the acinus houses a few **centroacinar cells**, the beginning elements of the pancreatic duct system. The presence of centroacinar cells is characteristic of the pancreas.

- Acinar cells resemble truncated pyramids whose apex is packed with zymogen granules containing proenzymes. The basal plasmalemma of each acinar cell possesses receptors for the hormone cholecystokinin and the neurotransmitter acetylcholine.
- The centroacinar cells of each acinus are continuous with the **intercalated ducts**, several of which join to form **intralobular ducts**, which unite with others to form **interlobular** and larger ducts that eventually drain into the **main pancreatic duct**. The common bile duct of the gallbladder and the main pancreatic duct join each other to pierce the wall of the duodenum, forming the **papilla of Vater**.

The **acinar cells** function in the synthesis of digestive proenzymes and enzymes that are stored and released when prompted by the binding of acetylcholine from parasympathetic postganglionic fibers in conjunction with cholecystokinin released from diffuse neuroendocrine system (DNES) cells of the duodenum.

- The **enzymes** released by the pancreatic acinar cells are RNase, DNase, lipase, and amylase, and the proenzymes released are elastase, chymotrypsinogen, trypsinogen, and procarboxypeptidase.
- The acinar cells protect themselves by synthesizing **trypsin inhibitor** to prevent the activation of trypsinogen while in the cytosol.
- The **bicarbonate-rich buffer** is released by cells of intercalated ducts and centroacinar cells in response to the binding to receptors of their basal plasmalemmae of acetylcholine, derived from postganglionic parasympathetic fibers and secretin, derived from DNES cells of the duodenum. The bicarbonate is manufactured within the striated duct cells that combine CO_2 and H_2O, which form H_2CO_3. This molecule dissociates into H^+ and HCO_3^-. The bicarbonate is released into the lumen of the duct along with Na^+ to maintain neutrality. H^+ is released into the connective tissue to enter the periacinar capillary bed.
- Because the **mechanism of release** of the enzymes and buffer depends on different signaling molecules, the enzymes and buffer are released independently, although sometimes simultaneously.

ENDOCRINE PANCREAS

The endocrine pancreas is composed of approximately 1 million **islets of Langerhans**, each encased in a thin, reticular fiber sheath that sends fibers into each islet to support its separate, rich vascular supply, the **insuloacinar portal system**. Veins leaving each islet meander by neighboring acini and bring signaling molecules released by the cells of the islets to control the function of the acini.

Five cell types constitute the 3000 or so cells of each islet of Langerhans. Each cell type manufactures a particular hormone: α cells manufacture **glucagon**, β cells synthesize **insulin**, δ cells form **somatostatin**, PP cells manufacture **pancreatic polypeptide**, and G cells manufacture **gastrin**. The frequency of these cells in the islets of Langerhans, the hormones that they produce, and the functions of the hormones are presented in Table 18.1.

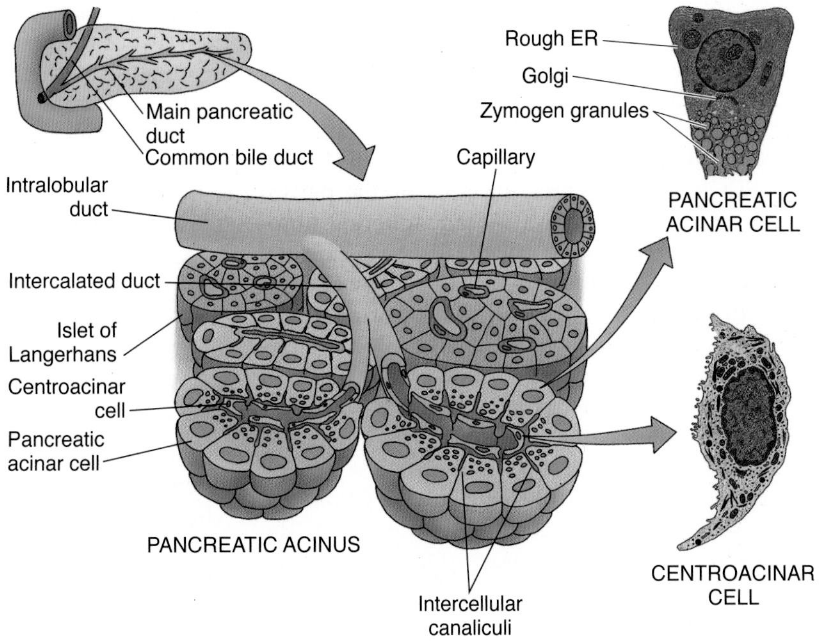

Figure 18.2 The pancreas displaying its tubuloacinar units and system of ducts and its endocrine components, the islets of Langerhans. ER, endoplasmic reticulum. *(From Gartner LP, Hiatt JL: Color Textbook of Histology, 3rd ed. Philadelphia, Saunders, 2007, p 418.)*

Table 18.1 CELLS AND HORMONES OF THE ISLETS OF LANGERHANS

Cells	Incidence	Hormone Produced	Function of Hormone
β cell	70%	Insulin	Decreases blood glucose levels
α cell	20%	Glucagon	Increases blood glucose levels
δ cell	5%		
D cell		Somatostatin	Inhibits release of hormones and exocrine products of pancreas
D$_1$ cell		Vasoactive intestinal peptide	Induces glycogenolysis; regulates intestinal motility; controls secretion of ions and H$_2$O by intestines
G cell	2%–3%	Gastrin	Stimulates HCl production by parietal cells of stomach
PP cell	2%–3%	Pancreatic polypeptide	Inhibits exocrine secretion by pancreas

Modified from Gartner LP, Hiatt JL: Color Textbook of Histology, 3rd ed. Philadelphia, Saunders, 2007, p 421.

CLINICAL CONSIDERATIONS

Diabetes mellitus is a condition in which the blood glucose level is higher than normal. There are two types of diabetes mellitus: **type 1**, which begins at a young age because the patient does not manufacture enough insulin, and **type 2**, which begins later in life when the patient produces enough insulin, but the body becomes resistant to its effects. The primary cause of type 2 diabetes mellitus is obesity, although chronic increased levels of corticosteroids and pancreatitis are also factors in the development of this disease. With the increasing incidence of obesity in children and in adults in the United States, the incidence of type 2 diabetes has been increasing. Initially, there are no overt symptoms of type 2 diabetes, but after years of living with this condition symptoms begin to be noted. The symptoms include increased urinary output, feeling of thirst, fatigue, dehydration, dizziness, confusion, blurred vision, and seizures. It is usually at this time that the patient sees a physician, and blood tests show very high blood glucose levels. The long-term sequelae may be very serious, involving circulatory problems, elevated blood pressure, damage to the heart, gangrene of the extremities, kidney failure, and blindness. The treatment is the reduction of blood glucose levels, which in type 2 diabetes can be accomplished with diet and exercise and medication in some cases.

Liver

The parenchymal cells of the **liver**, the largest gland of the body, are the **hepatocytes**, which manufacture the exocrine secretion—bile—and form myriad endocrine products that they release into the blood. The liver is almost entirely invested by the **peritoneum**, deep to which is a loosely adhering fibroelastic connective tissue called **Glisson's capsule**. Connective tissue elements, derived from the capsule, enter the substance of the liver at the **porta hepatis** and convey vascular, lymphatic, and bile duct elements into and out of the liver. The right and left hepatic arteries provide about 25% of the liver's oxygen supply, whereas the remaining 75% is received from the nutrient-laden blood carried by the **hepatic portal vein** that brings blood to the liver from the entire gastrointestinal tract and from the spleen. The **hepatic veins** carry blood away from the liver at its back, not at the porta hepatis, to deliver it into the **inferior vena cava** (Fig. 18.3).

CLASSIC LIVER LOBULE

The liver acts as a central depot, receiving blood that carries all the nutrients, except for chylomicrons, absorbed in the gastrointestinal tract. The liver also receives blood from the spleen bearing iron and degradation products of old red blood cells destroyed by that organ. Hepatocytes not only process these nutrients, store them, and convert them into products usable by the cells of the body, but also they eliminate toxic substances.

- The liver is organized into richly vascularized hexagonal solids, **classic lobules** that are 2 mm high and less than 1 mm across (see Fig. 18.3). In some animals, classic lobules are bounded by connective tissue, but in humans the connective tissue is too slim to define their borders clearly.
- These connective tissue elements are thickened, however, even in human livers, at the junction of three classic lobules into a **portal area (triad)** that houses slender branches of the portal vein, the hepatic artery, the interlobular bile duct, and a lymph vessel (see Fig. 18.3).
- Only three of the portal areas associated with the six longitudinal edges of the classic lobule are well defined. They are disposed so that they occupy every alternate edge of each lobule.
- A cylindrical **limiting plate**, composed of modified hepatocytes, surrounds each portal area but is isolated from the connective tissue by the **space of Moll**.
- Each branch of the hepatic artery at the portal area gives rise to numerous smaller branches, **distributing arterioles** that resemble the legs of

centipedes as they wrap around the adjacent walls of the hexagonal lobule, reaching toward the distributing arterioles from the adjacent portal area.
- Even smaller **inlet arterioles** arise from the distributing arterioles to serve the substance of each classic lobule. The branches of the portal vein emulate those of the hepatic artery, forming **distributing veins** and **inlet venules**.
- Interlobular bile ducts are supplied by the **peribiliary capillary plexus**. Bile, released into bile ducts, is delivered into the gallbladder for storage and eventual release.

The center of each classic lobule displays a longitudinally disposed **central vein**, the beginning of the **hepatic vein** (see Fig. 18.3). Anastomosing plates of liver cells radiate from the central vein, forming open vascular channels between them, known as **hepatic sinusoids**, which open into the central vein. Inlet arterioles and inlet venules deliver their blood into the hepatic sinusoids and then into the central vein. On leaving the lobule, the central vein drains into the **sublobular vein**, which receives numerous additional central veins from other classic lobules. Sublobular veins join each other to form **collecting veins** that eventually form the hepatic vein, taking blood away from the liver and into the inferior vena cava.

THREE CONCEPTS OF LIVER LOBULES

- As noted earlier, the **classic liver lobule** is a hexagonal solid in which the blood flows from the periphery of the lobule to the center, and bile flows in the opposite direction (Fig. 18.4).
- Generally, the flow of exocrine secretory product is toward the center of a lobule—hence another lobule was imagined in which, in a two-dimensional view of the liver, three adjoining central veins were imagined to form the apices of a lobule and the portal area then became the center of the lobule, called the **portal lobule**, where bile flows toward the center, as expected of an exocrine gland.
- The third model is based on blood flow. There are three concentric, diamond-shaped zones of hepatocytes observed, called the **acinus of Rappaport**: the zones closest to the central vein are zone 3, the zones closest to the periphery of the acinus of Rappaport are zone 1, and the zones in the region in between are zone 2. The boundaries of the acinus are formed by four imaginary lines, extending from a central vein to portal area to the adjoining central vein to the opposite portal area and back to the original central vein. The center of the acinus is the distributing arteriole.

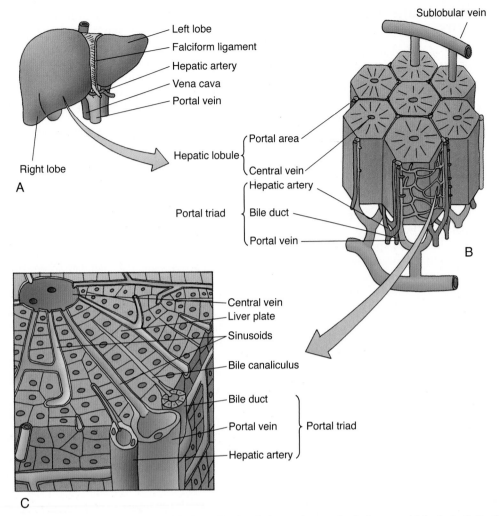

Figure 18.3 Liver. **A,** Gross anatomy. **B,** Classic lobules indicating their vascular supply, drainage, and bile ducts. **C,** Portion of a classic lobule displaying its various components. *(From Gartner LP, Hiatt JL: Color Textbook of Histology, 3rd ed. Philadelphia, Saunders, 2007, p 424.)*

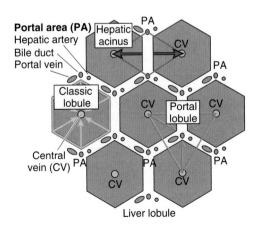

Figure 18.4 The three concepts of the liver lobule: classic lobule, portal lobule, and the acinus of Rappaport. *(From Gartner LP, Hiatt JL: Color Textbook of Histology, 3rd ed. Philadelphia, Saunders, 2007, p 425.)*

HEPATIC SINUSOIDS, PLATES OF LIVER CELLS, AND HEPATOCYTES

The plates of liver cells of an adult human, composed of a single layer of hepatocytes, anastomose with each other as they extend from the central vein, similar to spokes of a wheel, to the borders of a classic lobule. The spaces between the plates are occupied by **hepatic sinusoids** bounded by fenestrated **sinusoidal lining cells**. This endothelium is leaky because its cells have intercellular gaps as large as 0.5 μm. **Kupffer cells** (resident macrophages) are located on the sinusoidal aspect of the endothelial cells (Fig. 18.5).

- The sinusoidal lining cells are separated from the plate of hepatocytes by a 0.2- to 0.5-μm-wide space, the **perisinusoidal space of Disse**, where exchange of material between the **basolateral domain** of hepatocytes and the blood occurs, preventing hepatocytes from contacting the bloodstream. To increase their surface area, hepatocytes form microvilli on their surface that abuts the space of Disse.
- Additionally, this space contains collagen fibers, mostly type III but also some types I and IV, and two types of cells: **pit cells**, believed to be natural killer cells, and slender **Ito cells** (also known as **fat-storing cells** or **hepatic stellate cells**).
  - Ito cells store fats and vitamin A, manufacture type III collagen and other extracellular matrix components to be released into the space of Disse, and manufacture growth factors.
- In response to **tumor growth factor-β** (TGF-β) activation by hepatocytes and Kupffer cells, hepatic stellate cells not only increase their production and release of collagen, which reduces the leakiness of the endothelium, but they also transform into **myofibroblasts**, cells that reduce blood flow into the hepatic sinuses and facilitate cirrhosis-induced portal hypertension.

Hepatocytes are large, polygonal cells 20 to 30 μm in diameter that are closely packed within individual plates of liver cells. Each hepatocyte has:

- **Lateral domains**, where the hepatocyte comes in contact with other hepatocytes and forms narrow intercellular channels, **bile canaliculi**, into which hepatocytes deliver primary bile via active transport.
- **Sinusoidal domains**, where the hepatocyte comes in contact with the space of Disse to deliver its endocrine secretion and to endocytose material from the hepatic sinusoids (Fig. 18.6).

Three out of four hepatocytes have a single **nucleus**, whereas the other 25% of the cells possess two nuclei. Nuclei of 50% of hepatocytes are small, diploid nuclei, but some are larger and evidence polyploidy, attaining even 64 N.

The bile that hepatocytes manufacture is **primary bile**, which becomes concentrated and modified within the gallbladder to become the **bile** that is released into the duodenum.

- Because hepatocytes synthesize myriad proteins for their own use and for export, their cytoplasm is rich in **Golgi apparatus**, **ribosomes**, and **rough endoplasmic reticulum (ER)**.
- These cells also possess an abundance of **mitochondria** to serve their enormous adenosine triphosphate (ATP) needs. The mitochondria of zone 3 of the acinus of Rappaport are smaller but more abundant than the mitochondria of zone 1.
- Hepatocytes are also richly endowed by **smooth ER** because this organelle serves the detoxifying function of hepatocytes.
- Hepatocytes are also rich in inclusions such as **lipid deposits**, especially in the form of **very-low-density lipoproteins (VLDLs)**, and **glycogen (beta particles)** in large clumps surrounded by smooth ER in zone 1 hepatocytes and sparse deposits in zone 3 liver cells.
- Hepatocytes are also rich in **peroxisomes**, organelles that house oxidases that form H_2O_2 and **catalase** that breaks down H_2O_2. These organelles function in detoxification, β-oxidation of fatty acids, purine metabolism, and gluconeogenesis.

If the liver is injured either by toxic substances or because of mechanical injury (as by excision of a portion of the liver), Ito cells release various growth factors, such as TGF-α, TGF-β, hepatocyte growth factor, interleukin-6, and epidermal growth factor, which induce existing hepatocytes to undergo rapid mitotic activity. If the extent of the lesion is great, cholangioles and canals of Hering also participate in the **regeneration** of the liver.

Most of the myriad **functions** of the liver are carried out by hepatocytes.

- These functions include the formation of bile; metabolism, storage, and timely release of nutrients absorbed by the alimentary canal; detoxification of noxious substances; transfer of cholesterol and secretory IgA into bile; synthesis of albumins, nonimmune globulins, prothrombin, fibrinogen, factor VIII, complement proteins, and binding proteins for signaling molecules; and formation of urea.
- Other functions of the liver occur in Ito cells (storage of vitamin A) and Kupffer cells (phagocytosis).

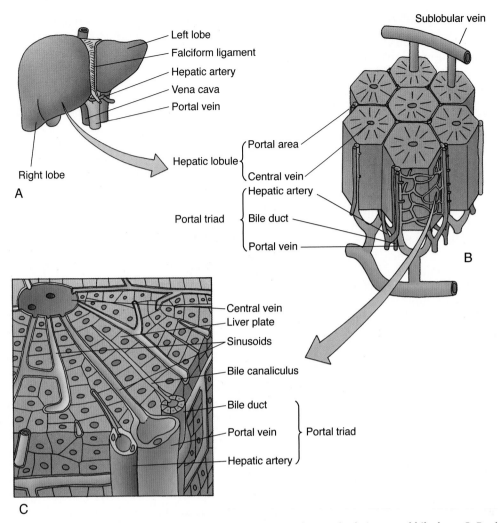

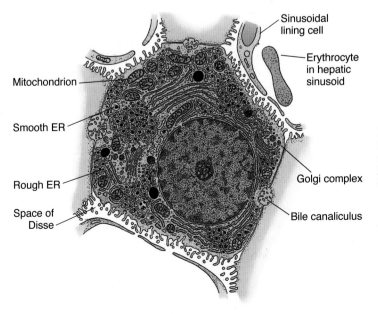

Figure 18.5 Liver. **A,** Gross anatomy. **B,** Classic lobules indicating their vascular supply, drainage, and bile ducts. **C,** Portion of a classic lobule displaying its various components. *(From Gartner LP, Hiatt JL: Color Textbook of Histology, 3rd ed. Philadelphia, Saunders, 2007, p 424.)*

Figure 18.6 Diagram of a hepatocyte displaying its sinusoidal and lateral domains. ER, endoplasmic reticulum. *(From Gartner LP, Hiatt JL: Color Textbook of Histology, 3rd ed. Philadelphia, Saunders, 2007, p 428.)*

BILE, BILIARY DUCTS, AND GALLBLADDER

Bile is composed of water, phospholipids, cholesterol, bile salts, bile pigments, lecithin, IgA, and electrolytes. **Bile salts (bile acids)** are formed in the hepatocyte smooth ER by conjugating **choline**, the metabolic by-product of cholesterol, to glycine or taurine, forming **glycocholic acid** or **taurocholic acid**, respectively. **Biliverdin**, a by-product of the conversion of heme derived from hemoglobin of erythrocytes destroyed by splenic macrophages, is reduced to the water-insoluble **bilirubin (bile pigment)** and released into the bloodstream, where it is bound to albumin. The albumin-bilirubin complex is uncoupled in hepatocytes, and the free bilirubin, complexed to the cytosolic carrier protein ligandin, enters the smooth ER, where it is uncoupled again. The **free bilirubin** enters the cytosol to be conjugated by the enzyme **glucuronyl transferase** to the water-soluble form **bilirubin glucuronide (conjugated bilirubin)**, which enters the bile canaliculi to reach the gallbladder or be released into the bloodstream (Fig. 18.7). From the gallbladder, it is released into the duodenum to become eliminated in the feces, and from the bloodstream, it enters the kidneys to be eliminated in urine.

HEPATIC DUCTS

The intercellular spaces bounded by adjacent hepatocytes form an anastomosing system of bile canaliculi that deliver their bile into **cholangioles** at the periphery of the classic lobules. These cholangioles are formed by hepatocytes contacting low cuboidal cells. Cholangioles empty into **canals of Hering**, slight branches of bile ducts composed of low cuboidal cells that parallel the inlet arterioles. **Bile ducts**, composed of a simple cuboidal epithelium, join other bile ducts to form larger and larger ducts terminating in the **right** and **left hepatic ducts**. The cuboidal cells of cholangioles, canals of Hering, and bile ducts form, in response to secretin released by DNES cells of the duodenum, a bicarbonate-rich buffer that is stored in the gallbladder for release into the duodenum along with the bicarbonate-rich buffer formed by the centroacinar cells and striated ducts of the exocrine pancreas.

The right and left hepatic ducts join each other to form the **common hepatic duct**, which joins the **cystic duct** of the gallbladder to form the 7- to 8-cm-long **common bile duct**. The **pancreatic duct** joins the common bile duct in the wall of the duodenum to form the **duodenal papilla (papilla of Vater)**, the common opening of the gallbladder and the pancreas into the lumen of the duodenum. This opening is controlled by a group of smooth muscle fibers, the **sphincter of Oddi**, which can open the two separate ducts independently of each other. Unless bile or pancreatic secretions are to be released into the duodenum, both ducts are closed. This closure of the common bile duct permits the entry of bile into the gallbladder because as the bile flows down the common bile duct and cannot enter the duodenum, the bile backs up, and at the junction of the common hepatic and cystic ducts the bile backs up into the cystic duct (flow of bile into the common hepatic duct is opposed by flow in the opposite direction from the right and left hepatic ducts).

Gallbladder

The **gallbladder**, attached to Glisson's capsule on the inferior aspect of the liver, can hold about 70 mL of bile; it is composed of a **body** that resembles a duffle bag whose opening, the **neck**, is continuous with the **cystic duct**. The function of the gallbladder is to concentrate the bile that it stores. The lumen is lined by a mucosa that is highly plicated when empty but smooth when the gallbladder is filled. Its simple columnar epithelium is composed mostly of **clear cells**, with numerous microvilli, whose function is to concentrate the bile by absorbing water via the **Na+,K+-ATPase** pump located in the basolateral plasmalemma of the cell. By actively pumping sodium out of the cell into the underlying connective tissue, Cl− and H$_2$O follow. The loss of these ions from the cell causes the same ions to enter the cell from the lumen, and the osmotic change drives water from the lumen into the cell, reducing the volume of the luminal content and concentrating bile.

The epithelium also has a few brush cells that may produce mucinogen. The fibroelastic **lamina propria** is a vascular connective tissue that houses small mucous glands, but only in the neck of the gallbladder, whose secretion lubricates the narrowed lumen of this region. The gallbladder has a two-layered, ill-defined **smooth muscle coat**, composed of an **internal oblique layer** and an **outer longitudinal layer**. The hormone **cholecystokinin** is released rhythmically by **DNES cells (I cells)** of the duodenum, and **acetylcholine** derived from the **vagus nerve** causes contraction of these smooth muscle fibers and intermittent emptying of bile from the gallbladder. Additionally, cholecystokinin and acetylcholine cause a concomitant relaxation of the sphincter of Oddi so that bile can enter the duodenum. The gallbladder has an **adventitia** where it adheres to Glisson's capsule and a **serosa** on its nonadherent aspect.

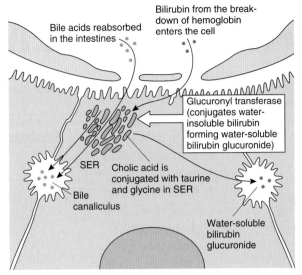

Figure 18.7 Secretion of bile acids and bilirubin by hepatocytes. SER, smooth endoplasmic reticulum. *(From Gartner LP, Hiatt JL: Color Textbook of Histology, 3rd ed. Philadelphia, Saunders, 2007, p 432.)*

CLINICAL CONSIDERATIONS

Fatty liver (steatohepatitis) may be of two types in the United States and Western countries: alcoholic and nonalcoholic. The first type is more common and is due to the excessive use of alcohol. The second type, **nonalcoholic steatohepatitis**, is due to syndromes such as diabetes mellitus, obesity, or elevated triglyceride levels. Both conditions result in an enlarged liver and can result in cirrhosis of the liver. Steatohepatitis in itself is not serious but should be controlled to prevent scarring of the liver and subsequent cirrhosis. The treatment is to control the underlying causes—eliminate excess alcohol consumption, dietary modification to reduce triglyceride levels, and lose weight in the case of obesity. The control of diabetes mellitus, when present, with insulin therapy or dietary regimen or both is essential.

The most common condition that affects the gallbladder and the biliary tract is the presence of cholesterol crystals, **gallstones**, that accumulate in that viscus (**cholelithiasis**) or along the extrahepatic bile ducts (**choledocholithiasis**) and obstruct the normal flow of bile. The presence of gallstones is gender related and age related:

More women and individuals older than 65 years have this condition. Usually, stones in the gallbladder are asymptomatic, but they can enter the biliary ducts and cause obstruction with associated inflammation and infection. When the extrahepatic bile ducts are obstructed, the patient experiences excruciating pain in the upper right of the abdomen and nausea and vomiting. Shortly after the obstruction, inflammation and infection can develop with fever and chills, and shortly thereafter the patient becomes jaundiced. The obstructed bile duct is treated either surgically or by an endoscopic procedure.

Cancers usually do not originate in the extrahepatic bile ducts, but occasionally the junction between the common bile duct and the hepatic duct develops a malignant tumor. When the mass obstructs the flow of bile, the patient becomes jaundiced without the presence of fever or chills, but with nausea, vomiting, abdominal tenderness or pain, weight loss, and generalized itching. Endoscopic treatment may permit the placement of stents to open the bile duct, but the chances of survival are not favorable.

19 URINARY SYSTEM

The two kidneys function to remove toxins from the bloodstream and to conserve water, salts, proteins, glucose, amino acids, and other essential substances. They also assist in regulating blood pressure, hemodynamics, and acid-base balance of the body fluids. Additionally, the kidneys produce hormones, such as erythropoietin and prostaglandins, and assist in the formation of vitamin D.

The hemisected view of the kidney in Figure 19.1A shows that the kidney is surrounded by a connective tissue **capsule** that covers the outer region of the substance of the kidney, known as the **cortex**, deep to which is the **medulla** with its **renal pyramids** and the intervening **cortical columns**. Each renal pyramid drains its urine into a:

- **Minor calyx**, and several minor calyces deliver their urine into a
- **Major calyx**, whose confluence forms
- The **renal pelvis**, the expanded region of the **ureter** located at the **hilum**.

Also at the hilum, the branches of the **renal artery** enter the kidney, and tributaries of the **renal vein** leave the kidney.

The basic unit of the kidney, known as the **uriniferous tubule** (Fig. 19.1B), is completely epithelial in structure and is separated from the connective tissue elements of the kidney by its **basal lamina**. It is composed of a **nephron** (**cortical** or **juxtamedullary**) and a **collecting tubule**. Several nephrons drain into a collecting tubule, and several collecting tubules join each other to form larger and larger collecting tubules. Each nephron has several component parts:

- **Bowman's capsule**
- **Proximal tubule**
- **Henle's loop**
- **Distal tubule**

About 15% of the nephrons—the juxtamedullary nephrons—have a long Henle's loop, and their renal corpuscle is located at the junction of the cortex and the medulla. About 85% of the nephrons—the corti-

cal nephrons—have a short Henle's loop, and their renal corpuscle is located closer to the kidney capsule.

Bowman's Capsule

Bowman's capsule (Fig. 19.1C), the expanded portion of the nephron, resembles a balloon during embryonic development and is composed of a simple squamous epithelium that is invaded by a cluster of fenestrated capillaries, the **glomerulus**, whose fenestrae have no diaphragms and are 70 to 90 nM in diameter. In this fashion, the space within Bowman's capsule is reduced and forms a narrow cavity, **Bowman's space** (**urinary space**), located between the outer and inner layers of Bowman's capsule (known as the **parietal** and **visceral layers of Bowman's capsule**, respectively). The glomerulus becomes invested by the visceral layer, all of whose cells become modified in shape and are known as **podocytes**. The glomerulus and Bowman's capsule collectively are known as the **renal corpuscle**. Where the podocytes and the endothelial cells of the glomerulus contact each other, the two **basal laminae** fuse. **Podocytes** (see Fig. 19.1C) bear numerous long, tentacle-like cytoplasmic extensions—**primary (major) processes**—each of which possesses many **secondary processes (pedicels)**, arranged in an orderly fashion. Pedicels completely envelop most of the glomerular capillaries by interdigitating with pedicels from neighboring major processes of different podocytes.

CLINICAL CONSIDERATIONS

During nephrogenesis and even at birth, the kidneys display signs of lobulations, but as the nephrons develop, a smooth, convex shape is formed. Occasionally, the lobes are recognizable externally in an adult, however, and this condition is known as a lobated kidney. This condition has no apparent functional consequences.

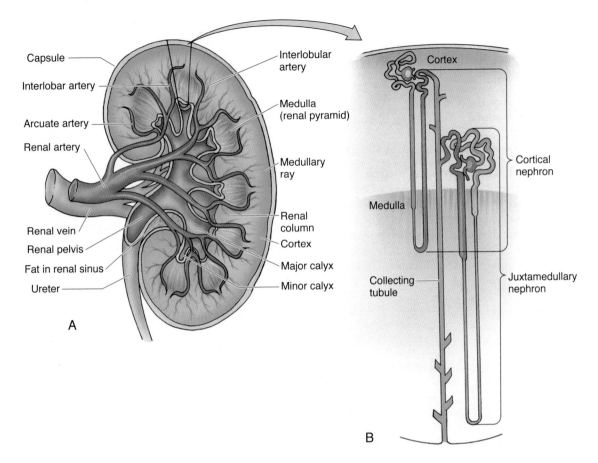

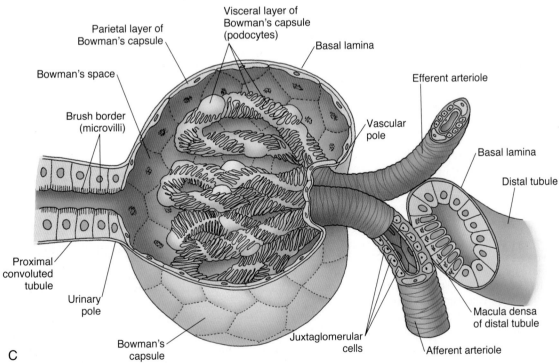

Figure 19.1 **A,** Hemisected kidney. **B,** Uriniferous tubules. **C,** Renal corpuscle. *(A–C, From Gartner LP, Hiatt JL: Color Textbook of Histology, 3rd ed. Philadelphia, Saunders, 2007, pp 438 [A and B] and 441 [C].)*

FILTRATION PROCESS

As the fluid leaves the capillary bed to enter Bowman's space, it has to pass through the filtration barrier, composed of the:

- Glomerular endothelium
- Fused basal laminae (which trap molecules >69,000 Da)
- Filtration slit diaphragm (Fig. 19.2A and *inset*)

The filtered fluid entering Bowman's space is called the **glomerular ultrafiltrate**. Because the basal lamina traps larger macromolecules, it would become clogged if it were not continuously phagocytosed by **intraglomerular mesangial cells** and replenished by the combined efforts of the visceral layer of Bowman's capsule (podocytes) and glomerular endothelial cells.

Proximal Tubule

The proximal tubule has two regions:

- Long, highly tortuous **pars convoluta (proximal convoluted tubule)** located near the renal corpuscle
- Shorter, straight **pars recta (descending thick limb of Henle's loop)** that dips into the medulla, where it joins the descending thin limb of Henle's loop (Fig. 19.2B)

Both regions of the proximal tubule are composed of a simple columnar epithelium with a well-developed apical striated border of densely packed microvilli, an endocytic apparatus richly endowed with endocytic vesicles, and intricately interleaved and interlocking lateral cellular processes.

The proximal tubule is responsible for resorbing 60% to 80% of the water, sodium, and chloride; 100% of the proteins, amino acids, and glucose; and toxins from the ultrafiltrate that enters its lumen from Bowman's space of the renal corpuscle. An adenosine triphosphate (ATP)–powered sodium pump, located in the basal cell membrane, drives sodium into the connective tissue stroma, and chloride follows passively to maintain electrical neutrality; water follows to maintain osmotic balance via **aquaporin-I channels**, reducing the volume but not affecting the osmolarity of the ultrafiltrate. The endocytic apparatus is responsible for the resorption of the larger macromolecules.

Thin Limb of Henle's Loop

The thin limb of Henle's loop, composed of a simple squamous epithelium, has three regions:

- Straight, descending thin limb
- Hairpin-shaped Henle's loop
- Straight ascending thin limb that joins the distal tubule (see Fig. 19.2B)

Although the thin limb may be absent in cortical nephrons, in juxtamedullary nephrons it is almost 1 cm long and may extend far into the medulla, reaching the renal papilla. The descending thin limb is completely permeable to water, urea, sodium, chloride, and other ions, whereas the ascending thin limb is relatively impermeable to water, but is permeable to urea and most ions.

Distal Tubule

The **distal tubule**, composed of a simple cuboidal epithelium, does not have as rich a supply of microvilli or as complex lateral interdigitations as do the cells of its proximal tubule. The distal tubule has three regions (see Fig. 19.2B):

- **Pars recta (ascending thick limb)**, which is the continuation of the ascending thin limb of Henle's loop
- Very short **macula densa**
- **Distal convoluted tubule**

CLINICAL CONSIDERATIONS

Minimal change disease is the most common kidney disorder in children. Adjacent pedicels seem to fuse with each other, resulting in proteinuria. In most cases, corticosteroid therapy successfully treats the condition.

Heroin-associated focal segmental glomerulosclerosis occurs subsequent to long-term intravenous use of heroin, resulting in significant proteinuria with irreversible uremia in 2 years. The syndrome occurs mostly in African American men younger than 50 years old. The disease attacks podocytes, causing some of them to degenerate and to lose contact with the basal lamina. The best treatment is elimination of heroin use, but in most patients progression to end-stage renal disease that would possibly require dialysis or renal transplant occurs.

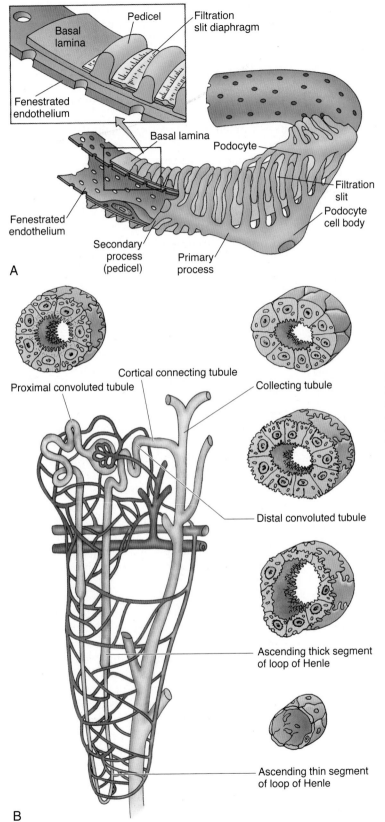

A

Pedicel
Basal
lamina
Filtration
slit diaphragm

Fenestrated
endothelium

Basal lamina
Podocyte
Filtration
slit
Podocyte
cell body

Fenestrated
endothelium

Secondary
process
(pedicel)

Primary
process

B

Cortical connecting tubule
Proximal convoluted tubule
Collecting tubule

Distal convoluted tubule

Ascending thick segment
of loop of Henle

Ascending thin segment
of loop of Henle

Figure 19.2 A, Segment of the glomerulus. **B,** Uriniferous tubule and cross sections of its component parts. *(A and B, From Gartner LP, Hiatt JL: Color Textbook of Histology, 3rd ed. Philadelphia, Saunders, 2007, pp 443 [A] and 446 [B].)*

Distal Tubule (cont.)

The pars recta of the distal tubule is almost 1 cm long, and its cells form very effective zonulae occludentes with their adjacent neighbors, forming an efficient barrier between the lumen and the surrounding connective tissue stroma and thus preventing material from taking the paracellular route. The pars recta is highly impermeable to water and urea, but its cuboidal cells possess basally located chloride (and perhaps sodium) pumps that deliver Na^+ and Cl^- into the connective tissue, reducing the Na^+ and Cl^- concentration of the ultrafiltrate in the lumen of the pars recta of the distal tubule to such an extent that by the time it reaches the corticomedullary junction, it is quite hypo-osmotic, but the concentration of urea remains high (see below).

The **macula densa**, located between the afferent and efferent glomerular arterioles in the vicinity of the distal tubule's own renal corpuscle, is part of the juxtaglomerular apparatus. The **distal convoluted tubules** (Fig. 19.3A) are less than 5 mm in length, are impermeable to water, and drain their ultrafiltrate into the collecting tubules. The columnar cells of the distal convoluted tubules possess **aldosterone receptors** and **Na+,K+-ATPase sodium-potassium exchange pumps**, both basally located. Binding of **aldosterone** to its receptors activates these cells to transfer sodium (and, passively, chloride) into the renal interstitium, reducing the osmolarity of the ultrafiltrate even further.

Juxtaglomerular Apparatus

The **juxtaglomerular apparatus** (function is described later) is composed of three parts: the macula densa, juxtaglomerular cells, and extraglomerular mesangial cells (Fig. 19.3B):

- Nuclei of the narrow, pale cells of the **macula densa** are very close to each other and appear as a dense spot—hence the name. The basal lamina is absent between the macula densa and the juxtaglomerular cells.
- **Juxtaglomerular cells** are modified smooth muscle cells of the afferent (and frequently) efferent glomerular arterioles. These cells synthesize and store **renin**, a proteolytic enzyme that converts angiotensinogen into angiotensin I. These cells also contain angiotensin-converting enzyme, angiotensin I, and angiotensin II.
- **Extraglomerular mesangial cells** occupy the space between the afferent and efferent glomerular arterioles. They may also enter the renal corpuscle, where they are known as intraglomerular mesangial cells.

Collecting Tubules

The second part of the uriniferous tubules, the **collecting tubules**, are approximately 2 cm long and have a different embryologic origin than the nephrons. The two become connected during embryonic development. Collecting tubules are composed of a simple cuboidal epithelium; they have three regions—cortical, medullary, and papillary—and during certain conditions, they modify the ultrafiltrate that they receive from nephrons.

- **Cortical collecting tubules** are located in the medullary rays, and their cuboidal epithelium is composed of principal and intercalated cells.
- **Principal cells** possess only a few, short microvilli, and their lateral cell membranes are smooth with only a few interdigitations with neighboring cells. Principal cells possess **aquaporin-2 channels** that are sensitive to antidiuretic hormone (ADH, vasopressin).
- **Intercalated cells** are of two types, **type A** and **type B**; both cell types possess numerous apically located microplicae and vesicles.
  - **Type A cells** transport H^+ into the lumen via apically located H^+-ATPase and acidify urine.
  - **Type B cells** have basolaterally located H^+-ATPase and resorb H^+ and secrete HCO_3^-.
- Several cortical collecting tubules join each other to form larger, **medullary collecting tubules** that increase in diameter as they progress deeper into the medulla. The tubules in the outer zone of the medulla have principal and intercalated cells, whereas tubules in the inner zone have only principal cells.
- Several medullary collecting tubules join each other to form the large (200 to 300 μm in diameter) **papillary collecting tubules (ducts of Bellini)** that open at the area cribrosa of the renal papilla to deliver their urine into the minor calyx. Papillary collecting tubules are formed by a simple columnar epithelium composed of **principal cells** only. These cells possess ADH receptors, and if ADH binds to these receptors, the cells place aquaporin-2 channels into their membrane and become permeable to water and to urea; as water leaves the lumina of these tubules and enters the renal interstitium, the urine becomes hyperosmotic and low in volume.

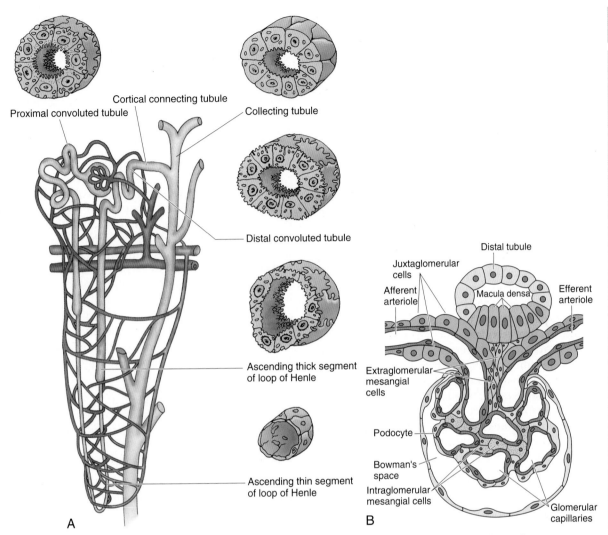

Figure 19.3 **A,** Uriniferous tubule and cross sections of its component parts. **B,** Renal corpuscle and juxtaglomerular apparatus. (**A** *and* **B,** *From Gartner LP, Hiatt JL: Color Textbook of Histology, 3rd ed. Philadelphia, Saunders, 2007, pp 446 [**A**] and 450 [**B**].)*

CLINICAL CONSIDERATIONS

Acute tubular necrosis, evidenced by engorged kidneys and focal necrosis of the kidney tubules, may be caused by nephrotoxins or ischemia, resulting in acute renal failure. Prompt correction of the insult can lead to rapid recovery as indicated by increased production of urine and reduction in serum creatinine.

Progressive, rapid, irreversible **renal failure** has been shown to be caused by the use of a weight reduction regimen that includes the Chinese herb *Aristolochia fangchi,* a family of plants that contain aristocholic acid. Renal cancers have also been

documented in patients using this herb to lose weight. Most of the patients involved were overweight, middle-aged women. Many health-conscious individuals use herbal supplements or remedies without informing their physician or other health professionals because the compounds they are ingesting are available over-the-counter, and they wrongly believe these are "natural." It is always wise for health professionals to inquire if patients are taking any over-the-counter supplements.

Renal Interstitium

The uriniferous tubules and the rich vascular supply of the kidney are completely surrounded by slender elements of connective tissue, known as the **renal interstitium**. Only 7% of the cortical volume and no more than 30% of the medullary volume is composed of connective tissue.

Renal Circulation

The **renal artery** (Fig. 19.4), a branch of the abdominal aorta, bifurcates into the anterior and posterior divisions, which in turn branch to form the five **segmental arteries** that enter the kidney at the hilum. Segmental arteries do not anastomose with each other; in a case of blockage, blood flow ceases to the region of the kidney supplied by that vessel.

Each segmental artery gives rise to **lobar arteries**, which branch to form two or three **interlobar arteries** that pass between the renal pyramids to ascend to the corticomedullary junction, where they form **arcuate arteries**. These remain at the junction of the cortex and the medulla as they distribute over the base of the renal pyramids to give rise to numerous **interlobular arteries**. The terminal branches of the arcuate arteries also become interlobular arteries.

Interlobular arteries ascend into the cortex about halfway between neighboring medullary rays and provide many branches that serve renal corpuscles. These branches are the **afferent glomerular arterioles** that are responsible for the formation of the capillary bed, or the **glomerulus**, of the renal corpuscle (see Fig. 19.4). The terminal branches of some interlobular arteries become afferent glomerular arterioles, whereas some terminate just deep to the renal capsule to participate in the formation of the **capsular plexus**. The glomerulus is drained by the **efferent glomerular arterioles (EFGs)**, which is why the blood pressure is higher within the glomerulus than in most other capillary beds (see Fig. 19.4).

- **EFGs of cortical nephrons** are responsible for the formation of the peritubular capillary network that supplies the tubules of the cortical labyrinth. These capillaries, whose endothelial cells manufacture **erythropoietin**, are drained by the **arcuate vein** (see Fig. 19.4).
- **EFGs of juxtamedullary nephrons** each branch to form 25 long, hairpin-like capillaries that extend into the medulla as far as the renal papilla. The descending limbs of these capillaries, the **arteriolae rectae**, have narrow lumina, whereas the ascending limbs, the **venae rectae**, have wider lumina, and they drain their blood into the **arcuate veins**. Together, the arteriolae

and venae rectae are known as the **vasa recta**, and they envelop the medullary regions of the uriniferous tubules. Their role in urine concentration is described subsequently.

Arcuate veins return their blood into the interlobular veins, which deliver their blood to interlobar veins and then to renal veins (see Fig. 19.4) that drain into the inferior vena cava.

Mechanism of Urine Formation

Every 5 minutes, the entire blood volume passes through the two kidneys; about 1250 mL of blood enters the glomeruli per minute. Because the glomerulus is an arterial capillary bed, blood pressure is much higher then in most other capillary beds. This and other factors exert an average of 25 mm of Hg (**filtration force**), compelling the fluid component of blood out of the capillaries and into Bowman's space, where it becomes known as the **glomerular ultrafiltrate**; 125 mL of ultrafiltrate enters Bowman's spaces per minute. The ultrafiltrate reaches Bowman's space by passing through the filtration barrier composed of:

- **Endothelial cells** of the glomerulus (stops particulate matter >90 nm in diameter)
- Fused **basal lamina** (stops macromolecules >69 kDa)
- **Filtration slits** of the podocytes

The basal laminae (similar to a filter paper in a Büchner funnel) would become rapidly clogged, but as intraglomerular mesangial cells phagocytose the basal lamina, the podocytes and endothelial cells replace it.

CLINICAL CONSIDERATIONS

Renal infarcts are common in patients with sickle cell anemia, in which smaller vessels become occluded by the malformed erythrocytes. The extent of the damage is determined by the vessel being occluded.

Fibrodysplasia (fibromuscular dysplasia) is a condition of unknown etiology that affects young women. The renal artery becomes narrowed because of the deposition of fibrous connective tissue at several sites in the wall of the artery. The stenosis is responsible for hypertension and should be suspected in young women who develop high blood pressure. This condition responds well to angioplasty and usually does not recur.

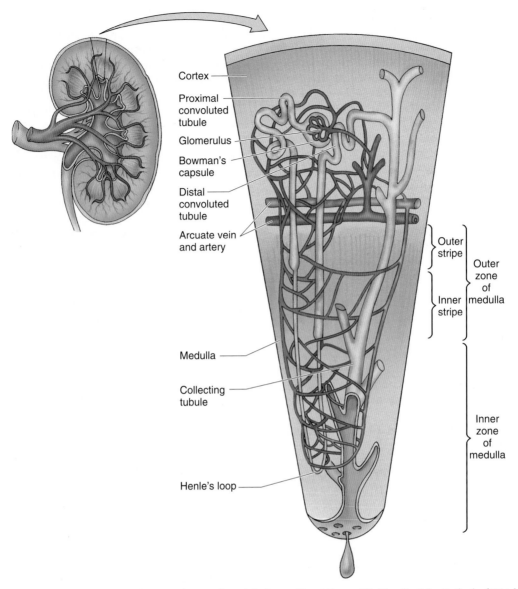

Figure 19.4 The uriniferous tubule and its vascular supply and drainage. *(From Gartner LP, Hiatt JL: Color Textbook of Histology, 3rd ed. Philadelphia, Saunders, 2007, p 439.)*

Mechanism of Urine Formation (cont.)

Most resorption occurs in the **proximal tubule**, and the recovered material enters the capillaries of the renal interstitium to be returned to the bloodstream (Fig. 19.5A and B). Most ions are resorbed secondary to the action of sodium pumps located in the basolateral cell membranes of the proximal tubules; 67% to 80% of Na^+, Cl^-, and H_2O is resorbed in the proximal tubule, reducing the volume without affecting the osmolarity of the ultrafiltrate. Additionally, almost 100% of HCO_3^- is resorbed, and 100% of the proteins, glucose, creatine, and amino acids is returned to the blood.

Juxtamedullary nephrons have a long Henle's loop and, via a **countercurrent multiplier system**, establish an increasing osmotic gradient extending from the corticomedullary junction to the renal papilla.

- The simple squamous epithelium of the **thin descending limb of Henle's loop** is permeable to water and partially permeable to salts. As the ultrafiltrate descends, it loses water, increasing its osmolarity (see Fig. 19-5A and B).
- The relatively short **thin ascending limb of Henle's loop** is mostly impermeable to water. As the ultrafiltrate flows toward the thick ascending limb, urea enters the lumen, and salts leave the lumen.
- The **thick ascending limb of Henle's loop** is composed of a simple cuboidal epithelium whose cells possess apical $Na^+/K^+/2Cl^-$ cotransporter and basally located Na^+,K^+-ATPase pump and chloride and perhaps sodium pumps that drive Cl^- and Na^+ into the renal interstitium from the lumen, establishing the gradient of salt concentration that is higher deep in the medulla and lower toward the cortex (see Fig. 19.5A and B). Consequently, the ultrafiltrate's volume remains constant, but its osmolarity decreases as the luminal fluid approaches the cortex.

MONITORING THE FILTRATE IN THE JUXTAGLOMERULAR APPARATUS

As the glomerular ultrafiltrate reaches the **macula densa**, whose cells are rich in **cyclooxygenase enzymes (COX-2)** and **nitric oxide synthase**, it is monitored for its sodium (or chloride) concentration and for its volume. At low sodium levels, the nitric oxide synthase synthesizes **nitric oxide**, which, when released, causes dilation of the afferent glomerular arteriole, increasing the flow of blood into the glomerulus. Concurrently, nitric oxide and **prostaglandin E₂**, a COX-2 product, prompt the **juxtaglomerular cells** to release **renin** into the bloodstream. This enzyme cleaves two amino acids from the circulating **angiotensinogen**, converting it to **angiotensin I**. The endothelial cells of most capillaries in the body, but especially those of the lung, are rich in **angiotensin-converting enzyme**, which cleaves two amino acids from angiotensin I to form **angiotensin II**. This molecule causes the constriction of blood vessels, including the efferent glomerular arteriole (increasing blood pressure within the glomerulus with a concomitant increase in glomerular filtration rate), and it causes the adrenal cortex to release aldosterone, a hormone that facilitates an increase in the resorption of Na^+ and Cl^- from the lumen of the distal convoluted tubule, making the ultrafiltrate more hypotonic.

MOVEMENT OF WATER AND UREA FROM AND INTO THE FILTRATE WITHIN COLLECTING TUBULES

Because the **collecting tubule** passes through the entire extent of the medulla, it encounters the identical osmotic gradients as did the limbs of Henle's loop (see Fig. 19.5A and B). The cells of the collecting tubule are impermeable to water in the absence of **ADH** (see Fig. 19.5A); however, if that hormone binds to **ADH receptors** of the cuboidal cells of the collecting tubule, it induces the cells to place **aquaporin** channels in their cell membrane. As the ultrafiltrate descends toward the **area cribrosa**, it loses water passively, and in the inner medulla loses **urea**, also passively. The urine is reduced in volume and becomes more concentrated (see Fig. 19.5B). Additionally, the urea concentration of the interstitium of the inner medulla is increased and is responsible for the high concentration gradient of the inner medulla (see Fig. 19.5B).

Vasa Recta

The **vasa recta**, composed of the narrow, descending **arteriolae rectae** and the wider, ascending **venae rectae**, are completely permeable to water and salts, and the blood in both limbs of this hairpin-shaped vessel reacts to the concentration gradient in the kidney medulla (Fig. 19.5C) and forms a **countercurrent exchange system**. The vasa recta not only maintain the osmotic gradient of the renal medulla but also take advantage of it by taking more water and salts away in the larger volume outflow of the venae rectae than are being brought in by the smaller caliber arteriolae rectae (see Fig. 19.5C).

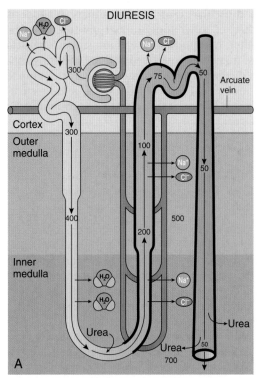

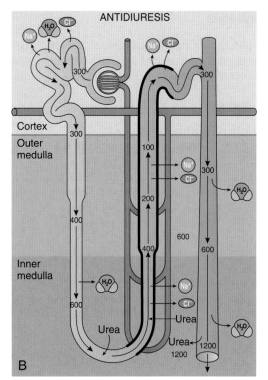

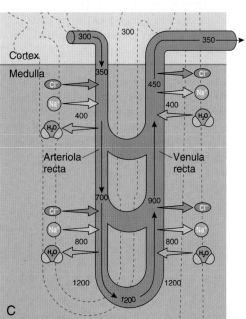

Figure 19.5 Histophysiology of the uriniferous tubule. **A,** In the absence of ADH. **B,** In the presence of ADH. **C,** Vasa recta. *(From Gartner LP, Hiatt JL: Color Textbook of Histology, 3rd ed. Philadelphia, Saunders, 2007, pp 456 [A and B] and 460 [C].)*

CLINICAL CONSIDERATIONS

Fanconi syndrome occurs in children whose proximal tubules do not resorb the proper amount of glucose, phosphate, bicarbonate, and amino acids, resulting in acidosis, dehydration, electrolyte imbalance, proteinuria, rickets, osteomalacia, and growth failure. This syndrome could have various causes, including a hereditary component, such as hereditary fructose intolerance. The use of expired tetracycline, whose decomposition product, anhydro-4-tetracycline, causes reversible tubular dysfunction, heavy metal poisoning, and glue sniffing, and certain over-the-counter Chinese herbal medicines have also been implicated in the development of Fanconi syndrome.

Excretory Passages

The excretory passages of the urinary system consist of the minor and major calyces, pelvis of the kidney, ureter, single urinary bladder, and single urethra.

CALYCES AND URETER

- Each **minor calyx**, lined by **transitional epithelium**, receives urine from the area cribrosa of the renal papilla. Deep to the epithelium is the lamina propria surrounded by a thin smooth muscle coat, whose contraction forces the urine into a **major calyx**. Except for their size, major calyces resemble the minor calyces and the **renal pelvis**.
- The **ureter**, approximately 30 cm long and 0.5 cm in diameter, is lined by a **mucosa** whose **transitional epithelium** lies on a lamina propria composed of fibroelastic connective tissue (Figs. 19.6 and 19.7). An inner longitudinal and an outer circular layer of smooth muscle cells form the muscular coat of the ureter, and its peristaltic contractions deliver urine into the urinary bladder.

URINARY BLADDER

As the **urinary bladder** becomes distended with its stored urine, its impermeable transitional epithelium becomes thinner and flatter (see Figs. 19.6 and 19.7). Its large dome-shaped cells also become flatter, and the plasma membranes unfold, so that the thick **plaque regions** are no longer folded into the cytoplasm but rather form a mosaic of thickened plaque and thinner **interplaque regions**, accommodating the increasing urine content of the bladder.

The **trigone**, the smooth triangular area of the bladder mucosa, has three apices:

- Openings of the two ureters
- The urethral orifice, where occasionally mucous glands reside in the fibroelastic connective tissue

The **muscular coat** of the urinary bladder is composed of **inner longitudinal**, **middle circular**, and **outer longitudinal** layers of smooth muscle that are frequently interlaced and are indistinguishable as distinct layers. The internal sphincter muscle of the urethra is formed by the thick, middle circular layer. A fibroelastic **adventitia** surrounds the muscle coat.

URETHRA

The urethra delivers urine from the urinary bladder for voiding. The female urethra is shorter than the male urethra.

- The **female urethra** is approximately 5 cm in length (see Fig. 19.6); it is lined by transitional epithelium in the vicinity of the urinary bladder and by nonkeratinized stratified squamous epithelium along the remainder of its length. Mucous **Littre glands** are present in its fibroelastic lamina propria.
- The **male urethra** is approximately 20 cm in length and has three regions: the **prostatic urethra**, the **membranous urethra**, and the **penile** (or **spongy**) **urethra** (see Fig. 19.7).
  - The prostatic urethra traverses the prostate gland and is lined by transitional epithelium.
  - The membranous urethra traverses the urogenital diaphragm and is lined by stratified columnar epithelium (with patches of pseudostratified columnar epithelium).
  - The penile urethra traverses the entire length of the penis and is lined by stratified columnar epithelium (with patches of pseudostratified columnar epithelium) until the glans penis, where its epithelium is stratified squamous keratinized.

The lamina propria is composed of a fibroelastic connective tissue with mucus-producing **Littre glands** in all three regions of the male urethra.

CLINICAL CONSIDERATIONS

Ten percent of renal cancers are **transitional cell carcinomas** of the calyces and pelvis of the ureter. Renal cancers are frequently associated with much more common transitional cell carcinomas of the urinary bladder.

Acute uncomplicated **urinary tract infection (UTI)** occurs frequently in women, involving 11 million women per year in the United States, but fewer than 10 per 10,000 men younger than age 50 per year. Most commonly, in healthy, young women, the cause of the infection is enteric bacteria (usually *Escherichia coli* from the rectum) entering the urinary bladder through the urethra. Clinical symptoms include dysuria, burning and pain sensation on urination, increase in the frequency of the urge for urination, and pain in the suprapubic regions.

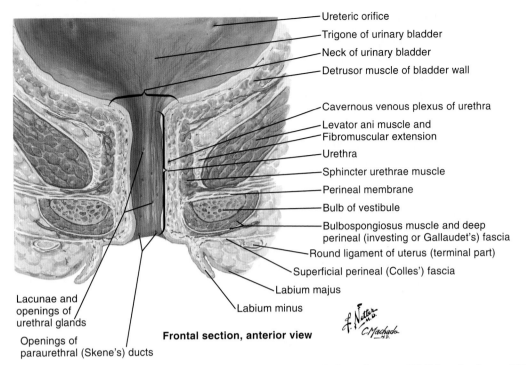

Frontal section, anterior view

Ureteric orifice
Trigone of urinary bladder
Neck of urinary bladder
Detrusor muscle of bladder wall
Cavernous venous plexus of urethra
Levator ani muscle and
Fibromuscular extension
Urethra
Sphincter urethrae muscle
Perineal membrane
Bulb of vestibule
Bulbospongiosus muscle and deep
perineal (investing or Gallaudet's) fascia
Round ligament of uterus (terminal part)
Superficial perineal (Colles') fascia
Labium majus
Labium minus
Lacunae and openings of urethral glands
Openings of paraurethral (Skene's) ducts

Figure 19.6 Female urinary tract. *(From Netter FH: Atlas of Human Anatomy, 3rd ed. Teterboro, NJ, ICON Learning System, 2003. © Elsevier Inc. All rights reserved.)*

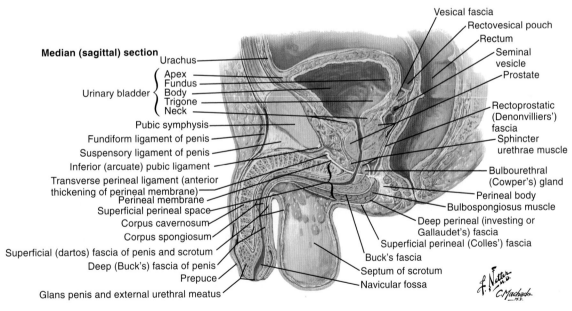

Median (sagittal) section

Urachus
Urinary bladder
  Apex
  Fundus
  Body
  Trigone
  Neck
Pubic symphysis
Fundiform ligament of penis
Suspensory ligament of penis
Inferior (arcuate) pubic ligament
Transverse perineal ligament (anterior thickening of perineal membrane)
Perineal membrane
Superficial perineal space
Corpus cavernosum
Corpus spongiosum
Superficial (dartos) fascia of penis and scrotum
Deep (Buck's) fascia of penis
Prepuce
Glans penis and external urethral meatus

Vesical fascia
Rectovesical pouch
Rectum
Seminal vesicle
Prostate
Rectoprostatic (Denonvilliers') fascia
Sphincter urethrae muscle
Bulbourethral (Cowper's) gland
Perineal body
Bulbospongiosus muscle
Deep perineal (investing or Gallaudet's) fascia
Superficial perineal (Colles') fascia
Buck's fascia
Septum of scrotum
Navicular fossa

Figure 19.7 Male urinary tract. *(From Netter FH: Atlas of Human Anatomy, 3rd ed. Teterboro, NJ, ICON Learning System, 2003. © Elsevier Inc. All rights reserved.)*

20 FEMALE REPRODUCTIVE SYSTEM

The **female reproductive system** comprises the ovaries, oviducts, uterus, vagina, and external genitalia as well as the mammary glands.

Before puberty, the germ cells of the ovary are in the resting stage. After the pituitary gland begins to release **gonadotropic hormones**, the reproductive system becomes activated, around 12 years of age, and menarche, the first menstruation, occurs. From then, the 28-day menstrual cycle continues for the entire reproductive life of the woman until **menopause** is reached.

> **KEY WORDS**
> - **Ovarian cortex**
> - **Ovarian follicles**
> - **Ovulation**
> - **Fallopian tubes**
> - **Uterus**
> - **Menstrual cycle**
> - **Placenta**
> - **Mammary glands**

Ovaries

Each **ovary** (3 cm × 2 cm × 1 cm) is attached to the broad ligament of the uterus by the **mesovarium** (Fig. 20.1). The ovary is covered by a simple squamous **germinal epithelium**, which overlies the connective tissue capsule, the **tunica albuginea**. The ovary has an outer **cortex** and an inner **medulla**.

The connective tissue **stroma (interstitial compartment)** of the cortex is populated by **ovarian follicles** and **stromal (interstitial) cells** that resemble fibroblasts and form the theca interna and externa of the ovarian follicles that house the **primary oocyte**.

- At fertilization, the sex of the embryo is determined by the presence or absence of the Y chromosome. If the Y chromosome is present, then the transcription factor of the *SRY* gene (sex-determining region on the Y chromosome), the **testis-determining factor**, induces the development of testes.
- The absence of the *SRY* gene causes the default condition—development of female gonads.
- Early in development, a pair of epithelially covered ridges, the **gonadal ridges**, forms and epithelial cells from their covering migrate into the gonadal ridges to form **primitive sex cords**.

- By the sixth week after fertilization, **primitive germ cells** migrate from the yolk sac into the gonadal ridges, induce further development of the gonads, and continue to divide to form numerous germ cells. At this point, the male and female gonads are identical and are known as **indifferent gonads**.
- In a **female**, the primitive sex cords migrate into the medulla of the gonadal ridges and form clusters of cells that degenerate soon, to be replaced by connective tissue. During the seventh week, other cells of the epithelial cover migrate into the cortex to form the cortical sex cords.
- During the **fourth month**, these cortical sex cords dissociate, and their cells surround primitive germ cells, become known as **follicular cells** (although follicular cells may also arise from the germinal epithelium), and the primitive germ cells become **oogonia**.
- By the end of the **fifth month** of fetal life, each ovarian cortex houses at least 3 million oogonia, but only 500,000 become surrounded by follicular cells; the others degenerate. The remaining oogonia enter the first meiotic division and become known as **primary oocytes**. Each primary oocyte with its surrounding follicular cells is known as a **primordial follicle**.
- **Follicular cells** surrounding the primary oocyte secrete **meiosis-preventing factor**, which arrests the primary oocyte in the diplotene stage of meiosis I until just before the oocyte is ovulated. In the first 10 years of life, two thirds of the primordial follicles undergo atresia.
- The remaining **primary oocytes** may continue to be in this arrested meiotic state until puberty or for the next 30 to 40 years.

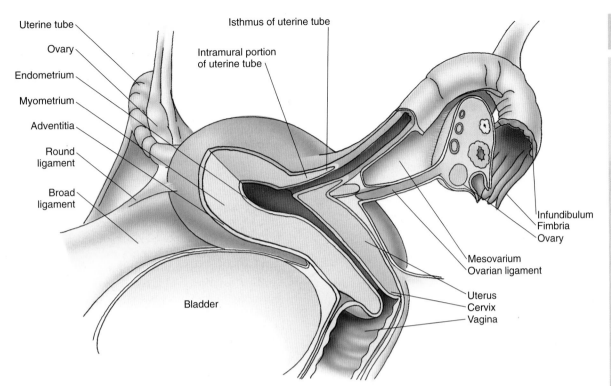

Figure 20.1 Female reproductive tract. The ovary is sectioned to display the developing follicles, and the fallopian tube, uterus, and vagina are open to show the continuity of their lumina. *(From Gartner LP, Hiatt JL: Color Textbook of Histology, 3rd ed. Philadelphia, Saunders, 2007, p 464.)*

CLINICAL CONSIDERATIONS

During development, in response to estrogens, the fallopian tubes, body and cervix of the uterus, and upper portion of the vagina are formed by the fusion of the right and left müllerian (paramesonephric) ducts. Around the ninth week after fertilization, the wall between the two fused ducts disintegrates, forming a single lumen. Occasionally, this fusion does not occur, and the individual has two, smaller uteri, known as **uterus didelphys**, and two cervices and two separate vaginas, each opening into its own uterus. More commonly, the wall between the two müllerian ducts remains intact, but the lumina of the two horns of the uterus open into a shared, single vagina; this condition is known as **uterus bicornis**.

The *WNT4* gene regulates genes that function in the development of the ovaries by suppressing the gene responsible for testis development (*SOX9*) and activating a series of genes, including *DAX1*, a member of the nuclear hormone receptor family that directs the development of the ovaries. Although it has not been shown in humans, in mice *DAX1* regulates a gene that codes for a part of the **TATA box** binding protein for RNA polymerase. In the absence of this protein, the mice cannot form ovaries.

During a woman's reproductive life, she ovulates every 28 days and releases about 450 oocytes. Since the female embryo does not manufacture testosterone or antimüllerian hormone, the mesonephric duct degenerates. Estrogens formed by the female embryo induce the **müllerian ducts (paramesonephric ducts)** to form the fallopian tubes, body and cervix of the uterus, and part of the vagina.

OVARIAN FOLLICLES

There are two categories of ovarian follicles, **primordial (nongrowing) follicles** and **growing follicles**; the latter have four stages—unilaminar primary follicle, multilaminar primary follicle, secondary (antral) follicle, and graafian (mature) follicle (Fig. 20.2 and Table 20.1). Of these, secondary and graafian follicles (but not the dominant follicle) require **follicle-stimulating hormone (FSH)** for development, whereas primordial and both types of primary follicles develop because of unknown local factors possibly manufactured by the follicular cells. During any one particular menstrual cycle, approximately 50 primordial follicles begin to develop; however, they begin their development at various times during the cycle, so that follicles at different stages of development are present in the ovary.

- The **primordial (nongrowing) follicle**, the smallest and least mature of the follicles, is a spherical cluster of cells composed of a small, 25-μm-diameter, primary oocyte (in prophase of meiosis I) surrounded by a single layer of flat follicular cells that adhere to each other by desmosomes. The follicle is enveloped by a basal lamina that isolates the follicle from the connective tissue stroma.

- **Unilaminar primary follicles** are composed of a primary oocyte (100 to 150 μm in diameter) whose nucleus is large and vesicular-appearing (and referred to as the germinal vesicle) surrounded by a single layer of cuboidal follicular cells (see Fig. 20.2 and Table 20.1). **Multilaminar primary follicles** resemble the unilaminar primary follicles except that mitotic activity of the follicular cells resulted in the formation of several layers of follicular cells (**granulosa cells**) around the oocyte. Additionally, a layer of amorphous material, the **zona pellucida**, composed of the glycoproteins ZP_1, ZP_2, and ZP_3, is formed by and surrounds the primary oocyte. Not only do filopodia of the granulosa cells invade the zona pellucida, contact the oocyte cell membrane, and form gap junctions with the primary oocyte, but the granulosa cells also form gap junctions with each other. The stroma surrounding the granulosa cells but separated from them by the basal lamina, become reorganized to form an inner vascularized cellular layer and an outer fibrous layer, known as the **theca interna** and the **theca externa** (see Fig. 20.2 and Table 20.1). The cells of the theca interna display membrane-bound **luteinizing hormone (LH)** receptors, and because they synthesize and release the male hormone **androstenedione**, they have the fine structural features of cells that manufacture steroid hormones. The released androstenedione crosses the basal lamina to enter the granulosa cells where the hormone is converted to **estradiol**, an estrogen, by the enzyme **aromatase**.

- **Secondary (antral) follicles** are similar to multilaminar primary follicles except that the primary oocytes are larger (200 μm in diameter [see Fig. 20.2 and Table 20.1]), the granulosa cell layer becomes thicker, and fluid-filled spaces (**Call-Exner bodies**) form among them. The fluid, liquor folliculi, is extracellular fluid enriched with steroid-binding proteins derived from the granulosa cells, glycosaminoglycans, proteoglycans, and hormones such as **progesterone, estradiol, inhibin, follistatin (folliculostatin)**, and **activin**. Activin is a hormone that induces basophils of the anterior pituitary to release **LH** and **FSH**. The continued development of the secondary follicle is FSH-dependent.

- **Graafian (mature) follicles** are recognizable by their large size and by the fact that the liquor folliculi that appeared in the secondary follicle as small, isolated pools of fluid are combined into a single, large, spherical fluid-filled compartment: the **antrum**. The wall of the antrum is composed of several layers of follicular cells, called the **membrana granulosa**, and at one point another cluster of granulosa cells, the **cumulus oophorus**, juts into the antrum, resembling Denmark jutting into the North Sea. The cumulus resembles a Popsicle in that its stalk, arising from the membrana granulosa, is cylindrical and its expanded free end is spherical. The center of the free end houses the primary oocyte, surrounded by numerous layers of granulosa cells, the innermost layer of which, bordering the zona pellucida, is known as the **corona radiata**. Two different types of granulosa cells may be distinguished: cells forming the wall of the antrum, known as **membrana granulosa cells**, and cells of the cumulus oophorus, known as **cumulus granulosa cells**. The theca interna and theca externa continue to develop into thicker layers (see Fig. 20.2 and Table 20.1).

- The **dominant follicle** refers to the one graafian follicle that continues to develop, becomes **FSH-independent**, and produces the hormone **inhibin**, which stems the release of FSH by the anterior pituitary, causing the degeneration, or **atresia**, of the other developing follicles. Usually, only the dominant follicle discharges its oocyte in ovulation.

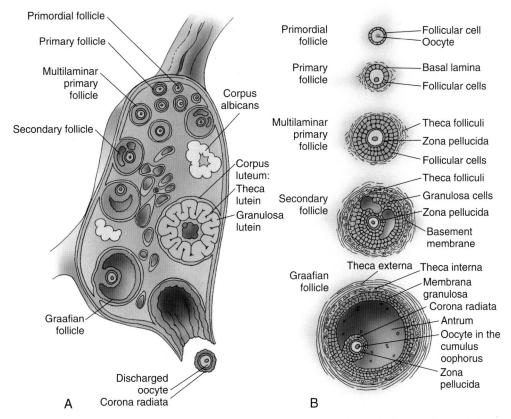

Figure 20.2 A and **B,** Follicle development in the ovary. *(From Gartner LP, Hiatt JL: Color Textbook of Histology, 3rd ed. Philadelphia, Saunders, 2007, p 465.)*

Table 20.1 STAGES OF OVARIAN FOLLICULAR DEVELOPMENT

Stage	FSH Dependent	Oocyte	Zona Pellucida	Follicular Cells or Granulosa	Liquor Folliculi	Theca Interna	Theca Externa
Primordial follicle	No	Primary	None	Single layer of flat cells	None	None	None
Unilaminar primary follicle	No	Primary	Present	Single layer of cuboidal cells	None	None	None
Multilaminar primary follicle	No	Primary	Present and microvilli of primary oocyte form gap junctions with filopodia of corona radiata cells	Several layers of follicular cells (now called granulosa cells)	None	Present	Present
Secondary follicle	Yes	Primary	Present with gap junctions	Spaces develop between granulosa cells	Accumulate in spaces between granulosa cells	Present	Present
Graafian follicle	Yes, until it becomes the dominant follicle	Primary, surrounded by corona radiata in cumulus oophorus	Present with gap junctions	Form membrana granulosa and cumulus oophorus	Fills the antrum	Present	Present

From Gartner LP, Hiatt JL: Color Textbook of Histology, 3rd ed. Philadelphia, Saunders, 2007, p 467.

OVULATION

Ovulation occurs on the 14th day before menstruation and is a function of decreased FSH and a sudden surge of LH levels in the blood. These hormonal changes are due to the elevated levels of estrogen produced by the graafian and secondary follicles (Figs. 20.3 and 20.4). **FSH-dependent follicles** that have been progressing through development no longer have access to FSH; they degenerate and are known as **atretic follicles**. The surge in LH levels is responsible for the following events:

- **Blood flow** to the ovaries is increased, leading to edema formation within the theca externa and the release of collagenase, histamine, and prostaglandin in the vicinity of the dominant follicle.
- The **membrana granulosa** of the dominant follicle undergoes proteolysis owing to the presence of LH-induced **plasmin** formation so that the dominant follicle can release its oocyte.
- **Follicular cells** manufacture and release **meiosis-inducing substance**, which stimulates the completion of the first meiotic division of the dominant follicle's primary oocyte, forming the **secondary oocyte** and the **first polar body**. The secondary oocyte begins its second meiotic division but cannot progress beyond **metaphase**.
- The **granulosa cells** continue to synthesize glycosaminoglycans and proteoglycans, resulting in continued accumulation of water and increasing the size of the dominant follicle, which increases its pressure on the tunica albuginea of the ovary, cutting off the blood supply at the place of greatest pressure. This avascular region of the ovary's capsule, known as the **stigma**, undergoes necrosis and, in conjunction with the proteolysis of the membrane granulosa in its vicinity, forms a channel leading from the lumen of the antrum to the peritoneal cavity.
- The **secondary oocyte**, surrounded by the corona radiata and accompanied by the first polar body, leaves the ovary, a process known as **ovulation**, and, normally, enters the **infundibulum** of the fallopian tube (oviduct).
- The remnant of the dominant follicle is converted into the **corpus luteum** (see Fig. 20.3).

CORPUS LUTEUM AND CORPUS ALBICANS

When ovulation occurs, the remnant of the dominant graafian follicle accumulates a little blood from the damaged blood vessels in the area, collapses on itself, and is known as the **corpus hemorrhagicum**. Within a couple of days, the blood is resorbed by macrophages, and, owing to the influence of LH, this structure is converted into a temporary endocrine gland, the **corpus luteum** (see Fig. 20.3). The corpus luteum comprises two principal cell types: 80% are granulosa lutein cells (derived from granulosa cells), and 20% are theca lutein cells (derived from theca interna). The basement membrane between the former theca interna and theca externa disintegrates, permitting vascularization of the region of granulosa lutein cells.

- **Granulosa lutein cells** are the larger of the two, and they synthesize **progesterone** and convert **androstenedione** (an androgen) into **estradiol** (an estrogen).
- The peripherally located **theca lutein cells** synthesize progesterone, androstenedione, and some estrogens.

The progesterone and estrogen secreted by the corpus luteum inhibit the basophils of the pituitary from releasing FSH and LH, the hormones necessary for the development of ovarian follicles and for the maintenance of the corpus luteum (see Fig. 20.4). If there is no pregnancy, the corpus luteum begins to degenerate and is referred to as the **corpus luteum of menstruation**. In the event of pregnancy, the forming placenta (but initially the **trophoblasts** of the developing embryo) releases **human chorionic gonadotropin (hCG)** that causes the corpus luteum to enlarge and sustains it for approximately 3 months, during which time it is referred to as the **corpus luteum of pregnancy**. After that time, the corpus luteum is no longer required because the placenta takes over the production of the hormones necessary to maintain the pregnancy, but it remains functional for several months.

Eventually, the corpus luteum (of menstruation and of pregnancy) becomes smaller because of **luteolysis** (regression), and invading fibroblasts manufacture type I collagen fibers to transform the corpus luteum into a **corpus albicans**, a fibrous connective tissue that continues to be resorbed until it becomes just a scar on the surface of the ovary. Luteolysis is initiated by **hypoxia** due to reduced blood flow, which causes the arrival of **T cells** whose product, **interferon-γ**, is responsible for macrophage recruitment. **Macrophages** release **tumor necrosis factor-α**, which drives cells of the corpus luteum into **apoptosis**.

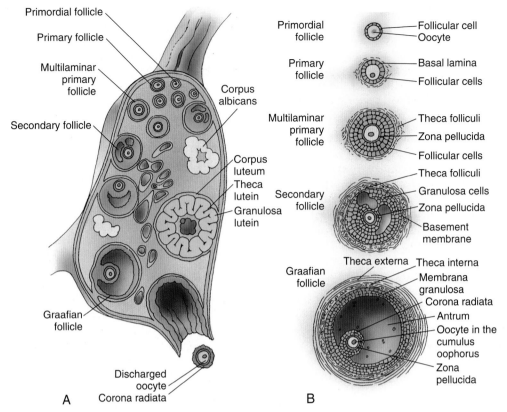

Figure 20.3 A and **B,** Formation of the corpus luteum and corpus albicans. *(From Gartner LP, Hiatt JL: Color Textbook of Histology, 3rd ed. Philadelphia, Saunders, 2007, p 465.)*

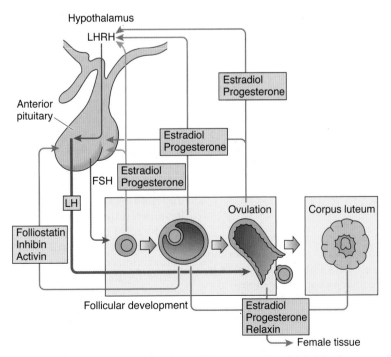

Figure 20.4 The interaction between hormones of the pituitary and the ovary. LHRH, luteinizing hormone–releasing hormone. *(From Gartner LP, Hiatt JL: Color Textbook of Histology, 3rd ed. Philadelphia, Saunders, 2007, p 472.)*

Oviducts (Fallopian Tubes)

Each **oviduct** is a narrow tubule that is open at both ends—at its free, peritoneal end, where it approaches the ovary, and at its other end, where it attaches to and pierces the wall of the body of the uterus. The oviduct has four well-defined regions, recognizable by features specific to each region (Fig. 20.5).

- The **infundibulum** is the free end of the oviduct, and its **fimbriae** press against the ovary during ovulation to trap the secondary oocyte, its attendant follicular cells, and the first polar body.
- The **ampulla** is the enlarged continuation of the infundibulum—normally the site of fertilization.
- The **intramural region** of the oviduct pierces the wall and opens into the lumen of the uterus.
- The **isthmus** is the narrow region between the intramural region and the ampulla.

The oviduct has three layers—the inner mucosa, the middle muscularis, and the outer serosa (absent in the intramural region).

The **mucosa** of the oviduct is highly folded, making its lumen very convoluted. It has a simple columnar epithelial lining, composed of peg cells and ciliated columnar cells.

- **Peg cells** are columnar, nonciliated cells; they secrete a fluid that not only is nutrient-rich, but also contains factors necessary for the **capacitation** of spermatozoa. Without these factors, spermatozoa are unable to fertilize the secondary oocyte. The nutrient-rich fluid nourishes not only the developing embryo as it travels along the oviduct, but also the spermatozoa.
- **Ciliated cells** are also columnar in shape and possess numerous cilia that propel the fertilized ovum toward the uterus.

The **lamina propria** is composed of a vascular, dense, collagenous connective tissue surrounded by the **muscularis**, composed of smooth muscle and arranged in a poorly defined inner circular and an outer longitudinal layer. Except for the intramural region, the muscularis is covered by a serosa.

Uterus

The **uterus** is a very muscular organ that houses the developing embryo and fetus until parturition. It is $7 \times 4 \times 2.5$ cm and is composed of three regions—the body, fundus, and cervix (see Fig. 20.5). The wall of the uterus has three layers—the endometrium, myometrium, and serosa or adventitia.

- The **endometrium** forms the mucosa of the uterus and is composed of a simple columnar epithelium with **nonciliated secretory cells** and **ciliated cells** that cover the vascular connective tissue housing fibroblasts, **decidual cells**, and branched, tubular **uterine glands**. The endometrium has two layers: the thicker outer **functionalis layer** that is sloughed off during menstruation and the deeper **basal layer** that is conserved during menstruation and whose tissue is occupied by the base of the uterine glands. The basal layer is vascularized by the **straight arteries**, whereas the functionalis layer is served by the **helical arteries**; both vessels arise from the **arcuate arteries** of the myometrium.
- The **myometrium** consists of smooth muscle arranged in three layers—innermost and outermost longitudinal layers and a middle circular layer. The middle circular layer is highly vascularized by the **arcuate arteries** and is often named the **stratum vasculare**. The muscle layers are replaced at the cervix by dense fibroelastic connective tissue. The size and number of the myometrial smooth muscle cells are directly affected by blood estrogen levels; the higher the estrogen levels, the larger and more numerous the smooth muscle cells. In the absence of estrogens, the smooth muscle cells of the uterus atrophy. During pregnancy, the opposite occurs: There is a hypertrophy and a hyperplasia of uterine smooth muscle cells. At parturition, **corticotropic hormone** induces the uterine smooth muscle cells and the cells of the membranes surrounding the fetus to release **prostaglandins**, which, in conjunction with **oxytocin** from the neurohypophysis, cause the myometrium to undergo contractions to expel the fetus. Continued release of oxytocin causes contraction of the uterine blood vessels to minimize blood loss that would otherwise result from the detachment of the placenta from the lining of the uterus.
- Much of the uterus is covered by a **serosa** except where the uterus adheres to the urinary bladder. In that region, there is an **adventitia** covering the uterus.

The **cervix** is a highly fibrous structure that protrudes into the vagina as the terminus of the uterus. Its lumen is lined by a **simple columnar epithelium** composed of mucus-secreting cells. Where it enters the vagina, it is covered by a stratified squamous nonkeratinized epithelium. The subepithelial connective tissue of the cervix houses mucus-secreting **cervical glands** whose secretion can either facilitate the entry of spermatozoa—as during ovulation—or form a thick mucous plug—as during pregnancy—to prevent the entry of spermatozoa into the lumen of the uterus. The change in consistency of the mucus produced by these glands is controlled by the blood level of progesterone.

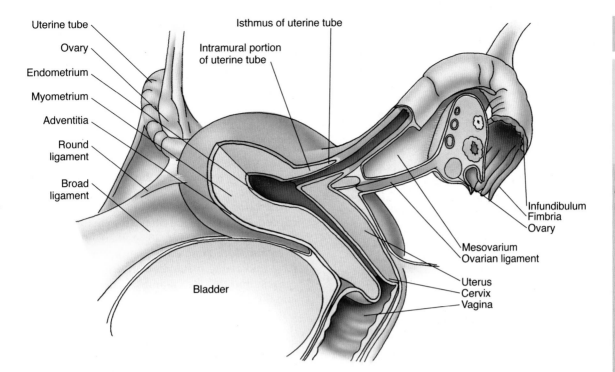

Figure 20.5 Female reproductive tract. The fimbriated infundibulum of the oviduct is in close association with the ovary. *(From Gartner LP, Hiatt JL: Color Textbook of Histology, 3rd ed. Philadelphia, Saunders, 2007, p 464.)*

CLINICAL CONSIDERATIONS

Acute endometritis—inflammation of the endometrium—is most frequently caused by *Staphylococcus aureus* or *Streptococcus* infection. Infection occurs if a portion of the placenta is retained, or if an abortion procedure was compromised. Other possible causes include instrumentation and even normal delivery. The patient presents with high fever and a vaginal discharge that contains pus. With antibiotic therapy, the condition resolves in about 14 days.

The **Papanicolaou smear technique (Pap smear)** is a diagnostic method. Vaginal aspirates or cervical scrapes are obtained, the specimens are prepared for histologic observations, and the slides are examined microscopically for the presence of cells exhibiting anaplasia, dysplasia, and carcinoma. The Pap smear is a very inexpensive tool that should be performed annually for sexually active women and by 21 years of age in non–sexually active women. New guidelines have been proposed that decrease the frequency of Pap smears in women older than 30 years who have not had abnormal cells 3 years in succession. This procedure has saved countless lives by early detection of precancerous and cancerous transformations that would have resulted in serious malignancies of the cervix. Annually, about 55 million Pap smears are done in the United States, and 6% of these display some abnormality requiring the attention of a physician.

Salpingitis, which is inflammation of the oviduct, is also referred to as *pelvic inflammatory disease*, although pelvic inflammatory disease is an infection that involves any pelvic organ, not just the oviducts. Salpingitis is usually a sexually transmitted bacterial infection that begins in the vagina and spreads into the cervix and uterus. From there it spreads to the oviducts. Rarely, it is caused by the insertion of an intrauterine device. The condition is manifested by the common symptoms of pain in the lower abdomen that is exacerbated by sexual intercourse and during vaginal examination, fever, frequent urination and a burning sensation during urination, and occasional nausea and vomiting. Diagnosis may involve a simple cervical swab that is cultured for bacterial growth or a laparoscopic examination of the uterus, oviducts, and ovaries. Antibiotic therapy normally alleviates salpingitis within 1 week. Frequently, the patient's sexual partner is also placed on antibiotic treatment.

Menstrual Cycle

The menstrual cycle is normally 28 days long and is divided into three continuous phases—menstrual phase, proliferative (follicular) phase, and secretory (luteal) phase. The cycle occurs when the woman is not pregnant; the menstrual cycle is interrupted in the case of pregnancy.

- The **menstrual phase** is about 3 to 4 days long. It begins with the onset of **menses** (vaginal bleeding) and is the result of reduced blood levels of estrogens and progesterone that cause initially sporadic, followed within 24 to 48 hours by continuous, constriction of the helical arteries (Figs. 20.6 and 20.7). The lack of blood supply to the functionalis layer causes necrosis and, as the helical arteries rupture, subsequent sloughing of the functionalis layer. The basal layer continues to receive a blood supply from the straight arteries and, although stripped of its epithelial cover, remains healthy. Epithelial cells of the base of the uterine glands begin the re-epithelialization of the denuded surface.
- The **proliferative (follicular) phase**, about 10 days long, begins at the end of menses and lasts until ovulation. This phase is characterized by the re-epithelialization of the denuded surface, rebuilding of the thickness of the endometrium and its helical arteries, and restoration of the glands, so that the functionalis layer is rebuilt until it becomes about 2 to 3 mm thick (see Fig. 20.6). By the time of ovulation, the glands, although not coiled, start to accumulate glycogen in their cells. The helical arteries are just beginning to twist into a tight helix and have reached about two thirds of the way into the functionalis layer. Just before ovulation, FSH, LH, and estrogen blood levels peak (see Fig. 20.7).
- The **secretory (luteal) phase**, about 2 weeks long, starts after ovulation and ends when menses begins. During this phase, the glands of the endometrium become highly coiled; the helical vessels reach all the way to the epithelially covered aspect of the functionalis layer, which has become about 5 mm thick; and the lumina of the endometrial glands are filled with their secretory product (see Fig. 20.6). By the 20th day of the menstrual cycle, the blood progesterone level has peaked, and the estrogen level is also quite high, although not at the high level it was during the proliferative phase (see Fig. 20.7). The helical arteries become surrounded by cells of the stroma that enlarge and become transformed into **decidual cells (decidual reaction)** that store glycogen and lipids anticipating implantation of the embryo. Decidual cell function in anticipating and during the process of implantation is discussed subsequently in the section on implantation.

Fertilization

When the secondary oocyte, its follicular cells, and the first polar body are released from the dominant graafian follicle, they enter the fimbriated infundibulum of the oviduct and are transported by the muscular action of the oviduct muscularis and by the concerted actions of the cilia of the ciliated columnar cells of the oviduct (Fig. 20.8). If spermatozoa have been introduced into the woman's reproductive tract, have undergone maturation in the epididymis and capacitation in the isthmus, and arrived at the ampulla of the oviduct, the sperm begins to press its way between the cells of the corona radiata to contact the zona pellucida.

When ZP_3 receptors in the cell membrane of the sperm bind ZP_3 in the zona pellucida, the sperm undergoes the **acrosomal reaction**, releasing the enzymes present in the sperm's acrosome—mostly **acrosin**—allowing the sperm to penetrate the zona pellucida and to contact the oocyte plasma membrane. This contact induces the oocyte to release its lysosomal enzyme, which modifies the zona pellucida, the **zona reaction**, and makes the zona impermeable to other spermatozoa. The cell membrane of the sperm possesses **fertilin** that interacts with **integrins** and **CD9** of the oocyte plasma membrane, permitting fusion to occur between the two membranes. The sperm enters the oocyte, a process known as **fertilization**. The oocyte then:

- Undergoes **cortical reaction**, preventing additional sperm from entering the oocyte
- Resumes its **second meiotic division**, forming the **ovum** and the diminutive **second polar body**
- Reforms its **haploid** nucleus, the **female pronucleus**, which moves toward the sperm's **haploid** nucleus (**male pronucleus**)

The two pronuclei duplicate their DNA, and the nuclear membranes of both pronuclei break down. The spindle apparatus that forms as the centrioles migrate to opposite poles of the ovum is now a **diploid** cell, known as the **zygote**. The zygote undergoes mitosis, known as **cleavage**, and the resulting cells migrate along the oviduct toward the uterus (see Fig. 20.8) and continue to divide, forming a cluster of cells known as the **morula**. If the oocyte is not fertilized, it degenerates within 24 hours.

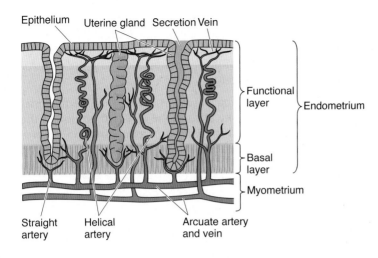

Figure 20.6 The two layers and vascularization of the uterine endometrium. *(From Gartner LP, Hiatt JL: Color Textbook of Histology, 3rd ed. Philadelphia, Saunders, 2007, p 477.)*

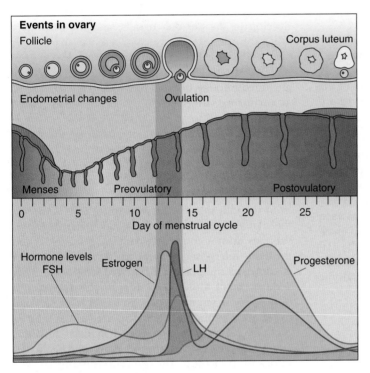

Figure 20.7 Relationships of ovarian events, phases of the uterine endometrium, and hormonal cycling. *(From Gartner LP, Hiatt JL: Color Textbook of Histology, 3rd ed. Philadelphia, Saunders, 2007, p 479.)*

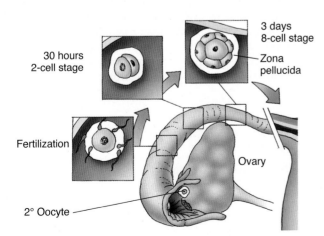

Figure 20.8 Fertilization and mitosis in the zygote. *(Modified from Gartner LP, Hiatt JL: Color Textbook of Histology, 3rd ed. Philadelphia, Saunders, 2007, p 481.)*

Implantation

As the morula travels along the oviduct, it is still surrounded by the zona pellucida, and its cells, known as **blastomeres**, continue to divide. About 4 to 5 days after fertilization, the morula reaches the uterus (Fig. 20.9). Uterine fluid penetrates the zona pellucida and rearranges the cells of the morula to form the **blastocyst**, whose lumen, the **blastocoele**, contains uterine fluid and a small cluster of cells, the **embryoblasts (inner cell mass)**. The peripheral cells that form the wall of the blastocyst are known as **trophoblasts** (see Fig. 20.9). The zona pellucida disintegrates, and the trophoblasts express **L-selectins** and **integrins** on their surfaces, which contact receptors of the uterine epithelium, beginning the process of **implantation**. The endometrium, in the **secretory (luteal) phase**, is ready to nourish the embryo as it is embedding itself into the wall of the uterus.

- The cells of the **embryoblasts** form the embryo and the amnion.
- **Trophoblasts** form the embryonic portion of the placenta and induce the **uterine endometrium** to form the placenta's maternal portion.

As the trophoblasts proliferate, they form an inner **cytotrophoblast** layer of vigorously dividing cells and an outer layer of nonmitotic **syncytiotrophoblasts**. As cells of the cytotrophoblasts divide, the newly formed cells are incorporated into the syncytiotrophoblast layer, which enlarges, becomes vacuolated forming interconnected **lacunae**, and penetrates the endometrial lining. By the end of the 11th day postfertilization, the embryo and its layers have become embedded into the vascularized endometrium (Fig. 20.10; see Fig. 20.9).

Placenta Development

As the syncytiotrophoblasts continue to infiltrate the vascular endometrium, they penetrate the walls of many of the blood vessels and blood flows into the lacunae, supplying the early embryo with nourishment and oxygen. As the **placenta** develops, the cells of the trophoblasts form the **chorion**. With further development, the chorion forms the **chorionic plate**, from which the **chorionic villi** develop (see Fig. 20.10). In response to the formation of the chorion, the endometrium of the uterus becomes known as the **decidua**. The decidua has three regions:

- **Decidua basalis** is the region of the decidua that becomes the maternal portion of the placenta.
- **Decidua capsularis** is the portion of the decidua located between the embryo and the lumen of the uterus; it does not contribute to the placenta and becomes known as the **chorion laeve**.

- **Decidua parietalis** is the portion of the decidua located between the myometrium and the lumen of the uterus—the regions of the endometrium that are not in close association with the embryo or the placenta.

The **decidua basalis** is invaded by the maternal vascular supply to form the maternal portion of the placenta, and the syncytiotrophoblasts and cytotrophoblasts of the chorionic plate respond by forming **chorionic villi**, known as the **primary villi (of the chorion frondosum)**. As the cores of the primary villi become populated by mesenchymal cells and by embryonic blood vessels, the primary villi become known as **secondary villi** (see Fig. 20.10). The cytotrophoblasts of the secondary villi are reduced in number as they become part of the expanding syncytium. As this is occurring, blood-filled **lacunae** develop in the decidua basalis, and the secondary villi protrude into these large, vascular spaces. The lacunae receive blood from and drain blood into maternal arterioles and venules. Some of the villi are anchored into the decidua basalis and are referred to as **anchoring villi**, whereas others are not anchored and are referred to as **free villi**.

Capillary beds of the villi approximate the syncytiotrophoblasts, and nutrients and oxygen from the maternal blood penetrate the tissues of the villi to enter their capillary beds. Waste products and carbon dioxide leave the fetal capillaries to make their way from the villi into the lacunae to be taken away by the maternal blood. The fetal and maternal blood supplies do not come into contact with each other; the tissue interposed between the two blood supplies is known as the **placental barrier** (Table 20.2).

Most small molecules can cross this barrier, but only a few macromolecules are capable of crossing it. Maternal antibodies are transported across the placenta by **receptor-mediated endocytosis**, and ions and glucose use active transport (ions) and facilitated diffusion (glucose). The syncytiotrophoblasts not only contribute to the formation of the placental barrier, but also secrete **hCG** (to maintain the corpus luteum), **estrogen**, **progesterone**, **chorionic thyrotropin**, and **chorionic somatomammotropin**. **Prostaglandins** and **prolactin** are synthesized by the **decidual** cells of the decidual stroma.

Table 20.2 COMPONENTS OF THE PLACENTAL BARRIER

Fetal capillary endothelium
Basal lamina of fetal capillary
Basal lamina of cytotrophoblasts
Cytotrophoblasts
Syncytiotrophoblasts

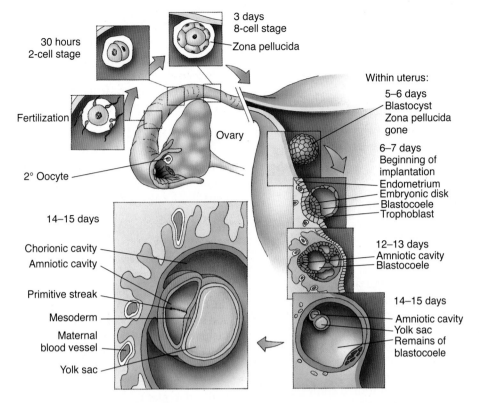

Figure 20.9 Process of implantation, and formation of cytotrophoblasts and syncytiotrophoblasts. *(From Gartner LP, Hiatt JL: Color Textbook of Histology, 3rd ed. Philadelphia, Saunders, 2007, p 481.)*

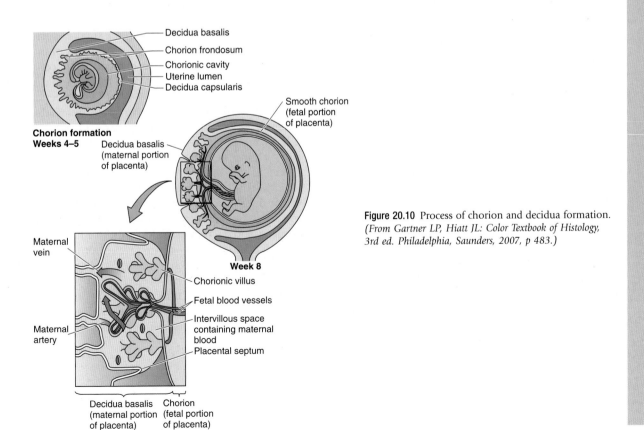

Figure 20.10 Process of chorion and decidua formation. *(From Gartner LP, Hiatt JL: Color Textbook of Histology, 3rd ed. Philadelphia, Saunders, 2007, p 483.)*

Vagina and External Genitalia

The **vagina** (Fig. 20.11), an 8- to 9-cm-long, three-layered fibromuscular sheath located between the vestibule and the uterus, is composed of the:

- **Mucosa**, lined by a **stratified squamous nonkeratinized epithelium** whose cells possess estrogen receptors, which, when occupied, induce these cells to form and store glycogen. The glycogen released into the vaginal lumen is metabolized by the indigenous bacterial flora to produce lactic acid, and by reducing the vaginal pH, it protects the vagina from pathogenic bacteria.
- **Lamina propria**, a highly vascular fibroelastic connective tissue richly endowed with lymphocytes and neutrophils. During sexual arousal, capillaries release plasma that diffuses into the lumen and combines with the cervical secretions to assist in lubricating the vaginal wall.
- Smooth muscle cells of the **muscularis**, which are longitudinally arranged intermingled with some circularly oriented fibers. The external orifice of the vagina possesses circularly arrayed smooth muscle fibers that form a **sphincter**.
- **Adventitia**, a dense fibroelastic connective tissue possessing a well-developed venous plexus and an abundance of sympathetic nerve fibers that originate from the pelvic splanchnic nerves.
- The **hymen**, a thin connective tissue sheath covered on both sides by an epithelium, which restricts the vaginal opening in virgins.

EXTERNAL GENITALIA

The **external genitalia (vulva)** consist of the:

- **Labia majora**, the homologue of the male scrotum, a pair of fat-padded folds of skin, well endowed with sweat and sebaceous glands. The internal aspect is hairless, whereas the external aspect is covered with pubic hair (see Fig. 20.11).
- **Labia minora**, couched between the labia majora, a pair of smaller folds of hairless skin whose connective tissue core is well innervated and richly vascularized (see Fig. 20.11).
- Space between the two labia minora, known as the **vestibule**. It is moistened by minor vestibular glands located in its walls and by the glands of Bartholin. Both the vagina and the urethra open into the vestibule (see Fig. 20.11).

- Two labia minora meet each other superiorly to form the prepuce over the small **glans clitoridis**, the external aspect of the small **clitoris**, which is the homologue of the penis (see Fig. 20.11). The two **erectile bodies** that compose the clitoris have a rich neurovascular supply and are highly sensitive to sexual stimulation.

Mammary Gland

The male and female **mammary glands** are identical until puberty, when ovarian **progesterone** and **estrogens** induce the further development of the female breasts by the appearance of **terminal ductules** and **lobules** (Fig. 20.12). The female mammary glands increase in size by accumulating adipose tissue and connective tissue proper until approximately 20 years of age. During pregnancy, estrogens and progesterone are produced by the placenta and prolactin from the anterior pituitary and glucocorticoids and somatotropin, which induce additional development to prepare the mammary glands for the production of milk to nourish the newborn. After parturition, the estrogens and progesterone originate from the ovaries. The mammary gland, a **compound tubuloalveolar gland**, is composed of 15 to 20 lobes, where the dilated portion of the **lactiferous duct** of each lobe, known as the **lactiferous sinus**, narrows as it passes through and opens at the surface of the nipple. The lactiferous duct and sinus are lined by a stratified cuboidal epithelium, and the smaller ducts are lined by a simple cuboidal epithelium. All of the ducts are surrounded by some **myoepithelial cells** that are ensconced between the basal lamina and the duct cells. The mammary glands of postpubertal women are in the **resting (inactive) state**, unless the woman is pregnant, and then they are said to be in the **lactating (active) state**. The resting glands have a small clump of cells, known as **alveolar buds**, at the end of the lactiferous ducts and their smaller branches. Under the influence of progesterone, the alveolar buds develop further, and during pregnancy the additional stimulation provided by placental **estrogens** and **lactogens** induces the formation of alveoli that produce **colostrum** (a thick protein-rich and immunoglobulin-rich secretion), and after a few days postpartum, maternal prolactin and estrogens induce the formation of **milk**. The formation of milk is continuous, and its release for the suckling infant, the milk ejection reflex, is induced by **oxytocin** from the posterior pituitary.

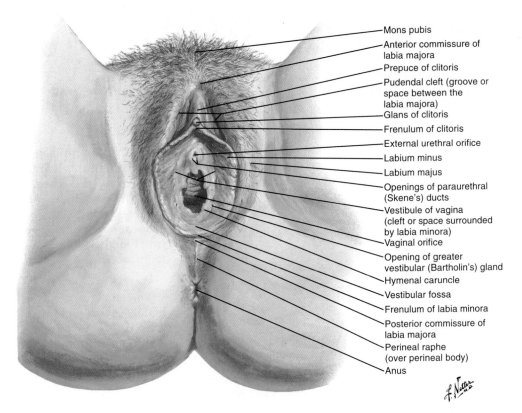

Figure 20.11 Peritoneum and external genitalia of the female. *(From Netter FH: Atlas of Human Anatomy, 3rd ed. Teterboro, NJ, ICON Learning System, 2003. © Elsevier Inc. All rights reserved.)*

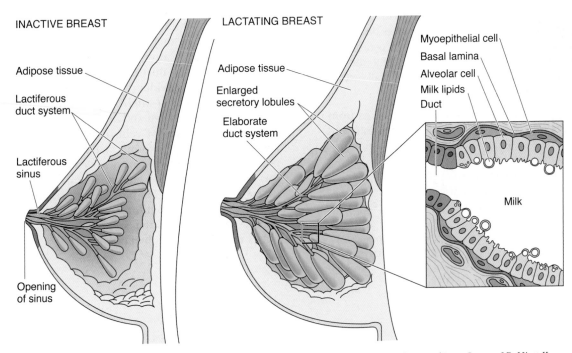

Figure 20.12 Comparison of the glandular differences between an inactive and a lactating breast. *(From Gartner LP, Hiatt JL: Color Textbook of Histology, 3rd ed. Philadelphia, Saunders, 2007, p 486.)*

21 MALE REPRODUCTIVE SYSTEM

The male reproductive system comprises the testes, genital ducts, scrotum, penis, and accessory glands—seminal vesicles, prostate gland, and bulbourethral glands (of Cowper). These accessory glands secrete the noncellular components of the semen that nourish the spermatozoa and provide a fluid medium for the delivery of the semen. The penis is not only the organ of delivery of semen into the female reproductive tract, but it also delivers urine outside the body. The testes form spermatozoa (the male gametes) and synthesize, store, and release testosterone, the male sex hormone (Fig. 21.1).

Testes

The **testes** (Fig. 21.2) are the paired male sex organs located in the scrotum that produce sperm and testosterone. Each testis of an adult is approximately 4 cm long, 2 to 3 cm wide, and 3 cm thick. During embryogenesis, the testes develop on the posterior abdominal wall behind the peritoneum and descend through the abdominal wall into the scrotum, taking coverings of the abdominal wall with them, which become tunicae of the testes.

- **Tunica vaginalis** is a serous sac derived from the peritoneum that nearly encases the testis and allows it to have a certain degree of mobility within the scrotum.
- **Tunica albuginea** is the collagenous connective tissue capsule of the testis.
- **Tunica vasculosa** is the vascular capsule of the testes.
- **Mediastinum testis** represents the posterior thickened portion of the tunica albuginea housing the **rete testis**.

> ### KEY WORDS
> - **Seminiferous tubules**
> - **Sertoli cells**
> - **Spermatogenic cells**
> - **Sperm formation**
> - **Interstitial cells of Leydig**
> - **Male genital ducts**
> - **Accessory male genital glands**
> - **Mechanism of erection**

- **Lobuli testis** consists of approximately 250 pyramid-shaped compartments housing a vascular connective tissue that envelops the **seminiferous tubules**, which produce spermatozoa, and the endocrine **interstitial glands (of Leydig)**, which produce testosterone.

One to four highly convoluted, blindly ending **seminiferous tubules** are located in each lobule, where each tubule is lined by a **seminiferous epithelium** whose function is the production of spermatozoa. When produced and released from the seminiferous epithelium, the spermatozoa enter the straight **tubuli recti** connecting the open ends of the seminiferous tubules to a series of labyrinthine spaces within the mediastinum known as **rete testis**. The spermatozoa enter 10 to 20 short tubules, the **ductuli efferentes**, and from there they enter the **epididymis**.

Paired **testicular arteries**, arising from the aorta, follow the testes and **ductus deferens (vas deferens)** into the scrotum, providing a vascular supply to each testis. As the testicular arteries approach the testes, they become convoluted and are surrounded by the **pampiniform plexus of veins**. These convolutions and the plexus of veins form a system of countercurrent heat exchange between these vessels that cools the temperature of the arterial blood to 95°F, a necessity for viable sperm production. Together, the testicular artery, pampiniform plexus of veins, and ductus deferens form the **spermatic cord**, which passes through the inguinal canal.

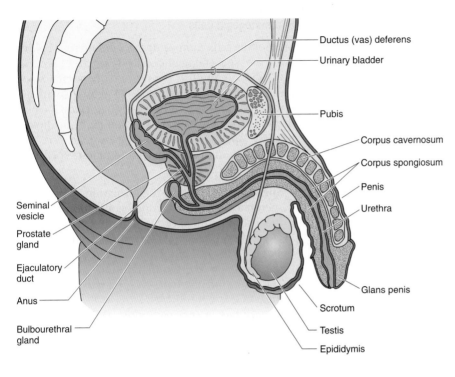

Figure 21.1 Male reproductive system. *(From Gartner LP, Hiatt JL: Color Textbook of Histology, 3rd ed. Philadelphia, Saunders, 2007, p 490.)*

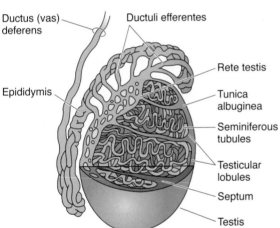

Figure 21.2 Testis and epididymis. Lobules and their contents are not drawn to scale. *(From Gartner LP, Hiatt JL: Color Textbook of Histology, 3rd ed. Philadelphia, Saunders, 2007, p 490.)*

CLINICAL CONSIDERATIONS

Hyperthermia is a major factor that results in sterility in men. More recent studies conducted with men using a laptop computer with the computer situated in their lap for an hour or more found that this contact with the computer caused an increase in intrascrotal temperature of 2.8°C. These studies are inconclusive, but it is advisable for boys and young men to avoid the use of laptop computers in their laps for an extended period.

Cryptorchidism is a developmental defect in which one or both testes fail to descend into the scrotum. When only one testis fails to descend,

the sperm in the descended testis usually is normal and fertile. When both testes fail to descend, the patient is sterile because normal body temperature inhibits spermatogenesis. Surgical procedures may be employed to correct this defect, but the sperm may be abnormal. Mutations in two genes, insulin-like factor 3 and *HOXA10,* are associated with bilateral cryptorchidism. There is a high incidence of testicular tumors associated with untreated cryptorchidism of the testis. Administration of hormones may induce descent, but when that fails, surgery is suggested.

SEMINIFEROUS TUBULES

Each testis possesses approximately 500 sperm-producing seminiferous tubules (30 to 70 cm long and 150 to 250 µm in diameter) embedded in a loose vascular connective tissue. The connective tissue wall of each seminiferous tubule, called the **tunica propria**, is surrounded by a basal lamina. The thick **seminiferous epithelium (germinal epithelium)** is composed of two different epithelial types: Sertoli (supporting) cells and spermatogenic cells that are in the process of differentiation to form spermatozoa.

Sertoli cells (Fig. 21.3) are tall columnar cells that possess large clear indented nuclei, abundant mitochondria, well-developed smooth endoplasmic reticulum, Golgi bodies, endolysosomes, and many cytoskeletal elements. The **occluding junctions** formed between adjacent Sertoli cells subdivide the lumen of the seminiferous tubule into:

- A **basal compartment**, basal to the tight junctions, which is exposed to the underlying vascular connective tissue
- An **adluminal compartment**, which is isolated from the vascular connective tissue, establishing a **blood-testis barrier** and protecting the developing gametes from being exposed to the immune system, which would otherwise mount an immune response against the developing gametes

The functions of Sertoli cells are to:

- Support, protect, and nourish developing spermatogenic cells
- Phagocytose cell remnants (residual bodies) discarded during the process of spermiogenesis
- Facilitate the release of mature spermatids into the lumen of the seminiferous tubules via actin-mediated contraction (**spermiation**)
- Secrete:
  - **Androgen binding protein (ABP)** into the seminiferous tubule lumen, increasing testosterone concentration in the seminiferous tubules
  - **Inhibin**, which hinders the release of FSH
  - **Fructose-rich fluid**, which nourishes and transports spermatozoa along the genital ducts
  - **Testicular transferrin** to assist in providing iron to maturing gametes
  - **Antimüllerian hormone**, during embryonic development, which prevents the formation of the female reproductive system and permits the development of the male reproductive system

Spermatogenic Cells

Most of the cells composing the seminiferous epithelium are **spermatogenic** cells (Fig. 21.4; see Fig. 21.3) that accomplish the process of spermatozoon formation via the following three phases: spermatocytogenesis, the formation of spermatocytes; meiosis, the formation of haploid spermatids from diploid primary spermatocytes; and spermiogenesis, the transformation of spermatids into mature spermatozoa (sperm).

- **Spermatocytogenesis**, the formation of primary spermatocytes from spermatogonia, occurs in the basal compartment of the seminiferous tubule. Diploid spermatogonia sit on the basal lamina, and the presence of the hormone testosterone induces them to begin their mitotic activity. The three different types of spermatocytes are the:
  - **Dark type A spermatogonia**, the least mature, are reserve cells whose oval nuclei are rich in heterochromatin, giving the cell a dark appearance. These cells enter the mitotic cycle to form more dark type A cells
  - **Pale type A spermatogonia**, whose oval nuclei are rich in euchromatin, giving them a paler appearance; testosterone prompts these cells to undergo rapid cell division forming more type A spermatogonia
  - **Type B spermatogonia**, whose round nuclei differentiate them from their precursors. These cells also enter the mitotic cycle to form primary spermatocytes.

As these cells are undergoing cell division, they maintain contact with each other via cytoplasmic processes, forming a large syncytium.

- **Meiosis** is a reduction division that forms haploid cells.
  - The large syncytium of diploid **primary spermatocytes** migrates from the basal compartment into the adluminal compartment of the seminiferous tubule and undergoes the first meiotic division.
  - **Secondary spermatocytes** are in the adluminal compartment, and they undergo the second meiotic division, forming spermatids.
  - **Spermatids**, haploid cells, are supported by Sertoli cells while they undergo the final phase of spermatogenesis.

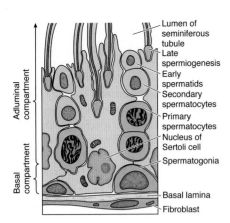

Figure 21.3 Seminiferous epithelium. *(From Gartner LP, Hiatt JL: Color Textbook of Histology, 3rd ed. Philadelphia, Saunders, 2007, p 492.)*

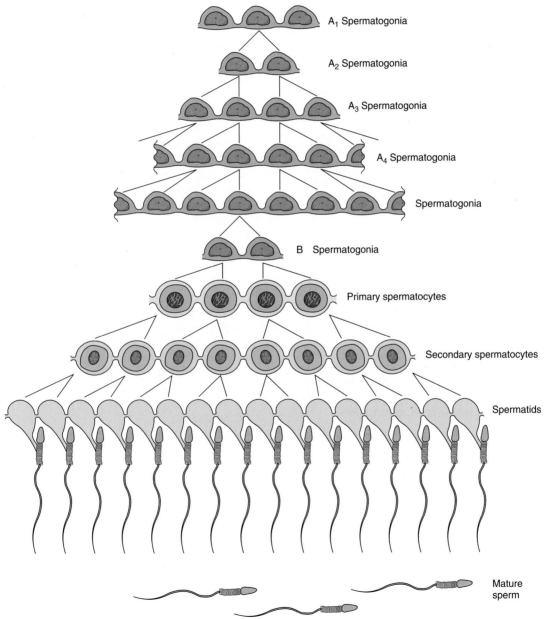

Figure 21.4 Spermatogenesis displaying the intercellular bridges that contain the syncytium during differentiation and maturation. *(Modified from Ren X-D, Russell L: Clonal development of interconnected germ cells in the rat and its relationship to the segmental and subsegmental organization of spermatogenesis. Am J Anat 192:127, 1991.)*

Spermatogenic Cells (cont.)

- **Spermiogenesis** is the phase of spermatogenesis in which the spermatids lose much of their cytoplasm and are transformed into spermatozoa. The four phases of spermiogenesis are the Golgi phase, cap phase, acrosomal phase, and maturation phase.
  - The **Golgi phase**, as its name implies, involves the packaging of hydrolytic enzymes by the Golgi apparatus into vesicles that fuse with each other to form the **acrosomal granule–containing acrosomal vesicle**; additionally, the flagellar **axoneme** and **connecting piece** are in the process of formation.
  - The acrosomal vesicle not only enlarges during the **cap phase**, but also attaches to and partially envelops the nuclear membrane and becomes known as the **acrosome**.
  - The nucleus of the spermatid becomes flattened and smaller, the entire cell becomes elongated, and the mitochondria collect in one location during the **acrosomal phase**. Additionally, a **manchette**, a temporary cylindrical collection of microtubules, is formed, causing the spermatid to increase further in length as it is being transformed into a spermatozoon. As the manchette disassociates, the **annulus**, which marks the junction between the developing spermatozoon's **principal** and **middle pieces,** is formed. Mitochondria assemble in the middle piece, and the **outer dense fibers** and the **fibrous sheath** are formed.
  - The final phase of spermiogenesis is the **maturation phase**, when the spermatids release their excess cytoplasm, freeing individual spermatozoa, from the syncytium. Spermatozoa are nonmotile until they undergo capacitation in the female reproductive tract. Sertoli cells phagocytose the cellular remnants; this process is known as **spermiation**.

Spermatozoa

Spermatozoa are haploid cells approximately 65 μm long that consist of a head and a long tail. The **head** of the spermatozoon (Fig. 21.5) is less than 5 μm in length and houses the haploid nucleus and enzyme-filled acrosome that contacts the nuclear envelope and the plasma membrane. As described in Chapter 20, when the spermatozoon contacts the ZP_3 molecule in the zona pellucida that surrounds the egg, the sperm undergoes the acrosome reaction, releasing the enzymes, neuraminidase, hyaluronidase, aryl sulfatase, acrosin (a trypsin-like enzyme), and acid phosphatase housed in the acrosome. These enzymes degrade the zona pellucida in the path of the spermatozoon, making it easier for the sperm to reach and fertilize the egg.

Tail of the Spermatozoon

Four separate regions constitute the tail of the spermatozoon (see Fig. 21.5):

- The **neck**, interposed between the head and the tail, consists of the **connecting piece** whose nine columns, surrounding the centrioles, persist as the nine **outer dense fibers**.
- The **middle piece** connects the neck with the principal piece and ends at the **annulus**. It is composed of the **mitochondrial sheath** surrounding the **outer dense fibers** and the central **axoneme**.
- The **principal piece** begins at the annulus and ends at the end piece. It is composed of the axoneme enclosed by the seven outer dense fibers that are encircled by a **fibrous sheath**. Near the distal terminus, the 45-μm-long principal piece constricts in diameter because the outer dense fibers and fibrous sheath are no longer present.
- The **end piece** is the caudal end of the spermatozoon. It is composed of the central axoneme, with its conventional nine doublets and two singlets, but becomes disorganized at the terminus into a cluster of individual microtubules.

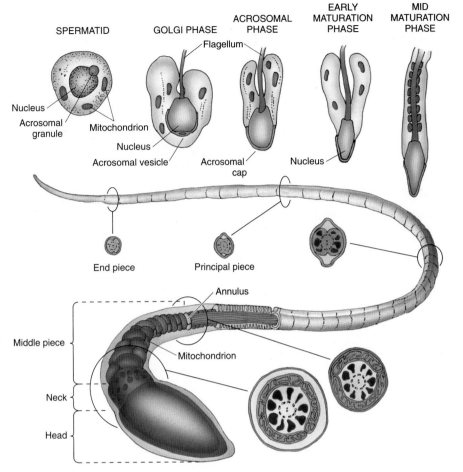

SPERMATID GOLGI PHASE ACROSOMAL PHASE EARLY MATURATION PHASE MID MATURATION PHASE

Figure 21.5 Spermatogenesis and a mature spermatozoon. *(From Kessel RG: Tissue and Organs: A Text Atlas of Scanning Electron Microscopy. San Francisco, Freeman, 1979.)*

CLINICAL CONSIDERATIONS

Mumps, a systemic viral infection, produces a 20% to 30% incidence of acute orchitis (inflammation of the testes) in postpubertal men. Generally, spermatogenesis is not affected by this disease.

Klinefelter syndrome results from an abnormality known as nondisjunction that occurs during meiosis, where the XX homologues fail to pull apart, producing an individual with an XXY genome (an extra X chromosome). These individuals have mental retardation, are infertile, are tall and thin, and display weakened masculine characteristics including small testes.

Cycle of the Seminiferous Epithelium

Germ cells derived from a pale type A spermatogonium are closely held together as a syncytium whose members communicate with each other and synchronize their development into **six stages of spermatogenesis** (Fig. 21.6) as they develop into spermatozoa. Each stage appears to last 16 days and is called the **cycle of seminiferous epithelium**. The completion of spermatogenesis requires the passage of four cycles (64 days).

INTERSTITIAL CELLS OF LEYDIG

The richly vascularized loose connective tissue surrounding seminiferous tubules also houses small groups of large polyhedral endocrine cells, the **interstitial cells of Leydig** (Fig. 21.7), which produce **testosterone**, the male sex hormone. The cells of Leydig are characteristic steroid-producing cells containing abundant smooth endoplasmic reticulum, numerous mitochondria with tubular cristae, and **crystals of Reinke**, whose function is unknown. Testosterone is believed to be released as it is being synthesized; these cells do not exhibit secretory vesicles.

CLINICAL CONSIDERATIONS

Chemotherapy treatments for cancer in young male patients may render them aspermatogenic because spermatogonia undergo mitosis and spermatocytes undergo meiosis, which can be affected. Dormant stem cells that are not currently involved in DNA synthesis and the cell cycle may be able to repopulate the seminiferous epithelium when anticancer chemotherapy is discontinued.

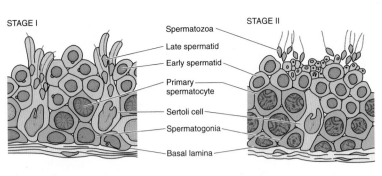

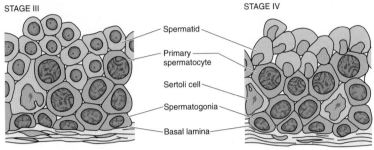

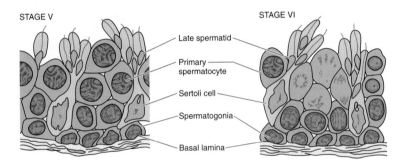

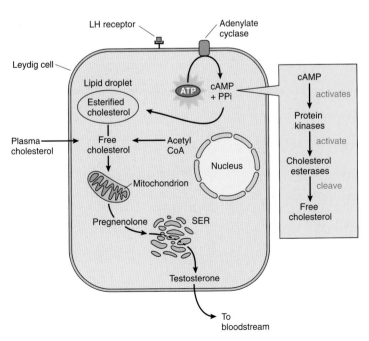

Figure 21.6 Six stages of spermatogenesis in the human seminiferous tubule. *(Redrawn from Clermont Y: The cycle of the seminiferous epithelium in man. Am J Anat 112:35-52, 1963.)*

Figure 21.7 Testosterone synthesis in the interstitial cells of Leydig. ATP, adenosine triphosphate; cAMP, cyclic adenosine monophosphate; CoA, coenzyme A; LH, luteinizing hormone; PPi, pyrophosphate; SER, smooth endoplasmic reticulum. *(From Gartner LP, Hiatt JL: Color Textbook of Histology, 3rd ed. Philadelphia, Saunders, 2007, p 500.)*

HISTOPHYSIOLOGY OF THE TESTES

Each testis produces approximately 100 million spermatozoa per day that are nourished and transported into the genital ducts by the fructose-rich medium produced by the Sertoli cells (Fig. 21.8). The process requires the actions of luteinizing hormone (LH) and follicle-stimulating hormone (FSH). The mechanism of hormonal control of spermatogenesis is illustrated in Figure 21.9.

- **LH** derived from the adenohypophysis activates the interstitial cells of Leydig to form the male androgen, testosterone. The mechanism of **testosterone** synthesis and release is illustrated in Figures 21.8 and 21.9.
- **FSH**, also derived from the adenohypophysis, stimulates Sertoli cells to manufacture and discharge **androgen-binding protein (ABP)**, which binds to testosterone and prevents it from leaving the seminiferous tubule. The increased level of testosterone in the region of spermatogenesis stimulates the process of spermatozoon production.
- The hormones **testosterone** and **inhibin**, secreted by Sertoli cells, stimulate a feedback mechanism to inhibit LH production. Testosterone is also:

- Necessary for the proper functioning of the seminal vesicles, the prostate gland, and the bulbourethral glands
- Responsible for the male sexual characteristics and appearance

CLINICAL CONSIDERATIONS

Testicular cancer is much more common among white men than men of African or Asian descent. Although a rare disease, testicular cancer is the most common form of cancer in men 20 to 34 years old. Testicular cancers arise from germ cells of the seminiferous epithelium 95% of the time and from the interstitial cells of Leydig approximately 5% of the time. There is no known cause, but the following conditions may predispose an individual to being affected by this disease: cryptorchidism, Klinefelter syndrome, and a family history of testicular cancer. Symptoms include size change in one or both testes, with or without pain; heavy feeling in the scrotum; and dull pressure or pain in lower back, stomach, or groin. Diagnosis is by blood tests and imaging tests. Treatment includes surgery, chemotherapy, and radiation therapy. Testicular cancer can be cured if treated early.

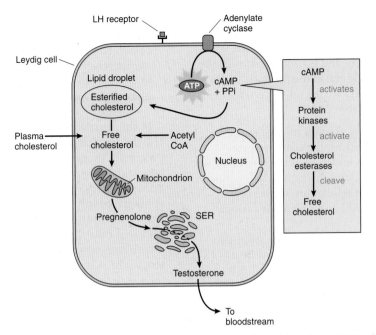

Figure 21.8 Testosterone synthesis in the interstitial cells of Leydig. ATP, adenosine triphosphate; cAMP, cyclic adenosine monophosphate; CoA, coenzyme A; LH, luteinizing hormone; PPi, pyrophosphate; SER, smooth endoplasmic reticulum. *(From Gartner LP, Hiatt JL: Color Textbook of Histology, 3rd ed. Philadelphia, Saunders, 2007, p 500.)*

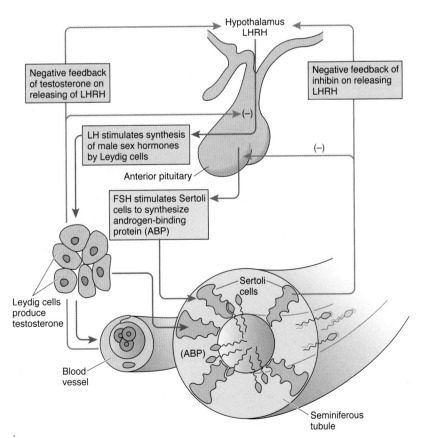

Figure 21.9 Hormonal control of spermatogenesis. LHRH, luteinizing hormone–releasing hormone. *(Adapted from Fawcett DW: Gloom and Fawcett's A Textbook of Histology, 10th ed. Philadelphia, Saunders, 1975.)*

Genital Ducts

The system of male genital ducts begins in the testis, with intratesticular ducts, and is continuous with the extratesticular ducts that end at the prostatic urethra. The **intratesticular ducts** are the tubuli recti and rete testis (Fig. 21.10 and Table 21.1).

- **Tubuli recti** are short, straight tubules that convey spermatozoa from the seminiferous tubules into the rete testes. Their proximal half is lined by Sertoli cells, and their distal half is lined by a simple cuboidal epithelium whose cells possess short microvilli and frequently a single cilium.
- **Rete testis** occupies the mediastinum testis and is a labyrinthine system of spaces lined by a simple cuboidal epithelium. The cells of this epithelium are similar to the ones that line the distal half of the tubuli recti.

The **extratesticular ducts** are the epididymis, ductus deferens (vas deferens), and ejaculatory duct (see Fig. 21.10 and Table 21.1).

- The **epididymis** is composed of two parts, the ductuli efferentes and the ductus epididymis.
  - The 10 to 20 **ductuli efferentes** are short tubules that convey spermatozoa from the rete testis into the ductus epididymis. These ducts are lined by a simple epithelium whose cells form a festooned appearance because of the alternating patches of simple cuboidal and simple columnar cells and reabsorb some of the fluid in which the spermatozoa are suspended. Deep to the epithelium is a basement membrane that separates it from the connective tissue, which is enveloped by a thin layer of circularly disposed smooth muscle cells.
  - The **ductus epididymis (epididymis)** is a tube approximately 4 to 6 m long lined by a **pseudostratified stereociliated** (long, nonmotile microvilli) epithelium. The wall of the epididymis houses circular layers of **smooth muscle** whose peristaltic contractions facilitate the delivery of spermatozoa into the ductus deferens. The epithelium is composed of two types of cells, regenerative **basal cells** and stereociliated **principal cells** that resorb fluid from the lumen, and secretes **glycerophosphocholine**, which makes the spermatozoa infertile until capacitation occurs in the female genital tract.

- The **ductus deferens (vas deferens)** has a small, irregularly shaped lumen and thick muscular wall and conveys the spermatozoa from the ductus epididymis to the ejaculatory duct. The epithelial lining is pseudostratified and resembles that of the ductus epididymis with shorter principal cells. The smooth muscle coat has inner longitudinal, middle circular, and outer longitudinal layers. The terminal portion of the vas deferens, the **ampulla**, is dilated and is joined by the duct of the seminal vesicle to form the ejaculatory duct.

- The short **ejaculatory duct**, lined by a simple columnar epithelium, has no muscle cells in its wall. It pierces the substance of the prostate gland and delivers its luminal content into the **colliculus seminalis** of the **prostatic urethra**.

CLINICAL CONSIDERATIONS

Vasectomy is chosen by more than 600,000 American men annually as a means of contraception. This brief surgical procedure is nearly 100% effective and is intended to be permanent. The vasectomy procedure is uncomplicated and commonly performed in a physician's office. The no-scalpel method is most often used, in which the scrotum is punctured, and a loop of the spermatic cord is retrieved, cut, and cauterized and then returned to the scrotum. Semen is collected and examined under a microscope after approximately 6 weeks and possibly later after surgery to ensure that no sperm remain. A few complications may be experienced, but most are transitory.

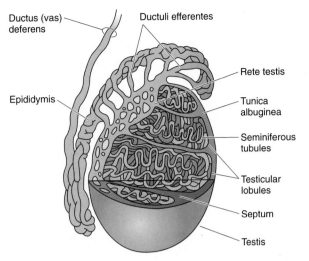

Figure 21.10 Testis and epididymis. Lobules and their contents are not drawn to scale. *(From Gartner LP, Hiatt JL: Color Textbook of Histology, 3rd ed. Philadelphia, Saunders, 2007, p 490.)*

Table 21.1 HISTOLOGIC FEATURES AND FUNCTIONS OF MALE GENITAL DUCTS

Duct	Epithelial Lining	Supporting Tissues	Function
Tubuli recti	Sertoli cells in proximal half; simple cuboidal epithelium in distal half	Loose connective tissue	Convey spermatozoa from seminiferous tubules to rete testis
Rete testis	Simple cuboidal epithelium	Vascular connective tissue	Conveys spermatozoa from tubuli recti to ductuli efferentes
Ductuli efferentes	Patches of nonciliated cuboidal cells alternating with ciliated columnar cells	Thin loose connective tissue surrounded by thin layer of circularly arranged smooth muscle cells	Convey spermatozoa from rete testis to epididymis
Epididymis	Pseudostratified epithelium composed of short basal cells and tall principal cells (with stereocilia)	Thin loose connective tissue surrounded by layer of circularly arranged smooth muscle cells	Conveys spermatozoa from ductuli efferentes to ductus deferens
Ductus (vas) deferens	Stereociliated pseudostratified columnar epithelium	Loose fibroelastic connective tissue; thick three-layered smooth muscle coat; *inner* and *outer* longitudinal, *middle* circular	Delivers spermatozoa from tail of epididymis to ejaculatory duct
Ejaculatory duct	Simple columnar epithelium	Subepithelial connective tissue folded, giving lumen irregular appearance; no smooth muscle	Delivers spermatozoa and seminal fluid to prostatic urethra at colliculus seminalis

From Gartner LP, Hiatt JL: Color Textbook of Histology, 3rd ed. Philadelphia, Saunders, 2007, p 502.

Accessory Genital Glands

The male **accessory genital glands** are the paired seminal vesicles, bulbourethral glands, and the single prostate gland.

- The right and left **seminal vesicles**, long coiled ducts located posterior to the bladder, join their respective ductus deferens to form the two ejaculatory ducts. The pseudostratified columnar epithelium of the seminal vesicles is composed of regenerative **basal cells** and **columnar cells**, whose height is a function of the local testosterone concentration. Each columnar cell possesses short microvilli and a single flagellum. The fibroelastic connective tissue that underlies the epithelium is enveloped by an inner circular and an outer longitudinal layer of smooth muscle tunic. These glands manufacture a yellow, fructose-rich fluid that also contains amino acids, proteins, citrate, and prostaglandins. The seminal vesicle secretion constitutes 70% of semen volume and provides nutrients for the spermatozoa.

- The two small **bulbourethral glands (Cowper's glands)**, lined by simple cuboidal to simple columnar epithelia, lie next to the membranous urethra and deliver their galactose-rich and sialic acid–rich viscous, slippery secretion into its lumen, lubricating it. The fibroelastic connective tissue capsule of the gland possesses smooth and skeletal muscle fibers.

- The single **prostate gland** (Fig. 21.11), normally the size of a horse chestnut, completely surrounds the ejaculatory ducts and the prostatic part of the urethra. Its fibroelastic capsule, interspersed with smooth muscle cells, invades the substance of the prostate to form the stroma, which also is enriched by smooth muscle cells. The glandular parenchyma is composed of 50 compound tubuloalveolar glands organized in three concentric layers:

- Innermost (immediately surrounding the urethra) **mucosal**, the shortest glands
- **Main** glands, which are the outermost glands and constitute most of the prostate
- **Submucosal** glands, which are intermediate in size and location, occupying the region between the mucosal and main glands

The parenchyma of the three glands comprises a simple to pseudostratified epithelium whose cells are well endowed with rough endoplasmic reticulum, Golgi apparatus, lysosomes, and secretory vesicles. These cells manufacture a watery secretion whose release is promoted by dihydrotestosterone and that is composed acid phosphatase, citrate, lipids, proteolytic enzymes, and fibrinolysin. Frequently, especially in older men, the lumina of these contain calcified glycoproteins, **prostatic concretions (corpora amylacea)**.

The release of the secretions of the accessory genital glands occurs after erection. The bulbourethral glands are the first to release their slippery lubricant shortly after erection, whereas release of the spermatozoa from the ampulla of the ductus deferens and the secretions from the seminal vesicles and the prostate occurs directly before ejaculation. The semen that is ejaculated is approximately 3 mL in volume and contains 200 to 300 million spermatozoa suspended in the secretions of the accessory glands.

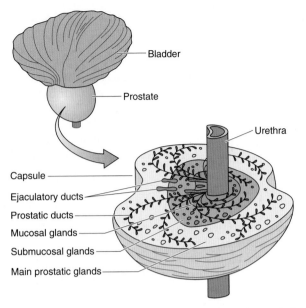

Figure 21.11 Human prostate gland. *(From Gartner LP, Hiatt JL: Color Textbook of Histology, 3rd ed. Philadelphia, Saunders, 2007, p 505.)*

Penis

The **penis** has a dual function—the delivery of urine to the outside and the conveyance of semen into the female reproductive tract. The penis is the **copulatory organ** and is composed of three masses of **erectile bodies** (Fig. 21.12):

- Two dorsally placed **corpora cavernosa**
- Single, ventrally positioned **corpus spongiosum urethrae**, whose distal terminus is the head of the penis, known as the **glans penis**, which displays a vertical slit, the external opening of the **urethra**

All three erectile bodies possess their own **tunica albuginea**, a fibrous connective tissue capsule, and the three structures are invested by a tubular sheath of thin skin that extends over the glans penis as a loose retractable sheath, the **prepuce**. The erectile tissues of the penis are composed of irregular, labyrinthine, endothelially lined vascular spaces that are bounded by connective tissue trabeculae enriched with smooth muscle cells. The two **corpora cavernosa**:

- Have vascular spaces of variable size that are smaller at the periphery and larger near the center
- Have fewer elastic fibers and more smooth muscle cells in their trabeculae
- Receive their blood supply from the deep artery and the dorsal artery of the penis, which pierce the trabeculae and form capillary beds and helical arteries. The helical arteries play a major role in the erection of the penis.

The **corpus spongiosum urethrae**:

- Has comparable sized vascular spaces centrally and peripherally
- Has fewer smooth muscle cells and more elastic fibers than the corpora cavernosa
- Is surrounded at its proximal terminus by the powerful **bulbospongiosus muscle** (skeletal muscle)

Venous drainage of the erectile tissues of all three erectile bodies and of the glans penis occurs via three sets of veins that are tributaries of the **deep dorsal vein**.

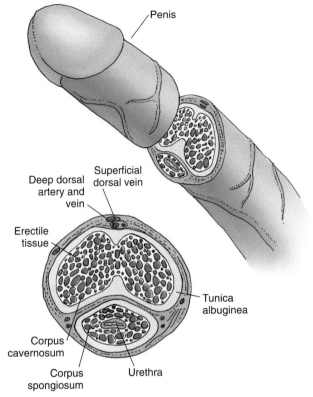

Figure 21.12 Penis in cross section. *(From Gartner LP, Hiatt JL: Color Textbook of Histology, 3rd ed. Philadelphia, Saunders, 2007, p 507.)*

CLINICAL CONSIDERATIONS

A normal single ejaculate contains approximately 70 to 100 million spermatozoa per milliliter. A man with a sperm count of less than 20 million spermatozoa/mL of ejaculate is considered to be **sterile**.

MECHANISMS OF ERECTION, EJACULATION, AND DETUMESCENCE

Blood flow in the flaccid penis is redirected to **arteriovenous anastomoses** between the arterial supply and the venous drainage, preventing the flow of blood into the vascular spaces of the erectile bodies (Fig. 21.13). When the blood flow is altered so that instead of entering the arteriovenous anastomoses it flows into the vascular spaces of the erectile tissues, the penis becomes **erect** and the tunica albuginea of the erectile bodies becomes stretched. Erection is achieved by:

- **Sexual stimulation**, whether tactile, visual, olfactory, or cognitive, which engages the **parasympathetic nervous system**
- Inducing the release of **nitric oxide** from the endothelia of the deep and dorsal arteries of the penis
- Causing a **relaxation** of the smooth muscles of the tunica media of these vessels, increasing blood flow into them

Simultaneously, the **arteriovenous anastomoses** become **constricted** and blood enters the **helical arteries**, which deliver their blood into the erectile tissues. The erectile tissues become turgid, compress the veins, and impede the outflow of blood, and erection is maintained.

If the **glans penis** remains stimulated, the bulbourethral glands release their slippery secretion, the secretory products of the seminal vesicles, along with the spermatozoa in the ampulla of the ductus deferens, into the ejaculatory ducts. The prostate releases its secretion into the prostatic urethra, and the semen is **ejaculated**, a process that is under the control of the **sympathetic nervous system**, as follows:

- Smooth muscles of accessory glands and genital ducts contract and convey semen into the urethra.
- Sphincter muscle of the urinary bladder contracts to prevent leakage of urine.
- Bulbospongiosus muscle contracts rhythmically, expelling the semen from the urethra.

Detumescence occurs after ejaculation because:

- The parasympathetic nerves no longer induce the release of nitric oxide in the deep and dorsal arteries of the penis.
- The reduced blood flow into these vessels permits the opening of the arteriovenous anastomoses.
- Drained blood from the vascular spaces of the erectile tissues results in the penis returning to the **flaccid** state.

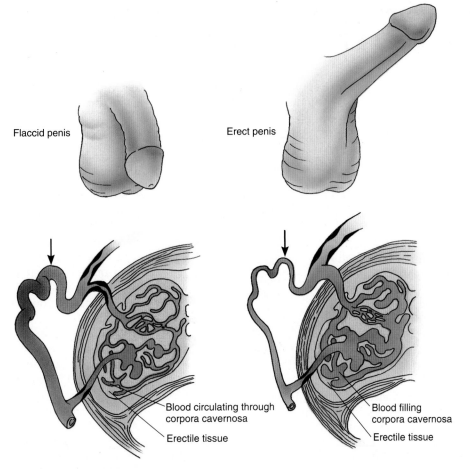

Figure 21.13 Blood circulation to the flaccid and erect penis. The arteriovenous anastomosis (*arrows*) in the flaccid penis is broad, diverting blood into the venous drainage. In the erect penis, the arteriovenous anastomoses are constricted and blood flow into the vascular spaces of the erectile tissue is increased, causing the penis to become turgid with blood. *(Adapted from Conti G: [The erection of the human penis and its morphologico-vascular basis.] Acta Anat (Basel) 5:217, 1952.)*

CLINICAL CONSIDERATIONS

Erectile dysfunction has nervous system involvements, including disturbances along the cerebral cortex—hypothalamus–spinal cord–autonomic nervous system pathways—and problems arising from vascular diseases. Additional causes include stroke, head injuries, spinal cord injuries, and anxiety disorders. Numerous systemic diseases, such as Parkinson's disease, diabetes, and multiple sclerosis, may also lead to erectile dysfunction.

Sildenafil (Viagra) was originally developed as a drug to treat heart failure. Patients who were previously impotent and were treated with this drug reported, however, that they were experiencing erections. From these observations and subsequent clinical studies, sildenafil became a drug of choice in the treatment of impotence. Numerous similar drugs have been developed that are also able to restore the ability to achieve erection in patients who are impotent.

22 SPECIAL SENSES

Sensory endings are specialized receptors at the terminals of dendrites that perceive stimuli that are transmitted to the central nervous system for processing. This chapter discusses these specialized receptors that are components of the general or special somatic and visceral afferent pathways. Three different classes of receptors are identified based on the stimulus received:

- **Exteroceptors** are located on the body surface and receive stimuli such as temperature, pressure, touch, and pain (general somatic afferent); light that permits vision and sound waves that permit the sense of hearing (special somatic afferent); and taste and smell (special visceral afferent; described in Chapters 16 and 15).
- **Proprioceptors** are located in tendons, in joint capsules, and in the muscle spindles of skeletal muscle and receive stimuli concerning the alertness of the body position in space.
- **Interoceptors** are located within the organs of the body and transmit information about these organs and are part of the **general visceral afferent** modality.

Specialized Peripheral Receptors

Dendritic specializations located in tendons, skin, muscles, fascia, and joint capsules respond to specific stimuli and are categorized as mechanoreceptors, thermoreceptors, and nociceptors; however, when a particular stimulus reaches a specific intensity, it can stimulate any receptor (Fig. 22.1).

   Mechanoreceptors become deformed by the stimulus or by the surrounding tissue and respond to stretch, vibrations, touch, and pressure. They may be either nonencapsulated or encapsulated. There are two types of **nonencapsulated mechanoreceptors**:

- **Peritrichial nerve endings** (see Fig. 22.1D) have neither a myelin sheath nor Schwann cells and enter the epidermis of the face and the cornea of the eye, providing a great deal of sensitivity to touch and pressure to those regions. Additional peritrichial nerve endings are associated with hair follicles and respond to hair movement. Some of the stimuli are interpreted as being tickled, as pain, or even as hot temperature.

> **KEY WORDS**
> - **Specialized peripheral receptors**
> - **Eyes**
> - **Retina**
> - **Rods and cones**
> - **Ears**
> - **Bony and membranous labyrinths**
> - **Organ of Corti**
> - **Vestibular function**

- **Merkel's disks** (see Fig. 22.1A) are mechanoreceptors discussed in Chapter 14.

   Encapsulated mechanoreceptors (see Fig. 22.1B, C, E, F, G, and H) consist of nerve fibers within a connective tissue capsule.

- **Meissner's corpuscles**, abundant in the dermal ridges of the fingertips, eyelids, lips, tongue, nipples, and skin of the foot and forearm, are specialized for tactile discrimination. Three or four nerve terminals along with their Schwann cells are encapsulated by connective tissue elements.
- **Pacinian corpuscles** are composed of a single unmyelinated axon surrounded by a complex of connective tissue sheaths of concentric layers of flattened cells. Pacinian corpuscles, located in the dermis, hypodermis, mesentery, and mesocolon, react to pressure, touch, and vibration.
- **Ruffini's endings** are highly branched nerve endings surrounded by a few layers of modified fibroblasts, located in the dermis of the skin, nail beds, periodontal ligaments, and joint capsules. Ruffini's endings perceive stretching and pressure.
- **Krause's end bulbs**, whose function is unknown, are spherical encapsulated endings in the subepithelial connective tissues of the oral and nasal cavities, peritoneum, papillary dermis, joints, conjunctiva, and genital regions.
- **Muscle spindles** and **Golgi tendon organs** are encapsulated mechanoreceptors specialized for proprioception. Muscle spindles perceive changes in muscle length and their rate of change, whereas Golgi tendon organs monitor tension and its rate of application to the joint.

   Thermoreceptors have not been identified, but it is assumed that naked nerve endings within the epidermis respond to heat and cold. **Nociceptors** are widely branched naked nerve endings in the epidermis that perceive pain. They function in one of three ways; they respond to:

- Mechanical stress or damage
- Extremes in heat or cold
- Chemical compounds including bradykinin, serotonin, and histamine

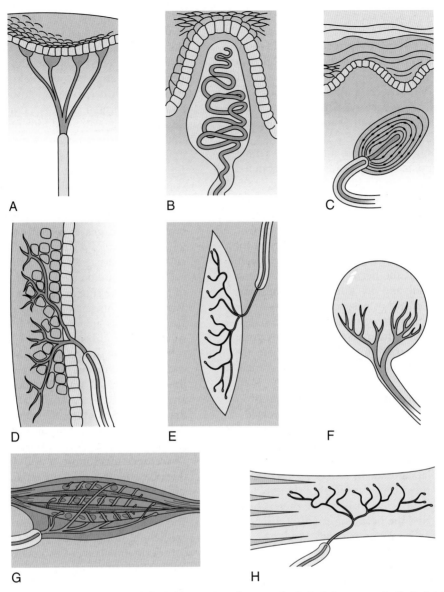

Figure 22.1 Various mechanoreceptors. **A,** Merkel's disk. **B,** Meissner's corpuscle. **C,** Pacinian corpuscle. **D,** Peritrichial (naked) nerve endings. **E,** Ruffini's corpuscle. **F,** Krause's end bulb. **G,** Muscle spindle. **H,** Golgi tendon organ. *(From Gartner LP, Hiatt JL: Color Textbook of Histology, 3rd ed. Philadelphia, Saunders, 2007, p 512.)*

Eye

The eyes are the **photosensory organs** of the body and are housed in the bony orbits of the skull. The **eyeball (bulb, globe)** (Fig. 22.2) and its associated structures function to receive light rays through the cornea and other refractory structures to focus the rays on the posterior wall of the bulb where the retina with its photosensitive rods and cones are located. When stimulated with light, a signal is transmitted to the brain for processing into a complex visual image that the individual perceives.

The eye develops from three sources. The retina and the optic nerve are outgrowths of the forebrain and may be observed at 4 weeks of development. The lens and some of the accessory structures in the anterior portion of the eyes are developed from surface ectoderm of the head. Associated structures within the eyeball and its tunics (coverings) are developed from adjacent mesenchymal tissues. The three layers are the outermost tunica fibrosa, the middle tunica vasculosa, and the innermost tunica nervosa.

The components of the **tunica fibrosa** are the opaque sclera, white sclera, and transparent cornea.

- The **sclera**, the opaque white of the eyeball, is composed of type I collagen fibers intermingled with elastic fibers, forming a strong fibrous coat that resists the pressure placed on it by the vitreous and aqueous humors. On its superior, inferior, medial, and lateral surfaces, it receives insertions of the extrinsic muscles of the eye. The deep aspect of the sclera displays the presence of melanocytes, and the posterior extent of the sclera is pierced by the optic nerve.
- The anterior transparent portion of the bulb, the **cornea**, bulges anteriorly, is avascular, and is profusely innervated with sensory nerve fibers. The cornea is composed of five layers:
  - **Corneal epithelium**, a stratified squamous nonkeratinized epithelium, is the continuation of the conjunctiva. The superficial layers of the epithelium display zonulae occludentes,

whereas cells of the deeper layer interdigitate with and are attached to each other by desmosomes. Pain fibers pierce the basal aspect of the corneal epithelium and arborize near the surface. The epithelial cells at the periphery of the cornea are mitotically active, and newly formed cells take 1 week to be desquamated. Water and ions from the underlying stroma penetrate the cornea and enter the conjunctival sac.
  - **Bowman's membrane**, a fibrous layer, is composed of type I collagen that separates the epithelium from the underlying stroma.
  - The **stroma**, also transparent, is the thickest layer of the cornea. It is composed of 200 to 250 lamellae of a regular arrangement of type I collagen bundles, where the collagen fibers of each lamella are parallel to each other but not to the lamellae superficial or deep to them. The collagen fibers and associated elastic fibers and fibroblasts are embedded in a chondroitin sulfate–rich and keratan sulfate–rich ground substance. The **trabecular meshwork** of endothelially lined spaces, known as the **limbus**, is located at the junction of the sclera and the cornea. These spaces are drained by the **canal of Schlemm**, the conduit that delivers the aqueous humor from the anterior chamber of the eye into a venous plexus.
  - **Descemet's membrane**, a well-developed, thick basement membrane separating the stroma from the corneal endothelium, becomes thicker and more fibrous with age.
  - The **corneal endothelium**, a simple squamous epithelium lining the deep aspect of the cornea, manufactures Descemet's membrane. Additionally, this endothelium actively transports sodium ions (followed passively by chloride ions and water) from the stroma into the anterior chamber, resulting in the dehydration of the stroma. This state maintains the characteristic transparency of the stroma.

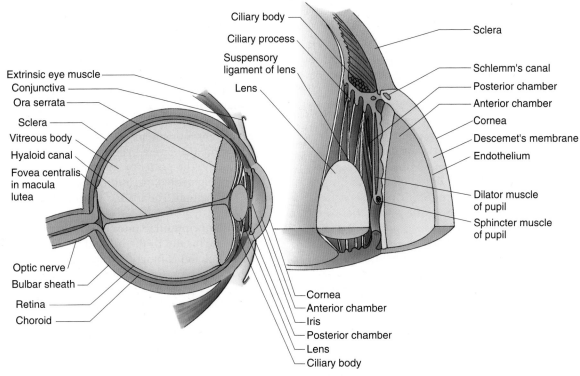

Figure 22.2 Anatomy of the eye (orb). *(From Gartner LP, Hiatt JL: Color Textbook of Histology, 3rd ed. Philadelphia, Saunders, 2007, p 515.)*

CLINICAL CONSIDERATIONS

Glaucoma, the leading cause of blindness in the world, results from prolonged intraocular pressure secondary to the blocking of aqueous humor from exiting the anterior chamber of the eye. Because aqueous humor is in constant production, blockage of its drainage from the anterior chamber of the eye over time builds pressure throughout the entire eye, first affecting the retina, causing a loss of peripheral vision, which leads ultimately to severe damage to the optic nerve and, if left unattended, blindness.

VASCULAR TUNIC (TUNICA VASCULOSA)

The components of the **tunica vasculosa** are the choroid, the ciliary body, and the iris (Fig. 22.3).

- The **choroid**, the highly vascularized pigmented layer of the posterior wall of the eyeball, is loosely attached to the tunica fibrosa. It is composed of loose connective tissue housing abundant fibroblasts, many blood vessels, and numerous melanocytes that impart the characteristic black color to the choroid. The inner regions of the choroid, the **choriocapillary layer**, is especially rich in capillaries and nourishes the retina, from which it is separated by **Bruch's membrane**, whose elastic fiber core is coated on both sides by collagen fibers.

- The **ciliary body**, located at the level of the lens, is a wedge-shaped extension of the choroid that surrounds the inner wall of the eye. The most anterior extension of the ciliary body adjoins the sclera at the limbus, whereas its most posterior extent abuts the vitreous body. The central (middle) portion juts toward the lens, and projecting from it are finger-like projections, the **ciliary processes**. The inner surface of the ciliary body and ciliary processes are lined with the **pars ciliaris of the retina** (a non–light-sensitive layer of the retina) composed of two strata: a nonpigmented layer facing the lumen of the bulb and an inner melanin-containing pigmented layer. **Zonule fibers**, composed of fibrillin, radiate out from the ciliary processes of the anterior portion of the ciliary body to insert into the lens capsule forming the **suspensory ligaments of the lens**. The inner nonpigmented layer of the pars ciliaris transports a plasma filtrate, the **aqueous humor**, which provides oxygen and nutrients to the lens and cornea, into the **posterior chamber of the eye**. The aqueous humor then flows through the **papillary aperture** into the **anterior chamber of the eye** and eventually exits the eye to enter the **canal of Schlemm** at the **limbus** to be drained into the venous system.
  - Three bundles of smooth muscles, known as the **ciliary muscle**, are located within the ciliary body. Because of its position, contractions of one of these muscles assist in opening the canal of Schlemm. The remaining two muscles by contracting release tension on the suspensory ligaments of the lens resulting in the lens becoming more convex and thicker, permitting the lens to focus on subjects that are close, a process known as **accommodation**. Relaxation of the ciliary muscles places tension on the lens resulting in its becoming flatter; most acute focusing is on distant objects.

- The choroid portion of the tunica vasculosa continues anteriorly as the **iris**, which lies between the anterior and posterior chambers of the eye and covers the entire lens except at the **pupil**. Its anterior surface possesses two rings: the **papillary zone** and the **ciliary zone**. The anterior surface is irregular with furrows at contraction sites. Its posterior surface is smooth and covered by the same two-layered epithelium covering the ciliary body. The posterior surface facing the lens is deeply pigmented, permitting light to pass only at the pupil. The iris has two intrinsic muscles:
  - The **dilator pupillae muscle**, which arises from the margin of the iris and radiates toward the pupil and is innervated by the sympathetic nervous system. Contraction of this muscle dilates the pupil in low light levels.
  - The **sphincter pupillae muscle**, which forms a concentric ring around the pupil and is innervated by the parasympathetic nervous system via the oculomotor nerve (CN III). Contractions constrict the pupil in bright light.

The color of the iris depends on the number of melanocytes in the epithelium. Dark eyes result from abundant melanocytes, whereas light blue eyes result from a low number of melanocytes being present.

LENS

The lens, a transparent flexible biconvex disk, is composed of several layers of flattened cells and their secretory products (see Fig. 22.3). The lens has three parts:

- The **lens capsule** represents a transparent basal lamina containing type IV collagen and glycoprotein. The capsule envelops the entire lens, being thickest anteriorly.
- The **subcapsular epithelium** lies immediately deep to the capsule and is located only anteriorly and laterally. It is composed of a single layer of cuboidal cells that communicate by gap junctions. Cell apices are directed to and interdigitate with the lens fibers.
- The **lens fibers**, approximately 200 or more elongated cells, arise from the subscapular epithelium and become highly specialized by losing their nuclei and organelles and becoming long (7 to 10 μm) hexagonal cells, a process continuing throughout life. These cells become filled with lens proteins called **crystallins** that increases their refractory index.

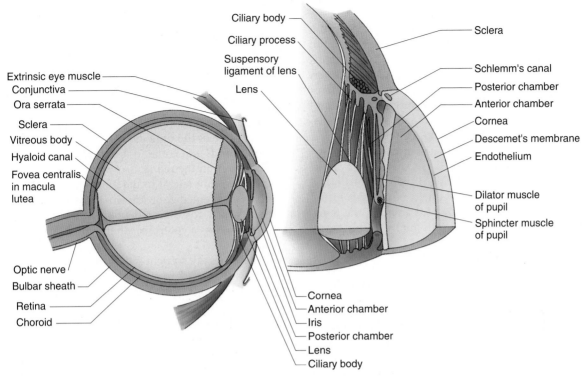

Figure 22.3 Anatomy of the eye (orb). *(From Gartner LP, Hiatt JL: Color Textbook of Histology, 3rd ed. Philadelphia, Saunders, 2007, p 515.)*

CLINICAL CONSIDERATIONS

Presbyopia is an age-related condition in which the eye exhibits a progressively diminished ability to focus on near objects. The exact cause is unknown; however, there is evidence that the lens loses its elasticity with age, and this may be coupled with the loss of the contractile strength of the ciliary muscles. Although there is no cure, most individuals can be fitted with prescription eyeglasses that accommodate for the loss of near vision.

Cataract is a clouding that develops in the lens of the eye, varying in degree from slight to complete opacity, obstructing the passage of light.

Cataracts typically progress slowly to cause vision loss and potentially can cause blindness if untreated. The condition usually affects both eyes, but almost always one eye is affected earlier than the other. Cataracts develop from various causes, including long-term exposure to ultraviolet light, exposure to radiation, advanced age, and secondary effects of diseases such as diabetes and hypertension. Cataracts may also be produced by eye injury or physical trauma. Cataracts do not respond to medications, but the affected lens can be removed and replaced with a corrective, artificial lens.

VITREOUS BODY

The transparent semigelatinous structure filling the posterior concavity behind the lens is known as the **vitreous body**. It is composed of 99% water containing a small amount of electrolytes, some collagen fibers, and hyaluronic acid. The vitreous body adheres to the retina principally at the **ora serrata** (the anterior border of the light-sensitive retina). Small cells, called **hyalocytes**, believed to synthesize collagen and hyaluronic acid, are located at the periphery of the vitreous body. A small channel, the **hyaloid canal**, located in the midline of the vitreous body, extends from the posterior aspect of the lens to the optic disk; it houses the hyaloid artery in the fetus, but in the adult it is filled with fluid.

RETINA (NEURAL TUNIC)

The innermost tunic of the eye, the **retina** (Fig. 22.4), is the neural portion that contains the rods and cones, specialized photoreceptor cells. The retina develops from neural tissue of the optic vesicle originating from the diencephalon of the brain. Later in development, the **optic vesicle** caves in to form the **optic cup**. The optic cup consists of two layers and is connected to the brain by the **optic stalk**. The outer layer of the optic cup becomes the **pigment layer of the retina**, the inner layer of the optic cup differentiates into the **neuronal layer of the retina (retina proper)**, and the optic stalk becomes the **optic nerve (CN II)**. The pigmented layer of the retina covers the interior surface of the orb, including the ciliary body and the posterior wall of the iris; however, the retina proper ends at the **ora serrata**.

- The optic disk on the posterior wall represents the exit site of the optic nerve, and because it is without rods and cones, it is considered the **blind spot** on the retina.
- About 2.5 mm lateral to the blind spot is a yellow pigmented zone known as the **macula lutea**, which possesses a depression in its center called the **fovea centralis**, where only cones are located.
  - The cones are so tightly packed within the fovea that other layers of the retina are crowded aside. Visual acuity is greatest in the fovea centralis.
  - As distance is increased from the fovea, fewer and fewer cones are present, whereas rods become prevalent.

The region of the retina that functions in photoreception is composed of 10 layers that face the inner surface of the choroid.

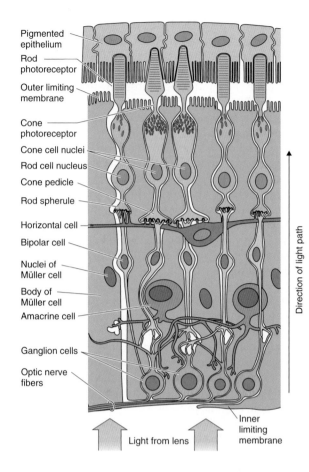

Pigmented epithelium
Rod photoreceptor
Outer limiting membrane
Cone photoreceptor
Cone cell nuclei
Rod cell nucleus
Cone pedicle
Rod spherule
Horizontal cell
Bipolar cell
Nuclei of Müller cell
Body of Müller cell
Amacrine cell
Ganglion cells
Optic nerve fibers
Inner limiting membrane
Light from lens
Direction of light path

Figure 22.4 Cellular layers of the retina. The space observed between the pigmented layer and the remainder of the retina is an artifact of development and does not exist in the adult except during detachment of the retina. *(From Gartner LP, Hiatt JL: Color Textbook of Histology, 3rd ed. Philadelphia, Saunders, 2007, p 520.)*

CLINICAL CONSIDERATIONS

Eye floaters that appear in one's vision, especially in older individuals, and seemingly move about are really shadows of small pieces of debris in the vitreous body that are cast on the retina. As the eye moves from side to side or up and down, these floaters also shift in position within the vitreous body, making the shadows move and appear to float. Eye floaters are associated with retinopathy of diabetes, retinal tears, retinal detachment, and nearsightedness. They occur more commonly in individuals who have had injury to the eyes or cataract surgery. Most eye floaters decrease in size and intensity with time because they may dissolve. The brain eventually disregards them, and the patient ceases to experience them.

CLINICAL CONSIDERATIONS

Detached retina may be caused by sudden blows around the eye, such as from a tennis ball, or jolts from falls on the head. Most often it is from the vitreous body drying and pulling away from the retina, causing a retinal tear as it pulls away from the pigmented layer. The vitreous body may leak fluid behind the retina and detach it further. Individuals with a detached retina need to see an ophthalmologist immediately because early diagnosis and repair provide the best outcome for vision. Delay may permit the detachment to expand to include the entire retina. If left untreated, blindness becomes complete in the affected eye. Current procedures for treating a detached retina include laser surgery and cryotherapy.

Layers of the Retina

The 10 layers of the retina, from the innermost pigment epithelium to the outermost inner limiting membrane, are very precisely arranged (Fig. 22.5).

- The **pigment epithelium** is composed of cuboidal to columnar cells, derived from the outer layer of the optic cup, and is attached to Bruch's membrane. Nuclei of the pigment cells are basally located; where the cells invaginate with Bruch's membrane, mitochondria are numerous, suggesting active transport. Microvilli extending from the free surface of these cells interdigitate with the tips of the rods and cones. The apical aspects of these cells are filled with granules of melanin, ensuring greater visual acuity. Also, the apical cytoplasm includes residual bodies containing phagocytosed tips shed by the rods. Pigmented epithelium functions to:
  - Prevent light reflections by absorbing the light after it has activated the rods and cones
  - Phagocytose spent tips of the rods and cones
  - Esterify vitamin A
- Two discrete types of photoreceptor cells are present in the **layer of rods and cones** (Fig. 22.6; see Fig. 22.5) of the retina. Rods number about 100 to 120 million, and cones number about 6 million. The apical portions of these highly specialized and polarized cells, called the **outer segments**, interdigitate with the apical regions of the cells of the pigmented layer. The basal aspects of rods and cones form synapses with the cells of the bipolar layer of the retina. Rods are specialized to perceive objects in dim light, whereas cones are specialized to perceive objects in bright light and to differentiate colors.
- The photosensitivity of **rods** (see Fig. 22.6) is so acute that they can produce a signal from a single photon of light, yet they cannot generate signals in bright light, and they cannot sense color. Rods are elongated cells (50 μm long × 3 μm in diameter) that are aligned parallel to each other situated perpendicular to the retina. These cells are divided into an outer segment, an inner segment, a nuclear region, and a synaptic region. The rod-shaped light-sensitive end (**outer segment**) is composed of 600 to 1000 flat, stacked membranous disks, each representing an invagination of the plasmalemma (detached from the cell surface). The membranes contain the light-sensitive pigment called **rhodopsin**

(**visual purple**). The speed of response to light is slower in rods than in cones, and rods are able to sum the reception collectively. Disks gradually migrate to the apical end of the outer segment and are shed and phagocytosed by pigmented epithelial cells. The **inner segment** is separated from the outer segment by a constriction, the **connecting stalk**. A modified **cilium** arises from the basal body located at the apical part of the inner segment and passes through the connecting stalk into the outer segment. Mitochondria that supply energy for the visual process are packed around the interface of the inner and outer segments. Proteins produced in the inner segment migrate to be integrated into the disks in the outer segment. The following occur in photoreception:

- Light is absorbed by **rhodopsin** (opsin bound to *cis* retinal) in the rod.
- Light absorption converts retinal to **all-*trans* retinal**, which dissociates from opsin.
- Bleaching produces activated opsin facilitating binding of guanosine triphosphate to the α-subunit of transducin, a trimeric G protein catalyzing the breakdown of 3′,5′-cyclic guanosine monophosphate (cGMP).
- Decreasing cytosolic cGMP concentration results in closure of Na^+ channels in the plasma membrane of the rod.
- Hyperpolarization of the rod results in inhibition of neurotransmitter release into the synapse with bipolar cells.
- In the next dark phase, the level of cGMP is regenerated, the Na^+ channels are reopened, and Na^+ flow resumes.
- Remaining all-*trans* retinal diffuses and is carried to the retinal pigment epithelium via retinal binding proteins. The all-*trans* retinal is recycled to its 11-*cis* retinal form.
- Finally, *cis* retinal is returned to the rod and is bound again to opsin, forming rhodopsin.

Na^+ channels in the plasmalemmae are maintained open when rods are not activated by light. During the dark phase, sodium ions are pumped out of the inner segment into the outer segment, triggering release of neurotransmitter substance into the synapse with bipolar cells. The signal is generated uniquely by light-induced hyperpolarization that is transmitted through the cell layers to the ganglion cells, where the signal generates an action potential along the axons on their way to the brain.

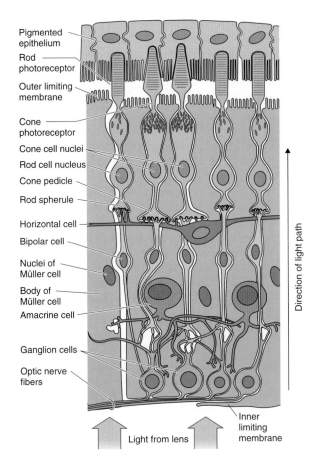

Pigmented epithelium
Rod photoreceptor
Outer limiting membrane
Cone photoreceptor
Cone cell nuclei
Rod cell nucleus
Cone pedicle
Rod spherule
Horizontal cell
Bipolar cell
Nuclei of Müller cell
Body of Müller cell
Amacrine cell
Ganglion cells
Optic nerve fibers
Direction of light path
Light from lens
Inner limiting membrane

Figure 22.5 Cellular layers of the retina. The space observed between the pigmented layer and the remainder of the retina is an artifact of development and does not exist in the adult except during detachment of the retina. *(From Gartner LP, Hiatt JL: Color Textbook of Histology, 3rd ed. Philadelphia, Saunders, 2007, p 520.)*

Figure 22.6 Morphology of a rod and cone. BB, basal body; C connecting stalk; Ce, centriole; IS, inner segment; M, mitochondria; NR, nuclear region; OS, outer segment; SR, synaptic region; SV, synaptic vesicles. *(Modified from Lentz TL: Cell Fine Structure: An Atlas of Drawings of Whole-Cell Structure. Philadelphia, Saunders, 1971.)*

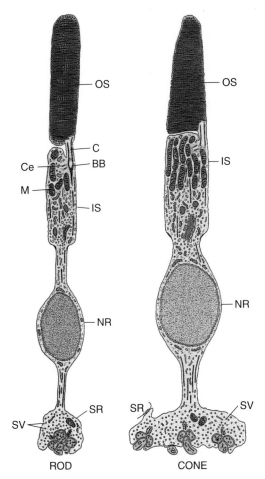

OS
C
Ce — BB
M
IS
NR
SR
SV

OS
IS
NR
SR
SV

ROD   CONE

Layers of the Retina (cont.)

- **Cones**, elongated cells approximately 60 μm long × 1.5 μm in diameter (Fig. 22.7), function in a similar fashion to rods except that they perform much better in bright light than in dim light, and they contain the photopigment **iodopsin**, of which there are three different varieties. Each variety of iodopsin has different opsin moieties, and each possesses a maximum sensitivity to one of three colors of the spectrum: red, green, and blue. The morphology of cones is similar to that of rods except in the following:
  - The outer segment is cone shaped.
  - The disks are attached to the plasmalemma.
  - Protein produced in the inner segment is inserted in all of the disks.
  - Cones are sensitive to color.
  - Recycling of the photopigment does not require pigment epithelial cells.
- The **external (outer) limiting membrane** is not a membrane; instead it is the region of zonulae adherentes formed between Müller cells (see later) and photoreceptor cells.
- The **outer nuclear layer** is a region occupied by the nuclei of the rods and cones.
- The **outer plexiform layer** consists of synapses between axons of photoreceptor cells and dendrites of bipolar and horizontal cells. Two types of synapses exist: flat synapses and invaginated synapses. In the latter, a dendrite of a bipolar cell and a dendrite from each of two horizontal cells form a **triad**. **Synaptic ribbons** are present within invaginated synapses that capture and assist in the distribution of neurotransmitter substances.
- The **inner nuclear layer** houses the nuclear regions of four cell types:
  - Each **bipolar neuron** may receive input from dozens of rods that permit the summation of signals, which permits enhancement of low light intensity information. Each cone provides signals to several bipolar neurons, however, augmenting visual information. Axons of bipolar cells synapse on ganglion cell dendrites.
  - **Horizontal cells** monitor and modulate the synaptic relationship between the photoreceptor cells and bipolar cells
  - Dendrites of **amacrine cells** maintain close contact with synapses between ganglion cells and bipolar cells and transmit their information to **interplexiform cells**, which influence the activities of horizontal and bipolar cells.
  - **Müller cells** extend between the vitreous body and the inner segment of the rods and cones where they form zonulae adherentes with photoreceptor cells at the external limiting membrane. These cells function as supporting cells.
- The **inner plexiform layer** is a complex region where axons and dendrites of bipolar, ganglion, and amacrine cells intermingle and synapse with each other, forming flat and invaginated synapses. Invaginated synapses consist of a bipolar cell axon and two dendrites of an amacrine cell and a ganglion cell or one dendrite from each of the two different cells, making a **dyad**.
- Cell bodies of large multipolar **ganglion cells** are located in the **ganglion cell layer**. Hyperpolarization of the rods and cones activates these cells to generate an action potential that is propagated along their axons to the visual areas of the brain.
- The **optic nerve fiber layer** is the region of the retina where unmyelinated axons of ganglion cells combine to form nerve fibers. As these axons pierce the sclera, they become myelinated.
- The **inner limiting membrane** is the innermost layer of the retina and consists of the basal lamina of the Müller cells.

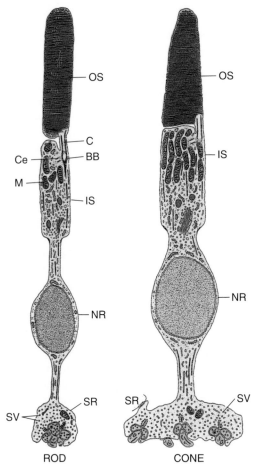

Figure 22.7 Morphology of a rod and cone. BB, basal body; C, connecting stalk; Ce, centriole; IS, inner segment; M, mitochondria; NR, nuclear region; OS, outer segment; SR, synaptic region; SV, synaptic vesicles. *(Modified from Lentz TL: Cell Fine Structure: An Atlas of Drawings of Whole-Cell Structure. Philadelphia, Saunders, 1971.)*

CLINICAL CONSIDERATIONS

There are two basic types of **macular degeneration**—wet and dry. Approximately 10% to 15% of cases of macular degeneration are the wet type that first manifested as the dry type. In the wet type of macular degeneration, abnormal blood vessels grow deep to the retina and macula, which may bleed or leak fluid that causes the macula to bulge, resulting in distorting or destroying central vision rapidly and severely. Different types of laser therapy have been used for treatment with only partial success at slowing the degenerative process. Also, scars from laser treatments may affect the macula, causing additional vision loss. More recently, a protein in the eye, called vascular endothelial growth factor (VEGF), was discovered. This encourages the development of blood vessels. Drugs are being developed to inhibit VEGF by trapping it or preventing it from binding with elements that would stimulate growth. Presently, three types of VEGF inhibitors are given for treatment by intraocular injections over an extended period. Early treatment has given positive results for slowing degeneration, and in some instances visual acuity has been improved.

ACCESSORY STRUCTURES OF THE EYE

The **accessory structures of the eye** include the conjunctiva, eyelids, and lacrimal apparatus.

- The **conjunctiva** is the transparent mucous membrane, consisting of a stratified columnar epithelium with goblet cells that overlies a loose connective tissue. It lines the internal aspect of the eyelids as the **palpebral conjunctiva**, and reflects over the sclera of the anterior surface of the eyeball as the **bulbar conjunctiva**. As the bulbar conjunctiva reaches the corneal-scleral junction, it no longer has goblet cells and becomes the stratified squamous epithelium of the cornea.
- The **eyelids** are folds of thin skin that seal over the anterior surface of the eye. The palpebral margins contain eyelashes that are arranged in rows of three or four; eyelashes are without arrector pili muscles. **Glands of Moll**, modified sweat glands, open into the follicles of the eyelashes. **Meibomian glands**, modified sebaceous glands, are within the **tarsal plates**. The tarsal plates are thickened connective tissue sheaths that support each lid, and meibomian glands form an oily secretion that mixes with and delays the evaporation of tears. Smaller modified sebaceous glands, the **glands of Zeis**, are associated with the eyelashes, and their secretions are emptied into the eyelash follicles.
- The **lacrimal apparatus** consists of the lacrimal glands, lacrimal canaliculi, lacrimal sac, and nasolacrimal duct.
    - The **lacrimal gland** is a serous, compound tubuloalveolar gland whose secretory acini are surrounded by myoepithelial cells. The gland is located outside the conjunctival sac; however, the secreted lacrimal fluid (tears) is emptied into the conjunctival sac via 6 to 12 secretory ducts. Tears, composed mostly of water containing **lysozyme**, an antibacterial agent, pass through secretory ducts into the conjunctival sac.
    - As the upper eyelid blinks, the tears are wiped medially to enter the **lacrimal punctum**, a small aperture near the medial margins of the upper and lower eyelids.
    - Each punctum leads to the **lacrimal canaliculi** that join into a common channel leading to the **lacrimal sac**, the superior dilated portion of the **nasolacrimal duct** that opens into the nasal cavity beneath the inferior meatus at the floor of the nasal cavity.

Ear (Vestibulocochlear Apparatus)

The **ear** serves as the organ of hearing and balance and is divided into three parts: external ear, middle ear (tympanic cavity), and inner ear (Fig. 22.8).

The **external ear** is composed of the auricle (pinna), external auditory meatus, and tympanic membrane (see Fig. 22.8).

- Irregularly shaped plates of elastic cartilage constitute the framework of the **auricle**, which is continuous with the cartilage of the external auditory meatus. The pinna is covered by tightly adhering thin skin.
- The **external auditory meatus** is covered with thin skin containing hair follicles, sebaceous glands, and **ceruminous glands** (modified sweat glands) that produce **cerumen** (earwax). The hair and the cerumen assist in thwarting objects from entering into the deep aspects of the meatus.
- The **tympanic membrane**, covering the deepest aspect of the external auditory meatus, represents the closing plate between the first pharyngeal groove and first pharyngeal pouch. Its external surface is composed of epithelium derived from ectoderm, whereas the internal surface is covered by epithelium derived from endoderm. A few scattered mesodermal connective tissue elements are located between these two surfaces. Sound waves are transmitted through the external auditory meatus, causing the tympanic membrane to vibrate. These vibrations are transmitted to the bony ossicles of the middle ear.

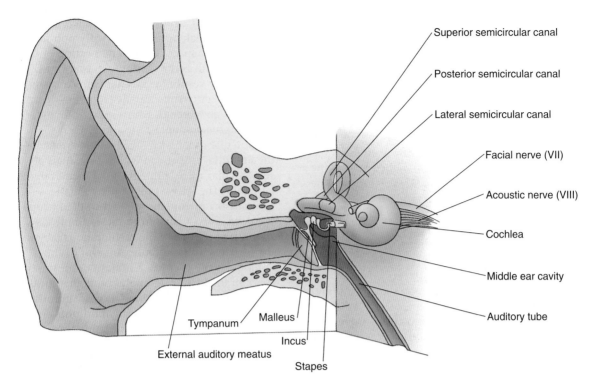

Figure 22.8 Anatomy of the ear. *(From Gartner LP, Hiatt JL: Color Textbook of Histology, 3rd ed. Philadelphia, Saunders, 2007, p 527.)*

CLINICAL CONSIDERATIONS

Conjunctivitis is an inflammation of the conjunctiva that may result from many sources, including bacterial and viral infections (then the condition is known also as pink eye) and from injury to the eye, but in most cases from exposure to allergens. Symptoms include redness of the sclera, irritation, itching, and watering of the eye with occasional puffiness of the eyelids. Cases of viral and bacterial conjunctivitis are contagious and require medical treatment, whereas conjunctivitis from other causes may resolve in a few days or 1 to 2 weeks. When the condition persists, the patient should be evaluated by a physician because some forms of conjunctivitis may cause blindness if untreated.

CLINICAL CONSIDERATIONS

The connection to the pharynx is opened during swallowing, yawning, and blowing the nose, permitting an equalization of the air pressure on the two sides of the tympanic membrane. The pressure differential can be felt during rapid descent when landing in an aircraft. Swallowing normally eases this pressure on the ear by opening the auditory tube at the pharynx.

MIDDLE EAR

The **middle ear (tympanic cavity)** (Fig. 22.9) is located within the petrous portion of the temporal bone and is an air-filled space between the tympanic membrane and the membrane covering the oval window. It communicates posteriorly with the mastoid air cells and anteriorly with the pharynx via the auditory tube (eustachian tube). The three ossicles occupy this space, which is lined by a simple squamous epithelium, a continuation of the lining of the internal surface of the tympanic membrane. The bony wall of the tympanic cavity is replaced with cartilage as it approaches the auditory tube, and the epithelial lining changes to a pseudostratified ciliated columnar epithelium. The lamina propria in this region contains numerous mucous glands that open into the lumen of the tympanic cavity, and, near the opening to the pharynx, goblet cells and lymphoid tissue are present.

Along the medial wall of the tympanic cavity are two membrane-covered gaps in the bony wall—the oval and round windows that connect the middle ear cavity to the inner ear.

- The inner surface of the tympanic membrane is connected to the membrane of the oval window by the three bony ossicles—the **malleus**, **incus**, and **stapes**. These bony ossicles transmit and amplify the vibrations of the tympanic membrane to the membrane of the oval window.
- Two small striated muscles—the **tensor tympani muscle** innervated by the trigeminal nerve (CN V) and the **stapedius muscle** innervated by the facial nerve (CN VII)—function in modulating the vibrations of the tympanic membrane and the movements of the bony articulations.

INNER EAR

The inner ear (see Fig. 22.9) is composed of the bony labyrinth and the membranous labyrinth that is suspended within it.

- The **bony labyrinth** (Fig. 22.10), housed within the petrous portion of the temporal bone, is lined with endosteum and is separated from the membranous labyrinth by the perilymph-filled perilymphatic space. The central portion of the bony labyrinth is the **vestibule**, posterior to which is the **vestibular mechanism**, consisting of the three **semicircular canals** (superior, posterior, and lateral), which arise from and return to the vestibule. One end of each semicircular canal is enlarged and is known as the **ampulla**. Suspended within the canals are the **semicircular ducts**, all part of the membranous labyrinth. The lateral wall of the vestibule contains the membrane-covered **oval** and **round windows**. Also arising from the vestibule are specialized regions of the membranous labyrinth, the **utricle** and the **saccule**. Anterior to the vestibule is the **cochlea**, a hollowed-out spiral space in the petrous temporal bone that turns on itself two and one-half times around a central column of bone known as the **modiolus** and its bony shelf, the **osseous spiral lamina**, providing a mode of entry for blood vessels and the spiral ganglion of the cochlear division of the vestibulocochlear nerve.
- The **membranous labyrinth** (see Fig. 22.10), composed of ectodermally derived epithelium, is suspended from the bony labyrinth by strands of connective tissue. The membranous labyrinth gives rise to the saccule, utricle, semicircular ducts, and cochlear duct. Endolymph, a viscous fluid, circulates within the membranous labyrinth. The **saccule** and **utricle** are connected to each other via a small duct. Also, each possesses small ducts that join to form the **endolymphatic duct**, whose blind end is known as the **endolymphatic sac**. Another small duct between the saccule and the cochlear duct is the **ductus reuniens**. Specialized regions of the saccule (**macula of the saccule**) and of the utricle (**macula of the utricle**) are receptors that monitor the orientation of the head in space and its acceleration. Both maculae possess non-neuroepithelial cells and neuroepithelial receptor cells.

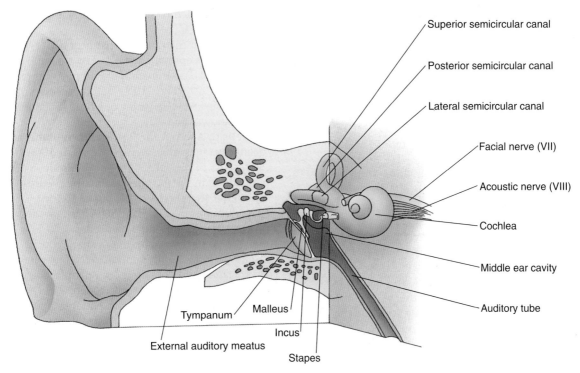

Figure 22.9 Anatomy of the ear. *(From Gartner LP, Hiatt JL: Color Textbook of Histology, 3rd ed. Philadelphia, Saunders, 2007, p 527.)*

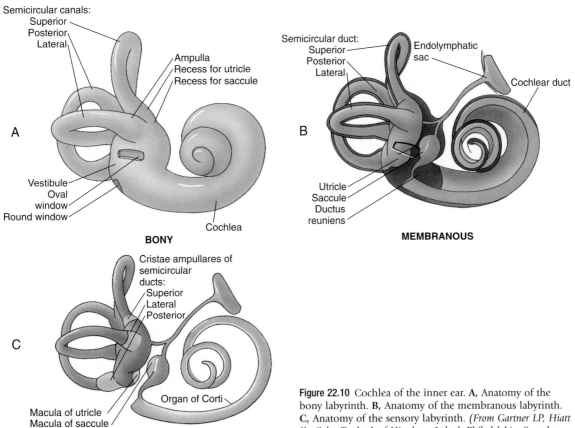

Figure 22.10 Cochlea of the inner ear. **A,** Anatomy of the bony labyrinth. **B,** Anatomy of the membranous labyrinth. **C,** Anatomy of the sensory labyrinth. *(From Gartner LP, Hiatt JL: Color Textbook of Histology, 3rd ed. Philadelphia, Saunders, 2007, p 528.)*

- Nonreceptor cells of both maculae are of two types, **light cells** and **dark cells**, whose functions are unknown, although it is suggested that the light cells may absorb endolymph, whereas dark cells may control the composition of endolymph.
- Two types of receptor cells (Fig. 22.11) are present in the two maculae—**types I** and **II hair cells (neuroepithelial cells)**. Both types of hair cells possess a single **kinocilium** and 50 to 100 **stereocilia** arranged in rows. Supporting cells sit on the basal lamina and are believed to maintain the hair cells or produce endolymph. The **vestibular division** of the vestibulocochlear nerve serves the hair cells (see Fig. 22.11). The stereocilia of the hair cells are embedded in a thick gelatinous mass, the **otolithic membrane**, whose surface contains **otoliths** or **otoconia (calcium carbonate crystals)**.
- The membranous labyrinth continues from the utricle as the three **semicircular ducts** (Fig. 22.12) housed in their respective semicircular canals. The expanded lateral ends of all three ducts are known as **ampullae** and contain specialized receptor sites known as **cristae ampullares**. Each crista ampullaris displays a crest containing neuroepithelial hair cells wedged between supporting cells, all sitting on a basal lamina. The hair cells are similar to the hair cells within the utricle and the saccule. A gelatinous mass overlying the cristae ampullares is the **cupula**, but it does not contain otoliths.
- The **cochlear duct (scala media)**, arising from the membranous labyrinth of the saccule, is a receptor organ housed within the bony cochlea. It is wedge shaped and surrounded on two sides by **perilymph**. Two membranes of the cochlear duct form the wedge. The membrane forming the roof of the cochlear duct is the **vestibular membrane**, whereas the membrane forming the floor of the cochlear duct is the **basilar membrane**. These two membranes isolate the cochlear duct from the surrounding perilymph. The perilymph-filled compartment above the vestibular membrane is the **scala vestibuli**, and the compartment below the basilar membrane is the **scala tympani**. Communication between these two perilymph-filled compartments occurs at the **helicotrema**.
- The vestibular membrane consists of two layers of squamous epithelia separated by a basal lamina. The basilar membrane supports the **organ of Corti** (Fig. 22.13), and it possesses various types of cells, some of whose functions are unknown, and others such as the **interdental cells** that secrete the **tectorial membrane**, a gelatinous mass that overlies the organ of Corti. Stereocilia of specialized receptor cells are embedded in the tectorial membrane. **Neuroepithelial (hair) cells** of the organ of Corti transduce impulses for hearing. These are the inner hair cells and outer hair cells.
- **Inner hair cells** are arranged as a single row of cells and surrounded by support cells. Inner hair cells are small and contain a centrally placed nucleus, copious mitochondria, rough endoplasmic reticulum, smooth endoplasmic reticulum, and small vesicles. Microtubules are located in the basilar area. Stereocilia, 50 to 60 arranged in a V shape, emanate from the apical surface. Stereocilia cores contain microfilaments, cross-linked with **fimbrin**. Also, microfilaments of the stereocilia merge with the terminal web. A basal body and a centriole are present in the apical region of the inner hair cells. The basal cell membranes of the inner hair cells synapse with afferent fibers of the cochlear division of the vestibulocochlear nerve.
- **Outer hair cells**, located near the outer boundary of the organ of Corti, are arranged in rows of three along the length of the organ. The outer hair cells are elongated cylindrical cells whose nuclei are located basally. Their cytoplasm contains rough endoplasmic reticulum and numerous basally located mitochondria. Just internal to the lateral cell membrane is a structure known as a **cortical lattice** composed of 5- to 7-nm filaments that are cross-linked with thinner filaments. It is assumed that this structure functions to support the hair cells and resist their deformation. About 100 stereocilia organized to form the shape of a W emanate for the apical surface of the outer hair cells. Also, because their length varies, they are arranged in gradations according to length. Outer hair cells are without a kinocilium but do possess a basal body. Afferent and efferent fibers of the cochlear division of the vestibulocochlear nerve synapse on the basilar portions of the hair cell.

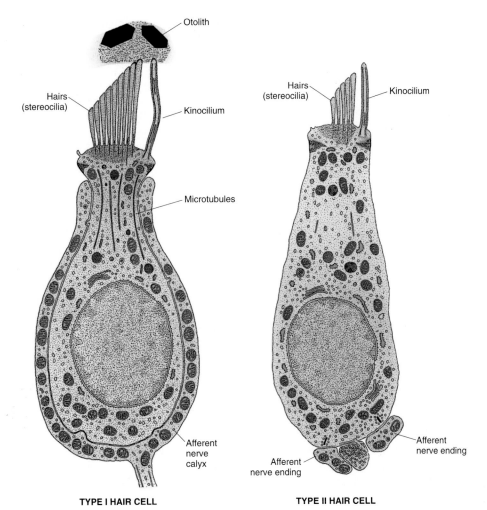

Figure 22.11 Morphology of types I and II neuroepithelial (hair) cells of the maculae of the saccule and utricle. *(Modified from Lentz TL: Cell Fine Structure: An Atlas of Drawings of Whole-Cell Structure. Philadelphia, Saunders, 1971.)*

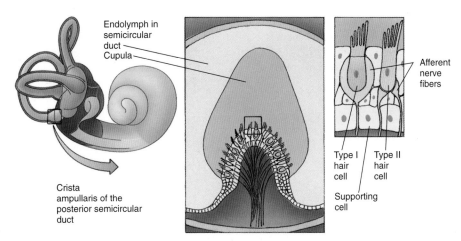

Figure 22.12 The hair cells and supporting cells in one of the cristae ampullares of the semicircular canals. *(From Gartner LP, Hiatt JL: Color Textbook of Histology, 3rd ed. Philadelphia, Saunders, 2007, p 531.)*

FUNCTIONS OF THE EAR

The dual functions of the ear are to monitor the body's position and movement in three-dimensional space (vestibular function) and the discernment of sound (cochlear function).

- **Vestibular function** of the inner ear monitors the changes in the velocity of the linear or circular movement of the head, a function that depends on the vestibular apparatus—the utricle, saccule, and semicircular ducts.
  - The **endolymph** of the **ampullae** of the utricle and saccule responds to **linear movements** of the head by causing the otoliths and the otolithic membrane to be displaced. As a consequence of the membrane displacement, the hair cells' stereocilia bend and the hair cells' membrane becomes depolarized. The change in resting membrane potential initiates action potentials that are transmitted to the vestibular division of the vestibulocochlear nerve that conveys the impulses to the brain for processing.
  - Neuroepithelial hair cells of the **cristae ampullares** of the **cupula** within the **semicircular ducts** react to **circular movements** of the head in a similar fashion as those of the utricle and saccule respond to linear movement. The **stereocilia** of the hair cells in the cristae ampullares become distorted in response to the movement of the **endolymph** in the semicircular ducts. Bending of the stereocilia results in the initiation of action potentials in the hair cells that are transduced to the vestibular division of the vestibulocochlear nerve for transmission to the brain for processing.
  - Linear and circular movements of the head require contraction of the skeletal muscles that are responsible for maintenance of balance. For that to occur, the brain must interpret the information it received from the hair cells of the vestibular apparatus and prepare an almost instantaneous response to prevent the individual from losing balance and falling down.
- **Cochlear function** (see Fig. 22.13) is the responsibility of all three regions of the ear—external, middle, and inner ears.
  - Sound waves received by the ear and passed through the external auditory meatus reach the tympanic membrane, setting it into motion.
  - This motion becomes translated into mechanical energy that sets the malleus and the two other bony ossicles of the middle cavity into motion.
  - The vibrations of the tympanic membrane are amplified by about 20 times as the energy is passed to the footplate of the stapes, where it impinges on the membrane of the oval window.
  - Two small skeletal muscles in the middle ear cavity modulate movements of the malleus and the stapes.
  - Movements of the membrane of the oval window create pressure waves in the perilymph within the scala vestibuli, through the helicotrema and into the scala tympani, causing wavelike movements of the basilar membrane.
  - This movement creates a shearing motion on the stereocilia of the hair cells embedded in the tectorial membrane.
  - As the stereocilia are deflected, the cell becomes depolarized and generates an impulse that is transmitted to afferent nerve fibers of the cochlear division of the vestibulocochlear nerve to the brain for processing.
  - High-frequency sounds are detected at the lower end of the organ of Corti (see Fig. 22.13), whereas low-frequency sounds are detected at the upper end of the organ of Corti, near its apex.

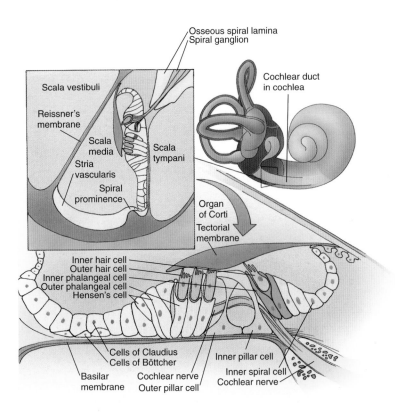

Figure 22.13 Organ of Corti. *(From Gartner LP, Hiatt JL: Color Textbook of Histology, 3rd ed. Philadelphia, Saunders, 2007, p 532.)*

CLINICAL CONSIDERATIONS

Ménière's disease is an episodic abnormality of the inner ear causing a host of symptoms, including severe dizziness, tinnitus (ringing sound in the ears), fluctuating hearing loss, and the sensation of pressure or pain in the affected ear. The disorder usually affects only one ear and is a common cause of hearing loss. The symptoms are associated with an increase in endolymph volume within a portion of the inner ear, causing the membranous labyrinth to balloon or dilate, a condition known as endolymphatic hydrops. Many experts believe that a rupture of the membranous labyrinth allows the endolymph to mix with perilymph, a condition that can cause the symptoms of Ménière's disease. Other experts are investigating several possible causes of the disease, including environmental factors and diet. Although there is no cure for Ménierè's disease, symptoms can be controlled successfully by reducing the retention of body fluids and dietary changes such as a low-salt or salt-free diet along with the abstaining from caffeine or alcohol.

Sensorineural hearing loss (nerve deafness) typically occurs in the organ of Corti when the hair cells are damaged or destroyed. Sensorineural hearing loss may have various causes, including heredity, aging, disease, infection, or prolonged exposure to loud noise. The nerve trunk to the brain is rarely damaged. Instead, damage most often occurs in the hair cells in the organ of Corti, which serve to send information, in the form of electrical signals, to the cochlear nerve. When a significant number of hair cells are damaged, an individual experiences severe or profound hearing loss, and hearing aids cannot alleviate the problem. In cases of profound hearing loss, a cochlear implant may be indicated.

Conductive deafness results when sound waves are impeded or prevented from being conducted through the outer ear or the middle ear or both and are prevented from being received by the inner ear. Conditions that may lead to conductive deafness include foreign objects, ruptured eardrum, impacted earwax, otitis media, and otosclerosis (where the footplate of the stapes becomes fixed to the oval window).

Otitis media is a common infection that occurs in the middle ear cavity, especially in young children, resulting from a respiratory infection that has involved the auditory tube. With otitis media, there is a fluid buildup in the middle ear cavity that restricts movement of the bony ossicles, restricting the ability to hear with the affected ear. The usual treatment for this condition is antibiotic therapy.

A antigens, 134
A band, 96
A kinase, 12
ABP. *See* Androgen-binding protein (ABP).
Absorption, small intestinal, 246, 247f
Accessory genital glands, male, 298, 299f
Accessory structures of eye, 316
Accommodation, visual, 308
Acellular cementum, 230
Acetyl coenzyme A (CoA), 20
Acetylcholine (ACh), 100, 121t, 124, 200
    arterial blood pressure and, 154
    gallbladder and, 258
    hydrochloric acid production and, 242
    interaction with secretin, 240
Acetylcholinesterase, 100
ACh. *See* Acetylcholine (ACh).
Acidophils, 190
Acinar cells, 252
Acinar exocrine glands, 60, 61f
Acini, 224
    of Rappaport, 254
Acne, 215b
Acquired immune system, 170
    cells of, 168, 169t, 172–178
Acquired immunodeficiency syndrome, CD4
    molecules in, 177b
Acromegaly, 89b
Acrosin, 280
Acrosomal phase of spermiogenesis, 290
Acrosomal reaction, 280
Acrosomal vesicles, 290
Acrosome, 290
ACTH. *See* Adrenocorticotropic hormone
    (ACTH).
Actin, 96, 140
Actin ring, 80
α-Actinins, 46, 96, 104, 106
Actin-linked cell-matrix adhesions, 52
Action potentials, 116–118, 117f, 119f
    olfaction and, 220
Activation agate, 116
Active fibroblasts, 64
Active sites, 118
    of G actin molecule, 98
    of presynaptic vesicles, 100, 101f
Active transport, 10, 11f
    gastric, 242
    secondary, 10
Activin, 274
Acute diarrhea, 239b
Acute myelogenous leukemia, 37b
Acute tubular necrosis, 265b
Acyl CoA synthetase in small intestine,
    246
Acyltransferases, 246
Adaptive immune system, 170
    cells of, 168, 169t, 172–178
Addison's disease, 201b, 209b
Adenocarcinoma(s), 57b
Adenohypophysis, 188, 189f, 189t, 190,
    191f
Adenoids, 186
Adenosine diphosphate (ADP), platelets and,
    140
Adenosine monophosphate (AMP), 66
Adenosine triphosphate (ATP), 96,
    100
    synthesis of, 20
Adenylate cyclase, 66
Adenylate cyclase system, 66
ADH. *See* Antidiuretic hormone (ADH).
Adhesive glycoproteins, 42, 62, 78

Adipocytes, 64–66, 65f
    fat storage and release by, 66, 67f
    multilocular, 62
    unilocular, 62
Adipose tissue, 72, 73f
    brown (multilocular), 72, 73b
    lymph nodes in, 182
    white (unilocular), 72, 73f
Aditus of larynx, 220
ADP. *See* Adenosine diphosphate (ADP),
    platelets and.
Adrenal glands, 200, 201f
Adrenocorticotropic hormone (ACTH), 190
    physiologic effects of, 194t
Adult obesity, 71b
Adventitia
    of digestive system, 238
    esophageal, 238
    of gallbladder, 258
    small intestinal, 244
    of tracheal lamina propria, 222
    of urinary bladder, 270
    uterine, 278
    vaginal, 284
Adventitial reticular cells, 142
Afadin-nectin complex, 54
Afferent components of peripheral nervous
    system, 108
Afferent lymphatic vessels, 166
Afferent nerve fibers, 120
Afferent neurons, 112
Aggrecan(s), 40, 76
Aggrecan composites, 76, 78
Agranulocytes, 136
AIDS, CD4 molecules in, 177b
Albinism, 23b, 209b
Albumin in plasma, 133t
Alcoholic hepatitis, 43b
Aldosterone, 104, 200, 203t
    binding of, 264
Aldosterone receptors of distal tubule,
    264
Alimentary canal, 238–248. *See also specific
    organs.*
    general organization of, 238, 239f
Alkaline phosphatase in osteoblasts, 79b
All-or-none law, muscle contraction and,
    98
All-*trans*-retinal, 312
Alpha chains of tropocollagen, 42
Alpha granules, 140
Alport syndrome, 47b
Alveolar bone proper, 234
Alveolar buds, 284
Alveolar cells, type I, 226
Alveolar damage, 235b
Alveolar ducts, 226, 227f
Alveolar exocrine glands, 60, 61f
Alveolar macrophages, 226
Alveolar sacs, 226
Alveolus(i)
    of lung, 226, 227f, 234, 235f
    of tooth, 230, 232
Alzheimer's disease, 129b
Amacrine cells of retina, 314
Ameloblasts, 230, 232, 233f
Amino acid derivative hormones, 188
Amino acid(s) in small intestine, 246
Amino sugars, 40–42
Aminoacyl tRNA, 14
Aminopeptidases, 246
    small intestinal, 244
AMP. *See* Adenosine monophosphate (AMP).

Ampulla(e)
    of oviduct, 278
    of saccule, 322
    of semicircular canal, 318
    of utrical, 322
    of vas deferens, 296
Anagen phase of hair growth, 214
Anal columns, 248
Anal sinuses, 248
Anal sphincters, 248
Anal valves, 248
Anamnestic response, 170
Anaphase, 36, 37f
Anaphase I of meiosis, 38, 39f
Anaphylactic reaction, 66
Anaphylactic shock, 70b
Anaphylaxis, systemic, 70b
Anchoring junctions, 52
Anchoring villi, 282
Androgen(s), 200, 203t
    bone repair and, 91b
Androgen-binding protein (ABP), 288, 294
Androstenedione, 203t, 274, 276
Anemia, sickle cell, 15b
Anencephaly, 109b
Aneurysms, 153b
Angiotensin I, 268
    arterial blood pressure and, 156
Angiotensin II, 158, 268
    arterial blood pressure and, 156
Angiotensin-converting enzyme, 268
    arterial blood pressure and, 156
    capillary production of, 158
Angiotensinogen, 268
    arterial blood pressure and, 156
Annulus in spermatogenesis, 290
Anterior chamber of eye, 308
Anterograde transport, 16
Antibodies, 68, 170, 171f, 171t
    membrane-bound, 170
Anticodons, 14
Antidiuretic hormone, 192
    arterial blood pressure and, 156
    physiologic effects of, 194t
    water and urea movement from and into
        collecting tubules and, 268
Antigen(s), 170, 183b
Antigen-presenting cells (APCs)
    macrophages as, 68, 136
    as migrating dendritic cells, 183b
    in splenic marginal zone, 184
    types of, 176
Anti-glomerular basement membrane
    antibody glomerulonephritis, 47b
Antimicrobial peptides, 168
Antimüllerian hormone, 288
Antiport transport, 10
Antral follicles, 275f, 275t
Antrostenedione, 200
Antrum, ovarian, 274
Aortic bodies, 154
Apaf1. *See* Apoptotic procapsace-activating
    adaptor protein (Apaf1).
APCs. *See* Antigen-presenting cells (APCs).
Aphthous ulcers, 231b
Apical domain of epithelial cells, 50, 51f
Apical foramen of root of tooth, 230, 232
Apocrine glandular secretion, 58, 59f
Apocrine sweat glands, 212
Aponeuroses, 94
Apoptosis, 38, 170, 174, 178, 180, 183b
Apoptosomes, 38
Apoptotic bodies, 38

Apoptotic procapsace-activating adaptor
     protein (Apaf1), 38
Appendices epiploicae, 248
Appendix, 248
Appetite center, 71b
Appositional growth, 76
Appositional stage of odontogenesis, 232
APUD cells, 60
Aquaporin(s), 10
Aquaporin channels, 268
     aquaporin-I, 262
     aquaporin-2, 264
Aqueous humor, 308
Arachidonic acid, 66
Arachnoid, 126, 127f
Arachnoid trabecular cells, 126
Arachnoid villi, 126
Arcuate arteries, 266, 267f, 278
Arcuate vein, 266, 267f
Area cribrosa, 268
Areolar connective tissue, 72
Argentaffin cells, 60
Argyrophil cells, 60
Aromatase, 274
Arrector pili, 214
Arteries, 152, 154–156, 155t. *See also specific*
     arteries.
     blood pressure regulation in, 154–156
     in bone marrow, 142
     sensory structures of, 154
Arteriolae rectae, 266, 268, 269f
Arteriosclerosis, 157b
Arteriovenous anastomoses, penile, 302
Arthritis
     osteoarthritis as, 93b
     psoriatic, 207b
     rheumatoid, 93b
Articular cartilage, 74, 75f, 75t, 92
     chondrocytes of, 76b
     histogenesis and growth of, 76, 77f, 77t
     hormone effects on, 76, 77t
     matrix of, 76
Artificial pacemakers, 105b
Aryl sulfatase, 69t
Aryl sulfate, 66
A-site, 12, 14
Asthma, 70b
Astrocytes, 112, 128
Atheromas, 157b
Atherosclerosis, 157b
ATP. *See* Adenosine triphosphate (ATP).
ATP synthase, 20
Atretic follicles, 276
Atria
     of heart, 164, 165f
     pulmonary, 226
Atrial granules, 104
Atrial natriuretic factor, 104
Atrial natriuretic polypeptide, 162
Atrioventricular anastomoses (AVAs), 158, 159f
Atrioventricular bundle, 162
Atrioventricular node, 162
Attachment plaques, 56
Auditory meatus, external, 316
Auerbach's plexus, 109b, 124, 238, 244, 246
Autocrine effects, 58
Autocrine hormones, 240
Autografts, 91b
Autoimmune diseases, 175b
Autonomic ganglia, 122, 124
Autonomic motor innervation, 122
Autonomic nervous system, 108, 122, 123f
Autonomic reflexes, somatic reflexes
     compared with, 109f
Autoradiography, 4
Autosomes, 28
AVAs. *See* Atrioventricular anastomoses (AVAs).
Axolemma, 114
Axon reaction, 130, 131f
Axon sprouts, 130
Axon terminals, 100, 116–118

Axoneme, 50, 290
Azurophilic granules, 138

B antigens, 134
B cells (lymphocytes), 136, 172, 173t
     activated, 183b
     splenic, 186
     in splenic marginal zone, 184
B memory cells, 176, 182, 183b
B7 molecules, 178
Backscatter electrons, 6
Bacteria, phagocytosed, T$_H$ cell-assisted killing
     of, 178, 179f
Bad breath, 235b
BALT. *See* Bronchus-associated lymphoid
     tissue (BALT).
Band 3 proteins, 134
Band 4.1, 134
Barbed end of microfilaments, 24
Baroreceptors, 154
Barr bodies, 138
Basal bodies, 22, 52, 53f
Basal cell(s)
     of epididymis, 296
     of olfactory epithelium, 218
     of respiratory epithelium, 222
     of seminal vesicles, 298
     of taste buds, 236
Basal cell carcinoma of skin, 211b
Basal lamina(e)
     of bone marrow, 142
     of Bowman's capsule, 260
     of capillaries, 156
     of epithelial cells, 46, 56
     of extracellular matrix, 46, 47f
     in splenic red pulp, 184
Basal layer
     of eccrine sweat glands, 212
     uterine, 278
Basal plasma membrane enfoldings, 56
Basal zone of osteoclasts, 80
Basement membrane
     of blood vessel walls, 152
     of extracellular matrix, 46, 47f
     of skin, 204
Basilar membrane, 320
Basolateral domain, 52–56
     basal surface specializations of, 56, 57f
     of epithelial cells, 52–56
     of hepatocytes, 256
     lateral membrane specializations of, 52–56,
          53f, 55f
Basophil(s), 70, 137t, 138, 190
Basophilic erythroblasts, 150t
Basophilic myelocytes, 150, 151t
BBB. *See* Blood-brain barrier.
Beta-particles of hepatocytes, 256
BFU-Es. *See* Burst-forming unit-erythrocytes
     (BFU-Es).
Bicarbonate
     gastric, 242
     salivary, 250
Bicarbonate-rich buffer, pancreatic, 252
Bicuspid valve, 164
Bile, 258
     primary, 256
Bile canaliculi, 256
Bile ducts, 246, 258
Bile pigment, 258
Bile salts (acids), 258
Biliary ducts, 258, 259f
Bilirubin, 258
     conjugated, 258
     free, 258
Bilirubin glucuronide, 258
Biliverdin, 258
Bilobed nucleus, 138
Bipolar neurons, 112, 113f, 314
Birbeck granules, 208
Bladder cancer, 37b
Blastocoele, 282

Blastocyst, 282
Blastomeres, 282
Bleeding
     from digestive tract, 239b
     subdural, 127b
Blind spot, 310
Blood, 132–140
     coagulation of, 132
     formed elements of, 132–140, 133f
     plasma of, 132, 133t
Blood clots, 140
Blood flow into capillary beds, regulation of,
     158, 159f
Blood islands, 144
Blood pressure, arterial, regulation of,
     154–156
Blood thymus barrier, 181b
Blood-brain barrier, 127b, 128
Blood-gas barrier, 226
Blood-testis barrier, 288
Bone(s), 78–92
     blood calcium levels and, 92
     calcification of, 88
     cancellous (spongy), 82
     cells of, 78–80, 79f, 81f
     compact, 82
          lamellar systems of, 82–84, 85f
     flat, 82
     formation of
          endochondral, 74, 86–88, 86t, 87f, 90
          intramembranous, 74, 84, 85f, 88
     gross observation of, 82, 83f
     histogenesis of, 84–88, 85f
     hormonal effects on, 92, 93t
     irregular, 82
     joints and, 92, 93f
     long, 82
     microscopic types of, 82–84
     primary (immature, woven), 82
     remodeling of, 90
     repair of, 90, 91f
     resorption of, mechanism of, 80
     secondary (mature, lamellar), 82
     sesamoid, 82
     short, 82
Bone marrow, 78, 84, 142–150, 143f, 183b
     cell-mediated immune response and, 170
     hematopoiesis and, 142, 144–150, 145t
     red, 82, 142
     yellow, 82, 142
Bone marrow phase of hematopoiesis, 144
Bone matrix, 78, 84
Bone morphogenetic proteins, 78, 232
Bone sialoproteins, 78, 88
Bone-lining cells, 78
Bony labyrinth, 318, 319f
Bony shelf of palate, 234
Bony union, 91b
Border cell layer of cranial dura mater, 126
Botulinum antitoxins, 119b
Botulinum toxin, 119b
Bowman's capsule, 260–262, 261f
Bowman's glands, 218
Bowman's membrane, 306
Bowman's space, 260
Bradykinins, 68, 69t
     capillary permeability and, 158
Brain natriuretic factor, 104
Brain sand, 202
Breasts, 284, 285f
Breathing, 218
     mechanism of, 228
Bronchi, 224
Bronchial tree, 224, 225f
Bronchioles, 224
     respiratory, 226, 227f
Bronchopulmonary segments of lungs, 224
Bronchospasm, 70b
Bronchus-associated lymphoid tissue (BALT),
     186
Brown adipose tissue, 72, 73b

Bruch's membrane, 308
Brunner's glands, 246
Brush cells of respiratory epithelium, 222
Bud stage of odontogenesis, 232
Buffy coat, 132
Bulbar conjunctiva, 316
Bulbospongiosus muscle, 300
Bulbourethral glands, 298
Bundle of His, 162
Burkitt's lymphoma, 37b
Burst-forming unit-erythrocytes (BFU-Es), 146

C antigens, 134
C cells, 196
C protein, 96
Cadherins, 54
Calcification
    of bone, 88
    zone of, 88
Calcitonin, 80, 90, 92, 196, 198, 203t
Calcitonin receptor, 80
Calcium, blood levels of, maintenance of, 92
Calcium carbonate crystals in inner ear, 320
Calcium channels, voltage-gated, 100
Calcium ions, 66
Calcium pumps, 88
Calcium release channels, 96, 104
Calcium tetani in DiGeorge's syndrome, 180
Calcium-sodium channels, 104
Caldesmon, 106
Call-Exner bodies, 274
Callus, 90
Calmodulin, 50
cAMP. See Cyclic adenosine monophosphate
    (cAMP).
cAMP response elements, 12
Canal of Schlemm, 306, 308
Canaliculi, 82, 84
Canals of Hering, 258
Cancellous bone, 82
Cancer. See also specific types of cancer.
    biliary, 259b
    of bladder, 37b
    of lung, 229b
    lymphatic spread of, 167b
    renal, 270b
    of skin, 211b
    testicular, 294b
Canker sores, 231b
Cap of microtubule, 22
Cap phase of spermiogenesis, 290
Cap stage of odontogenesis, 232
Cap Z, 96
Capacitation of spermatozoa, 278
Capillaries, 152, 156–158, 157f
    blood flow into, regulation of, 158, 159f
    continuous, 94, 156
    fenestrated, 156
    histophysiology of, 158, 159f
    lymphatic, 166, 167f
    sinusoidal, 156
Capillary beds, 156
    blood flow into, regulation of, 158, 159f
Capping proteins, 24
Capsaces, 38
Capsular plexus, 266
Carbaminohemoglobin, 134
Carbon dioxide
    delivery of, 218
    erythrocyte release of, 134
    erythrocyte transport of, 134
Carbonic anhydrase, 134
    gas exchange and, 228
    gastric, 242
Carcinoid syndrome, 60b
Carcinoid tumors, 60b
Carcinoma(s), 57b
    adenocarcinoma as, 57b
    basal cell, of skin, 211b
    of lung, 229b
    squamous cell

Carcinoma(s) (Continued)
    of oral cavity, 231b
    of skin, 211b
    transitional cell, renal, 270b
Cardiac glands, esophageal, 238
Cardiac muscle, 94, 95f, 105f, 162–164
    cells of, 104
Cardiac region of stomach, 240
Cardiocyte-specific troponin I (cardiocyte-
    specific TnI), 105b
Cardiodilatin, 162
Cardionatrin, 162
Cardiovascular system, 152–164
    aging of, 157b
    arteries and, 152, 154–156, 155t
        blood pressure regulation in, 154–156
        sensory structures of, 154
    capillaries and, 152, 156–158, 157f
        blood flow into, regulation of, 158, 159f
        histophysiology of, 158, 159f
    heart and, 162–164, 163f, 165f
    veins and, 152, 160, 161t
    vessel tunics and, 152–154, 153f, 155f
Cargo, 16
Cargo receptor proteins, 18
Carotid body, 154
Carotid sinus, 154
Carrier proteins, 10
Cartilage, 74–76, 75f, 75t
    elastic, 74, 75f, 75t
    hyaline (articular), 74, 75f, 75t, 92
        chondrocytes of, 76b
        histogenesis and growth of, 76, 77f, 77t
        hormone effects on, 76, 77t
        matrix of, 76
Catagen phase of hair growth, 214
Catalase
    of hepatocytes, 256
    in peroxisomes, 18
Cataracts, 309b
Catastrophe, 22
Catecholamines, 200, 203t
Cathepsin K, 80
Caveolae, 106
Caveolin, 106
C3b, 138
CD molecules, 172
CD regulatory T cells, 170, 174
CD4 molecules in AIDS, 177b
CD9, 280
CD40 ligands, 173b
CD95, 174, 178
CD95L molecule, 178
CDKs. See Cyclin-dependent kinases (CDKs).
Cell(s), 2, 8. See also specific types of cells.
    cytoskeleton of, 22–24, 23f, 25f
    inclusions of, 22
Cell cycle, 34–38, 35f
    apoptosis and, 38
Cell death, programmed, 38, 170, 174, 178,
    180, 183b
Cell membrane, 8, 9f
    E-face and P-face of, 8, 9f
    of erythrocytes, 134, 135f, 135t
    fluid mosaic model of, 8, 9f
    inner leaflet of, 8
    outer leaflet of, 8
    polarization of, 116
Cell signaling, 10, 12
Cell surface receptors, 188
Cell-mediated immune response, 136, 170
    TH1, 178, 179f
    TH2, 176, 177f
Cell-poor zone of dental pulp, 230
Cell-rich zone of dental pulp, 230
Cellular cementum, 230
Cellular respiration, 228, 229f
Cementing lines, 82–84
Cementoblasts, 230, 232
Cementoclasts, 230
Cementocytes, 230

Cementum, 230, 232
Central artery, 184
Central canal, 126
Central channels, 158
Central hyaline sclerosis, 43b
Central longitudinal vein, 142
Central lymphoid organs, 170, 178
Central memory T cells (TCM[s]), 172
Central nervous system (CNS), 108, 126–130
    blood-brain barrier of, 128
    cerebellar cortex of, 130
    cerebral cortex of, 128, 129t
    choroid plexus of, 128
    meninges of, 126, 127f
Central sheath in axonemes, 50
Central vein, 254, 255f
Centrioles, 9f, 22, 23f, 36
Centroacinar cells, 252
Centroblasts, 182
Centrocytes, 182
Centromeres, 36
Centrosomes, 22, 36
Cerebellar cortex, 130
Cerebellum, 130
Cerebral cortex, 128, 129t
Cerebrospinal fluid (CSF), 114, 126, 128,
    129t
Cerumen, 316
Ceruminous glands, 316
Cervical glands, 278
Cervical loop, 232
Cervix
    of tooth, 230
    uterine, 278
CFU-Basophils, 146
CFU-Eosinophils, 146
CFU-Es, 146
CFU-GMs, 146, 150
CFU-Gs, 146
CFU-LYs. See Colony-forming unit-
    lymphocyte cells (CFU-LYs).
CFU-M(s), 146, 150
CFU-Megs, 146, 150
CGN. See cis-Golgi network (CGN).
Channel(s). See also specific types of channels.
    gated, 10
    ungated, 10
Channel proteins, 10
Checkpoints, 34
Chemokines, innate immune system and, 168
Chemotherapy, 115b, 292b
    cell cycle and, 35b
Chiasmata, 38
Chief cells, 198, 240
Chloride, gastric, 242
Chloride shift, 134, 228, 229f
Choanae, 218
Cholangioles, 258
Cholecystokinin, 242
    duodenal release of, 258
Choledocholithiasis, 259b
Cholelithiasis, 259b
Cholera, 249b
Choline-O-acetyltransferase, 100
Chondrification centers, 76
Chondroblasts, 74, 76
Chondrocytes, 74, 76, 76b
Chondrogenic cells, 76, 78, 90
Chondroitin sulfate, 66, 69t
Chondroitin 4-sulfate, 41t
Chondroitin 6-sulfate, 41t
Chondronectin, 42, 62, 76
Choriocapillary layer, 308
Chorion, 282
Chorion frondosum, 282
Chorion laeve, 282
Chorionic plate, 282
Chorionic somatomammotropin,
    syncytiotrophoblast secretion of, 282
Chorionic thyrotropin, syncytiotrophoblast
    secretion of, 282

Chorionic villi, 282, 283f
Choroid, 308
Choroid plexus, 114, 128
Chromaffin cells, 200
Chromatids, sister, 36
Chromatin, 28–32, 29f
  nucleolus-associated, 32
Chromatolysis, 130
Chromophils, 190
Chromophobes, 190
Chromosomes, 28, 29f
  sex, 28
Chronic diarrhea, 239b
Chronic obstructive pulmonary disease
    (COPD), 226b
Chyle, 246
Chylomicrons, 66, 246
  plasma, 133t
Chyme, 240
Ciliary body, 308
Ciliary muscle, 308
Ciliary processes, 308
Ciliary zone, 308
Ciliated cells
  endometrial, 278
  of oviduct, 278
Ciliated columnar cells of respiratory,
    epithelium, 222
Cilium(a), 50, 51f
  movement of, 52
  primary, 52
  retinal, 312
Circular DNA, 20
Circular movements of head, vestibular
    function and, 322
Circulatory system. *See* Cardiovascular system;
    Lymphatic system.
Circumanal glands, 248
Circumferential lamellar system, 82–84
Circumvallate papillae, 236
cis-face of Golgi appratus, 16
cis-Golgi network (CGN), 16
Cistern, 16
Clara cells, 224
Class II human leukocyte antigens (class II
    HLA), 136
Class II-associated invariant protein (CLIP),
    176
Clathrin, 16
Clathrin coat, 118
Clathrin-coated vesicles, 16, 158
Claudins, 54, 114
Clear cells, 196
  of eccrine sweat glands, 212, 213f
  of gallbladder, 258
Clear zone of osteoclasts, 80
Cleavage, 280
Cleavage furrow, 36
CLIP. *See* Class II-associated invariant protein
    (CLIP).
Clonal deletion, 170, 180
Clonal expansion, 170
Clones, 170, 183b
Clostridium botulinum, 119b
Clostridium tetanae, 101b
Clotting mechanism, 158
Clotting proteins, 133t
Cluster of differentiation proteins (CD
    molecules), 172
CNS. *See* Central nervous system (CNS).
CoA. *See* Acetyl coenzyme A (CoA).
Coagulation, 132
  splenic red pulp and, 184
Coagulation factors, 140
Coated vesicles, 16
Coatomer I (COP I), 16
Coatomer II (COP II), 16
Cochlea, 318
Cochlear duct, 320
Cochlear function, 322, 323f
Codons, 14

Cofilin, 24
Cohesin, 36
Coiled tubular glands, simple, 212
Colchicine, 35b
Colitis, collagenous, 43b
Collagen, 42
  platelet adhesion and, 140
  synthesis of, 44, 45f
  type I, 63t, 72
  type II, 63t, 76
    capillary production of, 158
  type III, 63t, 70, 72
    of spleen, 184
  type IV, 46, 47f, 56, 63t
    capillary production of, 158
  type V, 63t
    capillary production of, 158
  type VII, 63t
Collagen fibers, 62, 63t
Collagen-like proteins, 42
Collagenous colitis, 43b
Collecting tubules, 264
  filtrate within, movement of water and urea
    from and into, 268
Collecting veins, 254
Colliculus seminalis, 296
Colony-forming unit-lymphocyte cells
    (CFU-LYs), 146
Colony-stimulating factor(s) (CSF), 148, 149t
  CSF-1, 90, 92
  innate immune system and, 168
Color of hair, 214
Colostrum, 284
Columnar cells of seminal vesicles, 298
Columnar epithelium, 49f, 49t
  pseudostratified, 49f, 49t
Common bile duct, 258
Communicating junctions, 52, 53f, 55f, 56, 57f
Compact bone, 82
  lamellar systems of, 82–84, 85f
Complement, 168
Complement proteins, 133t
Complement receptor, 138
Compound microscope, 2, 3f
Compound multicellular exocrine glands, 60
Condenser lenses, 4
Conducting portion of respiratory system,
    218–224, 219t, 221f
Conductive deafness, 323b
Cones, retinal, 312, 313f, 314, 315f
Confocal microscopy, 6, 7f
Congenital megacolon, 109b
Conjugated bilirubin, 258
Conjunctiva, 316
Conjunctivitis, 317b
Connecting piece, 290
Connecting stalk of retina, 312
Connective tissue, 62–72
  adipose tissue as, 72, 73f
  cells of, 62, 64–70, 64t
    fixed, 64–68, 65f
    transient, 64, 68–70
  classification of, 70–72, 71t
  dense, 72
  embryonic, 70
  functions of, 62
  loose (areolar), 72
  mesenchymal, 70
  mucoid, 70
  reticular, 72
  subepithelial, of oral cavity, 230
Connective tissue proper, 62, 72
  adipose tissue as, 72
  composition of, 62, 63t
  dense, 72
  loose (areolar), 72
  reticular, 72
Connexins, 56
Connexons, 56, 57f
Constipation, 239b
Constitutive pathway of secretory proteins, 16

Continuous capillaries, 94, 128, 156
Continuous conduction, 122
Continuous exocytosis, 16
Contractile bundles, 24
Contractile ring, 36
COP I. *See* Coatomer I (COP I).
COP II. *See* Coatomer II (COP II).
COPD. *See* Chronic obstructive pulmonary
    disease (COPD).
Cornea, 306
Corneal endothelium, 306
Corneal epithelium, 306
Corona of lymph nodes, 182
Corona radiata, 274
Coronary heart disease, 165b
Corpora amylacea, 298
Corpora arenacea, 202
Corpora cavernosa, 300, 303f
Corpus albicans, 276
Corpus hemorrhagicum, 276
Corpus luteum, 276, 277f
  of pregnancy, 276
Corpus spongiosum, 300
Corpus spongiosum urethrae, 300
Cortex of hair shaft, 214
Cortical collecting tubules, 264
Cortical lattice, 320
Cortical nephrons, efferent glomerular
    arterioles of, 266, 267f
Cortical plate of alveolar bone, 234
Corticosterone, 200, 203t
Corticotrophs, 190
Corticotropic hormone, 278
Corticotropin, 190
Cortisol, 200, 203t
Costamere, 96
Costimulatory signals, 176
Cough reflex, 221b
Countercurrent exchange system, 268
Countercurrent multiplier system, 268
Coupled transport, 10
Coupling, 90
Cowper's glands, 298
COX-2. *See* Cyclooxygenase-2 enzymes.
CR7+ cells, 172
CR7− cells, 172
Cranial dura mater, 126
Cranial motor nerves, 122
CRE(s). *See* cAMP response elements.
Creatine kinase, 96, 105b
Creatine kinase-MB isoenzyme, 105b
Creatine phosphate, 96
CRE-binding protein, 12
Cretinism, 199b
C-rings, 222
Cristae ampullares, 320, 322
Crohn's disease, 249b
Crown of tooth, 230
Crypt(s)
  of Lieberkühn, 244, 248
  of tonsils, 186
Cryptorchidism, 287b
Crystal(s), 22
  of Reinke, 292
Crystallins, 308
  αβ-crystallin as, 96
CSF. *See* Cerebrospinal fluid (CSF);
    Colony-stimulating factor(s) (CSF).
CTLs, 170, 174, 178
Cuboidal epithelium, 49f, 49t
Cumulus granulosa cells, 274
Cumulus oophorus, 274
Cupula, 320, 322
Cushing's syndrome, 201b
Cuticle
  of hair, 214
  of internal root sheath, 214
  of nails, 216, 217f
Cyclic adenosine monophosphate (cAMP), 12,
    66, 188
Cyclin-dependent kinases (CDKs), 34

Cyclooxygenase-2 enzymes (COX-2), 268
Cystic duct, 258
Cystinuria, 11b
Cytochemistry, 4
Cytocrine secretion, 208
Cytokines, 58
    hematopoiesis and, 144
    innate immune system and, 168
    origin and functions of, 175t
Cytokinesis, 36, 37f, 150
Cytomorphosis, 204
Cytoplasm, 8
Cytoplasmic peptidases, 246
Cytoplasmic ring, 26, 27f
Cytoskeleton, 22–24, 23f, 25f
Cytotrophoblast, 282

D antigens, 134
Dark cells
    of eccrine sweat glands, 212, 213f
    of inner ear, 320
    of taste buds, 236
Deafness
    conductive, 323b
    nerve, 323b
    nonsyndromic, 57b
Death ligand, 174, 178
Death receptors, 38, 174, 178
Decidua basalis, 282, 283f
Decidua parietalis, 282
Decidual capsularis, 282
Decidual cells (reaction), endometrial, 278,
    280
Deciduous teeth, 230
Decorin, 40
Dedifferentiated liposarcomas, 71b
Deep brain stimulation, 121b
Defensins, 168
    small intestinal, 244, 244b
Dehydration for light microscopy, 2
Dehydroepiandrosterone, 200, 203t
Delta granules, 140
Dendritic cells, 183b
    of lymph nodes, 182
    of thymus, 180
Dense bars, 100
Dense bodies, 106, 107f
Dense irregular collagenous connective tissue,
    72
Dense regular collagenous connective tissue,
    72
Dense regular elastic connective tissue,
    72
Dense tubular system, 140
Dental lamina, 232, 233f
Dental papilla, 232
Dental sac, 232
Dentin, 230, 232
    radicular, 232
Dentinal tubules, 230
Dentinoenamel junction, 232
Deoxycorticosterone, 200, 203t
Deoxyhemoglobin, 134
Depolarization, 116–118
Depolymerization, 36
Dermal papillae, 214
Dermal ridges (papillae), 204, 210
Dermatan sulfate, 41t
Dermatoglyphs, 204
Dermis, 204, 210
Descemet's membrane, 306
Desmin, 96, 106, 156
    binding of, 24
Desmocollin, 54
Desmoglein, 54
Desmoplakins, 54
Desmosine cross-links, 44
Desmosomes, 52, 53f, 54, 55f, 57f
Detached retina, 311b
Detumescence, 302, 303f
α-Dextrinase, 246

DHSRs. See Dihydropyridine-sensitive
    receptors (DHSRs).
Diabetes insipidus, 192b
Diabetes mellitus, 253b
Diakinesis, 38
Diapedesis, 136, 138, 158
Diaphyses, 82
Diarrhea, 239b
Diarthrosis joints, 92, 93f
Diffuse neuroendocrine system (DNES) cells,
    60, 188
    gastric, 240, 242
    of respiratory epithelium, 222
    small intestinal, 244, 258
DiGeorge's syndrome, 180
Digestion, 246
Digestive system. See also Alimentary canal;
    Oral cavity; specific organs.
    bleeding from, 239b
    glands of, 250–258. See also specific glands.
Dihydropyridine-sensitive receptors (DHSRs),
    96
Diiodinated tyrosine (DIT), 196
Dilator pupillae muscle, 308
2,3-Diphosphoglycerate, 134
Diploë, 82
Diploid cells, 280
Diplotene, 38
Direct method of immunocytochemistry, 4, 5f
Distal convoluted tubule, 262, 264, 265f
Distal ring, 26, 27f
Distal tubule, 260, 262, 264, 265f
Distributing arterioles, hepatic, 254
Distributing veins, hepatic, 254
DIT. See Diiodinated tyrosine (DIT).
DNA, 28, 30
    circular, 20
DNES cells. See Diffuse neuroendocrine
    system (DNES) cells.
Docking proteins, 14, 15f
Dolichol phosphate, 12
Domains of epithelial cells, 50
Dominant follicle, ovarian, 274
Dopamine, 121t
Dorsal horns, 126
Dorsal root ganglia, 124
Dorsal vein, deep, 300
Double negative thymocytes, 180
Double positive thymocytes, 180
Doublets in axonemes, 50
Down syndrome, 39b
Ducts of Bellini, 264
Ductuli efferentes, 286, 296, 297t
Ductus deferens, 286, 296, 297t
Ductus epididymis, 296
Ductus reuniens, 318–320
Duodenal glands, 246
Duodenal papilla, 246, 258
Dura mater, 82, 126, 127f
Dust cells, 226
Dwarfism, 89b
Dynamic instability, 22
Dynamic muscle fibers, 102
Dynamic sensory ending nerve fibers, 102,
    103f
Dynein, 22, 36
Dynein arms, 50
Dysphagia, 239b
Dystroglycans, 46
Dystrophin, 46, 96

E antigens, 134
Ear(s), 316–322, 317f
    external, 316, 317f
    functions of, 322
    inner, 318–320, 319f, 321f, 323f
    middle, 318, 319f
Early endosomes, 18
Earwax, 316
Eccrine sweat glands, 212, 213f

ECM. See Extracellular matrix (ECM).
ECP. See Eosinophil cationic protein (ECP).
Ectoderm, 48
Edema
    capillary permeability and, 158
    mechanism of, 70b
E-face, 8, 9f
Effector cells, 170
Effector memory T cells (TEM[s]), 172
Effector organs, 108, 122
Effector T cells, 172, 174, 175t
Efferent components of peripheral nervous
    system, 108
Efferent glomerular arterioles (EFGs), 266
Efferent lymph vessels, 182
Efferent lymphatic vessels, 166
Efferent nerve fibers, 120
Efferent neurons, 112
EFGs. See Efferent glomerular arterioles
    (EFGs).
EGF. See Epidermal growth factor (EGF).
Ehlers-Danlos syndrome, 63b
Ejaculation, 302
Ejaculatory duct, 296, 297t
Elastic cartilage, 74, 75f, 75t
Elastic fibers, 44, 45f, 62
Elastic membranes, 156
Elastic sheet of tracheal lamina propria, 222
Elastin, 44, 45f, 62
Electron microscope
    scanning, 3f
    transmission, 3f
Electron microscopy, 6, 7f
Eleidin, 206
Elicited macrophages, 68
Embedding for light microscopy, 2
Embryoblasts, 282
Embryonic connective tissue, 70
Enamel, 230, 232
    age-related changes of, 231b
Enamel knot, 232
Enamel matrix, 232
Enamel organ, 232
Enamel rods (prisms), 230
Enamelins, 230
Encapsulated mechanoreceptors, 304, 305f
Encephalomyopathy, mitochondrial, 21b
End piece of spermatozoa, 290
End-feet, 128
Endocardium, 162–164
Endochondral bone formation, 74, 86–88,
    86t, 87f, 89f, 90
Endocrine effects, 58
Endocrine glands, 58, 60
    diffuse neuroendocrine system and, 60
Endocrine hormones, 240
Endocrine pancreas, 252, 253t
Endocrine system, 188–202. See also
    Hormone(s); specific glands; specific
    hormones.
Endocytosis, 18, 19f
Endoderm, 48
Endogenous proteins, 176
Endolymph, 322
Endolymphatic duct, 318–320
Endolymphatic sac, 318–320
Endolysosomes, 18, 19f
Endometritis, acute, 279b
Endometrium, 278
    implantation and, 282
Endomitosis, 150
Endomysium, 94, 95f
Endoneurium, 120, 123f
Endoplasmic reticulum (ER), 12
    rough, 9f, 12
        of hepatocytes, 256
    smooth, 9f, 12
        of hepatocytes, 256
    transitional, 16, 17f
Endorphin(s), 121t
β-Endorphin, 190

Endosomes, 18, 19f
 early, 18
 late, 18
 recycling, 18
Endosteum, 78, 84
Endothelial cells
 of glomerulus, 266
 of lymph nodes, 182
Endothelin, 140
Endothelium
 arterial, 152
 corneal, 306
Enkephalins, 121t
Entactin, 42, 46
Enteric nervous system, 238
Enterokinases, 246
 small intestinal, 244
Enzymes. *See also specific enzymes.*
 bone calcification and, 88
 capillary production of, 158
 pancreatic, 252
Eosinophil(s), 70, 137t, 138
Eosinophil cationic protein (ECP), 138
Eosinophil chemotactic factor, 66, 68, 69t
Eosinophilic myelocytes, 150, 151t
Ependymal cells, 114, 126
Epicardium, 162, 164
Epidermal growth factor (EGF), 204, 232
Epidermal ridges (papillae), 204
Epidermis, 204–208, 205t
 as defense, 168
 keratinocytes in, 204, 205f
 layers of, 206, 207t, 209f
 nonkeratinocytes in, 208, 209f
Epidermolysis bullosa, 207b
Epididymis, 286, 296, 297t
Epidural space, 126
Epiglottis, 220
Epilepsy, 109b
 myoclonus, 21b
Epimysium, 94, 95f
Epinephrine, 66, 200, 203t
Epineurium, 120, 123f
Epiphyseal plate, 82, 89f
Epiphyses, 82
Epistaxis, 221b
Epithelial layer of digestive system lumen,
 238
Epithelial reticular cells, 180
Epithelial tissue, 48–56
 classification of, 48, 49f, 49t
 functions of, 48
 polarity and cell surface specializations of,
 50–56
Epithelium
 columnar, simple, cervical, 278
 corneal, 306
 as defense, 168
 gastric, 240
 germinal, ovarian, 272
 junctional, gingival, 234
 nonkeratinized, squamous, stratified,
 vaginal, 284
 olfactory, 220, 221f
 basal cells of, 218
 globose cells of, 218
 sustentacular cells of, 218
 pigment, of retina, 312, 313f
 pseudostratified stereociliated, of
 epididymis, 296
 respiratory, 222, 223f
 seminiferous, 286
 cycle of, 292–294, 293f
 seminiferous (germinal), 288
 subcapsular, of lens, 308
 transitional
 of renal calyces, 270
 ureteral, 270
Epitope(s), 18, 136, 170, 176
Epitope-MHC II complex, 178
Eponychium, 216

ER. *See* Endoplasmic reticulum (ER).
Erectile bodies of penis, 284, 300,
 301f
Erectile dysfunction, 303b
Erythroblast(s), 144
Erythroblastosis fetalis, 135b
Erythrocytes, 132, 134, 144, 150t
 carbon dioxide and oxygen transport by,
 134, 135t
 cell membrane of, 134, 135f, 135t
Erythrokeratodermia variabilis, 57b
Erythropoiesis, 150, 150t
Erythropoietin, 148, 149t, 266
Escherichia coli, urinary tract infections due to,
 270b
E-site, 12
Esophageal glands proper, 238
Esophagus, 238
Estradiol, 274, 276
Estrogens
 acne and, 215b
 bone repair and, 91b
 mammary glands and, 284
 syncytiotrophoblast secretion of, 282
Euchromatin, 28
Excitatory postsynaptic potentials, 118
Executioner, 38
Execution, 38
Exhalation, 228
Exocrine glands, 58–60, 59f
 multicellular, 58, 60, 61f
 unicellular, 58, 59f
Exocrine pancreas, 252
Exocytosis, 18
 continuous, 16
 discontinuous, 16
Exogenous proteins, 176
Exons, 30
Exportins, 28, 29f
External anal sphincter, 248
External auditory meatus, 316
External callus, 90
External ear, 316, 317f
External elastic lamina, arterial, 152
External genitalia
 female, 284, 285f
 male, 300–302, 301f
External laminae
 of extracellular matrix basement membrane,
 46
 of postsynaptic membrane, 100
 of smooth muscle cells, 106
External limiting membrane of retina, 314
External mesaxon, 114
External respiration, 218
External root sheath, 214
Externum, 138
Exteroceptors, 304
Extracellular fluid, 2, 72, 132
Extracellular materials, 8
Extracellular matrix (ECM), 2, 40–46, 41f, 62,
 74
 basement membrane of, 46, 47f
 fibers of, 42–44
 ground substance of, 40–42, 41t
 integrins and dystroglycans of, 46
Extracellular space, 114
Extrafusal muscle fibers, 102
Extraglomerular mesangial cells, 264
Extramural glands, 250
Extrapulmonary bronchi, 224
Extratesticular ducts, 296, 297f, 297t
Extrinsic pathway of apoptosis, 38
Eye(s), 306–316, 307f
 accessory structures of, 316
 lens of, 308, 309f
 retina of, 310–314, 311f
 tunica vasculosa of, 308, 309f
 vitreous body of, 310
Eye floaters, 311b
Eyeball, 306, 307f
Eyelids, 316

F actin, 98
F_0 portion of ATP synthase, 20
F_1 portion of ATP synthase, 20
Factor XIII, 140
$FADH_2$, 20
Fallopian tubes, 276, 278, 279f
Fanconi syndrome, 269b
Fas ligand, 178
Fas protein, 178
Fascia occludentes, 156
Fasciae adherentes, 54
Fascicles, 94, 120
Fast sodium channels, 104
Fat cells. *See* Adipocytes.
Fat-storing cells, 256
Fatty acid(s), 66
Fatty acid derivative hormones, 188
Fatty liver, 259b
Fc fragment, 170
Fc receptor, 138
Feedback mechanism, 188
Female reproductive system, 272–284. *See also
 specific organs.*
 fertilization and, 280, 281f
 implantation and, 282, 283f
 menstrual cycle and, 280, 281f
 ovulation and, 276, 277f
 placenta development and, 282, 282t
Fenestrated capillaries, 156
Fenestrated membranes, 156
Fertility, male, 287b, 301b
Fertilization, 280, 281f
FGF-4. *See* Fibroblast growth factor-4 (FGF-4).
Fibril-associated collagens, 42
Fibril-forming collagens, 42, 43f
Fibrillin, 44
Fibrin, 140
Fibrinogen, 140
Fibroblast(s), 64, 64b, 65f, 94
 active, 64
 inactive, 64
Fibroblast growth factor-4 (FGF-4), 232
Fibrocartilage, 74, 74b, 75f, 75t
Fibrodysplasia, 266b
Fibromuscular dysplasia, 266b
Fibronectin, 42, 62
 capillary production of, 158
Fibrous astrocytes, 112
Fibrous layer, 92
Filaggrins, 24
Filiform papillae, 236
Filopodia, thyroid, 196
Filtration force, 266
Fimbriae, 278
Fimbrin, 24, 50, 320
Fingerprints, 204
First polar body, 276
Fixation for light microscopy, 2
Fixed macrophages, 68
Flagella, 52
Flat bones, 82
Fluid mosaic model of cell membrane, 8, 9f
5-Fluorouracil, 35b
Foliate papillae, 236
Follicles, ovarian, 272, 274, 275f, 275t
 atresia of, 274
 atretic, 276
 FSH-dependent, 276
 primordial, 272
Follicle-stimulating hormone (FSH), 190
 follicles dependent on, 276
 ovarian follicles and, 274
 physiologic effects of, 194t
 testes and, 294
Follicular cells, 272, 276
Follicular dendritic cells, 183b
 of lymph nodes, 182
Follicular exocrine glands, 60
Follicular phase of menstrual cycle, 280
Folliculostatin, 274
Folliculostellate cells, 190

Follistatin, 274
Fontanelles, 84
Foramen cecum, 236
Foreign body giant cells, 68, 136
Formed elements of blood, 132–140, 133f
Fovea centralis, 310
Foveolae, 240
Free bilirubin, 258
Free macrophages, 68
Free villi, 282
FSH. See Follicle-stimulating hormone (FSH).
Function, structure related to, 2
Functionalis layer, uterine, 278
Fundic glands, cellular composition of, 240–242, 241f
Fundic region of stomach, 240
Fundus of stomach, 240
Fungiform papillae, 236
Fusion strands, 54

G actin, 24, 98
G protein(s), 12, 188
G protein-gated ion channels, 10
G protein-linked receptors, 12, 13f
G_0 phase, 34
G_1 cyclins, 34
G_1 (gap) phase, 34, 35f
G_2 phase, 34, 35f
GABA. See Gamma-aminobutyric acid (GABA).
GAGs. See Glycosaminoglycans (GAGs).
Gallbladder, 258
Gallstones, 259b
GALT. See Gut-associated lymphoid tissue (GALT).
Gamma granules, 140
Gamma-aminobutyric acid (GABA), 121t
Ganglia, 124, 125f
    autonomic, 124
    dorsal root, 124
    sensory, 124
Ganglion cell layer of retina, 314
Ganglion cell(s) of retina, 314
Gap junctions, 52, 53f, 55f, 56, 57f, 80
Gastric glands, 240
Gastric inhibitory peptide, 242
Gastric intrinsic factor, 240
Gastric lipase, 240
Gastric pits, 240
Gastrin, 242, 252, 253t
    hydrochloric acid production and, 242
Gate(s), 10
Gated channels, 10
G-CSF. See Granulocyte colony-stimulating factor (G-CSF).
Gelatinase, 138
Gell-like networks, 24
Gelsolin, 24
General visceral afferent modality, 304
Genital ducts, male, 296, 297f, 297t
Genital glands, accessory, male, 298, 299f
Genitalia, external
    female, 284, 285f
    male, 300–302, 301f
Genome, 28
Germ cells, primitive, 272
Germinal centers
    of lymph nodes, 182, 183b
    in splenic white pulp, 184
Germinal epithelium
    ovarian, 272
    of seminiferous tubules, 288
Ghrelin, 71b, 240
Giemsa stain, 3t, 132
Gigantism, pituitary, 89b
Gingiva, 234, 235f
Glands, 58–60, 188. See also specific glands.
    endocrine, 58, 60
        diffuse neuroendocrine system and, 60
    exocrine, 58–60, 59f
        multicellular, 58, 60, 61f

Glands (Continued)
        unicellular, 58, 59f
    of Moll, 316
    of skin, 212, 213f
    small intestinal, 246
    of von Ebner, 236
    of Zeis, 316
Glans clitoridis, 284, 285f
Glans penis, 300, 302
Glassy membrane, 214
Glaucoma, 307b
Glial fibrillar acidic protein, 112
Glial scars, 113b
Glisson's capsule, 254
Globin, 134
Globose cells of olfactory epithelium, 218
Globulins in plasma, 133t
Glomerular arterioles, afferent, 266
Glomerular ultrafiltrate, 266
Glomerular ultrafiltration, 262
Glomerulosclerosis, focal segmental, heroin-associated, 262b
Glomerulus(i)
    in olfactory bulb, 220
    renal, 260
Glomus cells, 154
Glucagon, 252, 253t
Glucocorticoids, 203t
Glucuronyl transferase, 258
Glutamic acid, 121t
Glycerol, 66
Glycerophosphocholine, 296
Glycine, 42, 62, 121t
Glycocalyx, 8
Glycocholic acid, 258
Glycogen, 22
    of hepatocytes, 256
Glycogen storage disorders, 23b
Glycolipids, 8
Glycophorin A, 134
Glycoproteins, 8, 42, 114
    adhesive, 62, 78
Glycosaminoglycans (GAGs), 40–42, 41t, 62, 74
G_2/M checkpoint, 34
GM-CSF. See Granulocyte-macrophage colony-stimulating factor (GM-CSF).
Goblet cells
    small intestinal, 244
    of tracheal epithelium, 222, 223f
    as unicellular exocrine gland, 58, 59f
Goiter
    nontoxic, 195b
    simple, 199b
Golgi apparatus (complex), 9f, 14, 16, 17f, 256
Golgi phase of spermiogenesis, 290
Golgi tendon organs, 102, 304, 305f
Gonadal ridges, 272
Gonadotrophs, 190
Gonadotropic hormones, 272
Goodpasture syndrome, 47b
Goose bumps, 214
Graafian follicles, 274, 275t
Granular layer of cerebellar cortex, 130
Granulation tissue, 90
Granulocyte(s), 136
Granulocyte colony-stimulating factor. (G-CSF), 148, 149t
Granulocyte-macrophage colony-stimulating factor (GM-CSF), 148, 149t
Granulocytopoiesis, 150, 151t
Granulomeres, 140
Granulosa cells, 274, 276
Granulosa lutein, 276
Granzymes, 174
Graves' disease, 175b, 199b
Gray matter, 126
Ground substance, 40–42, 41t, 70, 72
Group Ia nerve fibers, 102, 103f
Group II nerve fibers, 102, 103f

Growth factors, hematopoiesis and, 144
G_1/S cyclins, 34
G_S proteins, 12
GTP, 12
Guillain-Barré syndrome, 115b
Gums, 234, 235f
Gut-associated lymphoid tissue, 186
Gyri, 128

H band, 94, 96, 97f
Haemophilus influenzae, halitosis caused by, 235b
Hair, 214, 215f
    arrector pili and, 214
    color of, 214
    growth of, 214
Hair bulb, 214
Hair cells of inner ear, 320, 321f
Hair follicles, 214
Hair root, 214
Hair shaft, 214
Halitosis, 235b
Hard palate, 234
Hassall's corpuscles, 180
Haustra coli, 248
Haversian canal(s), 82–84, 85f
Haversian canal systems, 82–84
Hay fever, 70b
hCG. See Human chorionic gonadotropin (hCG).
HCO_3^-
    gastric, 242
    salivary, 250
H&E. See Hematoxylin and eosin (H&E).
Head movements, vestibular function and, 322
Head of ATP synthase, 20
Hearing loss
    conductive, 323b
    sensorineural, 323b
Heart, 162, 164, 163f, 165f
    fibrous skeleton of, 162
Heart failure cells, 229b
Heavy chains, 170
Helical arrangement, 82–84
Helical arteries, 278, 302
Helicotrema, 320
Hematocrit, 132
Hematopoiesis, 78, 132, 142, 144–150, 145t
    cells of, 144, 145t
    postnatal, 144
    prenatal, 144
Hematopoietic compartment, 142
Hematopoietic cords, 142
Hematopoietic growth factors, 148, 149t
Hematopoietic islands, 142
Hematoxylin and eosin (H&E), 2, 3t
Heme groups, 134
Hemidesmosomes, 52, 53f, 55f, 56, 57f
Hemoglobin, 134, 135t
Hemopoiesis, 78, 132, 142, 144–150, 145t
    cells of, 144, 145t
    postnatal, 144
    prenatal, 144
Hemorrhage
    from digestive tract, 239b
    subdural, 127b
Hemorrhagic disease of the newborn, 141b
Hemorrhoidal venous plexi, 248
Henle's loop, 260
    thick limb of
        ascending, 262, 268
        descending, 262
    thin limb of, 262
        ascending, 268
        descending, 268
Henley's layer, 214
Heparan sulfate, 41t, 46
Heparin, 41t, 66, 69t
Heparin-like molecule, 140
Hepatic ducts, 258
Hepatic phase of hematopoiesis, 144

Hepatic portal vein, 254
Hepatic sinusoids, 254, 255f, 256
Hepatic stellate cells, 256
Hepatic veins, 254, 255f
Hepatitis, alcoholic, 43b
Hepatocytes, 254, 256
  basolateral domain of, 256
Hereditary nephritis, 47b
Hereditary spherocytosis, 135b
Heroin-associated focal segmental
    glomerulosclerosis, 262b
Herring bodies, 192
Hertwig's epithelial root sheath (HERS), 232
Heterochromatin, 28
Heterogeneous nuclear ribonucleoprotein
    particles (hnRNPs), 30
Heterografts, 91b
HEVs. *See* High endothelial venules (HEVs).
Hiatal hernia, 241b
High endothelial venules (HEVs), 182
Hirschsprung's disease, 109b
Histamine, 66, 68, 69t
  capillary permeability and, 158
Histamine$_2$, hydrochloric acid production
    and, 242
Histochemistry, 4
Histodifferentiation stage of odontogenesis,
    232
Histone(s), 28
Histone H$_1$, 28
H$^+$,K$^+$-ATPase, 240
hnRNPs. *See* Heterogeneous nuclear
    ribonucleoprotein particles (hnRNPs).
Holocrine glands, 212
Holocrine glandular secretion, 58, 59f
Homografts, 91b
Horizontal cells of retina, 314
Hormone(s), 188. *See also* Neurohormones;
    specific hormones.
  affecting hyaline cartilage, 76, 77t
  binding to receptors, 188
  bone formation and, 91b, 92, 93t
  classification of, 188
  gastric, 240, 242
  pituitary, physiologic effects of, 194t
Hormone receptor complex, 188
Hormone-sensitive lipase, 66, 67f
Howship's lacunae, 80
Human chorionic gonadotropin (hCG), 276
  syncytiotrophoblast secretion of, 282
Human epidermal growth factor, 246
Humorally mediated immune response, 136,
    170
Humorally mediated immune system, 172
Huntington's chorea, 121b
Huxley sliding filament theory, 98
Huxley's layer, 214
Hyaline cartilage, 74, 75f, 75t, 92
  chondrocytes of, 76b
  histogenesis and growth of, 76, 77f, 77t
  hormone effects on, 76, 77t
  matrix of, 76
Hyaline cartilage model of bone formation,
    86
Hyalocytes, 310
Hyaloid body, 310
Hyaluronic acid, 40, 41f, 41t, 47b, 70, 76, 92
Hydration shell, 78
Hydrocephalus, 129b
Hydrochloric acid, 240
  gastric production of, 242
Hydrogen ion, gastric, 242
Hydrogen peroxide, 138
Hydrolytic enzymes, 140
Hydroxyapatite crystals, 78
Hydroxylysine, 42
Hydroxyproline, 42
Hymen, 284
Hyperallergic individuals, 70b
Hypercellular obesity, 71b
Hyper-IgM syndrome, 173b

Hyperparathyroidism, primary, 198b
Hyperplastic obesity, 71b
Hyperthermia, male sterility due to, 287b
Hypertrophic obesity, 71b
Hypervitaminosis A, bone development and,
    93t
Hypocalcemia in DiGeorge's syndrome, 180
Hypochlorous acid, 138
Hypodermis, 204, 210
Hyponychium, 216
Hypoparathyroidism, 198b
Hypophysis, 188–192, 189f, 189t, 191t
  anterior, 188, 189f, 189t, 190, 191f
  posterior, 188, 189f, 189t, 190, 192, 193f,
    195f
Hypothalamic neurosecretory hormones, 190
Hypothalamohypophyseal tract, 192
Hypothalamus, 71b
  nuclei of, 192
  releasing hormones of, 191t
Hypothyroidism, 199b
Hypoxia, luteolysis and, 276

I bands, 94, 96, 97f
Ia nerve fibers, 102, 103f
ICAMs. *See* Intracellular adhesion molecules
    (ICAMs).
IdA dimers, 250
IEE. *See* Inner enamel epithelium (IEE).
Immature bone, 82
Immediate hypersensitivity reaction, 66
Immune response
  cell-mediated, 136, 170
    T$_H$1, 178, 179f
    T$_H$2, 176, 177f
  humorally mediated, 136, 170
  primary, 170
  secondary, 170
Immune system, 168–186
  acronyms associated with, 169t
  adaptive (acquired), 170
    cells of, 168, 169t, 172–178
  clonal selection and expansion and, 170
  humorally mediated, 172
  innate (natural), 168, 169t
    cells of, 168, 169t, 172–178
  lymphoid organs and, 178–186
    lymph nodes as, 168, 182, 183f
    mucosa-associated lymphoid tissue as,
    186
    spleen as, 168, 184–186, 185f
    thymus as, 168, 180, 181f
Immunocytochemistry, 4
Immunogens, 170
Immunoglobulin(s), 170, 171f, 171t
  IgA, 230
  surface, 170
Implantation, 282, 283f
Importins, 28, 29f
Inactivation gate, 116
Inactivation of voltage-gated Na$^+$ channels,
    116
Inactive fibroblasts, 64
Inclusions of cells, 22
Incus, 318
Indian hedgehog, 88
Indifferent gonads, 272
Indirect method of immunocytochemistry, 4,
    5f
Inducible T reg cells, 174
Inferior hypophyseal arteries, 190
Inferior vena cava, 254, 255f
Inflammation
  acute, 136b
  chronic, 136b
Inflammatory myopathies, 95b
Inflammatory responses, 138
Infundibulum
  of fallopian tube, 276, 278
  of neurohypophysis, 192, 193f
Inhalation, 228

Inhibin, 274, 288, 294
Inhibitory hormones, pituitary, 190
Inhibitory output of Purkinje cells, 130
Inhibitory postsynaptic potentials, 118
Inhibitory responses, 188
Initiator, 38
Initiator tRNA, 14
Inlet arterioles, hepatic, 254
Inlet venules, hepatic, 254
Innate immune system, 168, 169t
  cells of, 168, 169t, 172–178
Inner cellular layer
  of cartilage, 76
  of periosteum, 78, 82
Inner circumferential lamellar system, 82, 84
Inner ear, 318–320, 319f, 321f, 323f
Inner enamel epithelium (IEE), 232
Inner hair cells, 320
Inner limiting membrane of retina, 314
Inner nuclear layer of retina, 314
Inner nuclear membrane, 26, 27f
Inner plexiform layer of retina, 314
Inner segment of retina, 312
Inner table of compact bone, 82
Insulin, 71b, 252, 253t
Insulin-like growth factors, 92
Insuloacinar portal region, 252
Integral proteins, 8
Integrins, 46, 78, 138, 280
  implantation and, 282
Integument, 204–216. *See also* Hair; Nail(s)
    (nail plates); Skin.
Interalveolar septa, 226, 227f
Intercalated cells of collecting tubules, 264
Intercalated disks, 104, 105f
Intercalated ducts
  pancreatic, 252
  of salivary glands, 250
Intercellular pockets, small intestinal, 244
Interchromatin granules, 32
Intercristal space, 20, 21f
Interdental cells, 320
Interdigitating dendritic cells
  splenic, 186
  in splenic marginal zone, 184
Interfascicular oligodendrocytes, 112
Interferon(s)
  IFN-α, origin and functions of, 175t
  IFN-β, origin and functions of, 175t
  IFN-γ, origin and functions of, 175t
  IFN-τ, 92, 149t
    luteolysis and, 276
  innate immune system and, 168
Interleukin(s)
  IL-1, 68, 90, 92, 138
  IL-1α, 204
  IL-2, 148, 149t
    origin and functions of, 175t
  IL-3, 148, 149t
  IL-4, origin and functions of, 175t
  IL-5, 148, 149t
    origin and functions of, 175t
  IL-6, 92, 148, 149t
    origin and functions of, 175t
  IL-7, 148, 149t
  IL-8, 139b
  IL-10, origin and functions of, 175t
  IL-11, 148, 149t
    innate immune system and, 168
  IL-12, 148, 149t
    origin and functions of, 175t
Interlobar arteries, 266
Interlobular ducts, pancreatic, 252
Intermediate cells of taste buds, 236
Intermediate faces of Golgi apparatus, 16
Intermediate fibers, 94
Intermediate filament(s), 22–24, 23f, 25f, 54
Intermediate filament binding proteins, 24
Intermembrane space, 20, 21f
Internal callus, 90
Internal elastic lamina, arterial, 152

Internal mesaxon, 114
Internal respiration, 218
Internal root sheath, 214
Interneurons, 112, 126
Internodal segment, 114
Interoceptors, 304
Interphase, 34, 35f
Interplaque regions of urinary bladder, 270
Interplexiform cells, 314
Interstitial cells
    ovarian, 272
    of pineal gland, 202
Interstitial cells of Leydig, 292, 293f
Interstitial cell-stimulating hormone,
        physiologic effects of, 194t
Interstitial glands of Leydig, 286
Interstitial growth, 76
Interstitial lamellae, 82–84
Interterritorial matrix, 76
Intestinal gas, 249b
Intracellular adhesion molecules (ICAMs)
    ICAM-1, 138, 139b
    ICAM-2, 138, 139b
Intracellular canaliculi, 240
Intracellular receptors, 188
Intrafusal muscle fibers, 102
Intraglomerular mesangial cells, 262
Intralobar ducts, pancreatic, 252
Intramembranous bone formation, 74, 84, 85f
Intramural glands, 250
Intramural region of oviduct, 278
Intraperiod gap, 114
Intraperiod line, 114
Intrapulmonary bronchi, 224
Intratesticular ducts, 296, 297f, 297t
Intrinsic pathway of apoptosis, 38
Introns, 30
Involucrin, 206
Iodide
    oxidation of, 196
    thyroid function and, 196
Ion(s), movement of, 242
Ion channels, 10
    receptor-associated, 118
Iron hematoxylin, 3t
Irregular bones, 82
Islands of hematopoietic cells, 142
Islets of Langerhans, 188, 252
Isogenous groups, 76
Isthmus, 240
    of oviduct, 278
    Ito cells, 256

J chains, 250
Jaw-jerk reflex, 235b
Joint(s), 92, 93f
Joint capsule, 92
Junctional complexes, 52, 53f, 55f, 57f
Junctional epithelium, gingival, 234
Junctional feet, 96
Junctional folds, 100
Juxtaglomerular apparatus, 264, 265f
    filtrate in, monitoring of, 268
Juxtaglomerular cells, 264, 268
Juxtamedullary nephrons, 268
    efferent glomerular arterioles of, 266

K+ channels, voltage-gated, 116, 118
K+ leak channels, 10, 116
Karyokinesis, 36
Karyoplasm, 8
Kearns-Sayre syndrome, 21b
Keratan sulfates, 41t
Keratin filaments, 206, 214
Keratin intermediate filaments, 56
Keratinized epithelium, 49f, 49t
Keratinocytes, 204, 205f
Keratohyalin, 206
Kidneys, 260, 261f
    arterial blood pressure and, 156
    lobulations of, 260b

Kiesselbach's area, 221b
Killer-activating receptors, 168
Killer-inhibitory receptors, 168
Kinesin, 22
Kinetochores, 36
Klinefelter syndrome, 291b
Krause's end bulbs, 304, 305f
Kupffer cells, 256

L cells, 71b
Labia majora, 284, 285f
Labia minora, 284, 285f
Labyrinth
    bony, 318, 319f
    membranous, 318–320, 319f
Lacrimal apparatus, 316
Lacrimal canaliculi, 316
Lacrimal glands, 316
Lacrimal punctum, 316
Lacrimal sac, 316
Lactase, 246
Lactating state, 284
Lacteals, 66
    small intestinal, 244, 245f
    of small intestine, 244
Lactiferous duct, 284
Lactiferous sinus, 284
Lactoferrin, 230
Lactogens, 284
Lacunae
    of cementum, 230
    chondroblasts in, 76, 77f
    chondrocytes in, 74
    in dicidua basalis, 282
    osteoblasts in, 78, 84
    osteocytes in, 82
    in syncytiotrophoblasts, 282
Lambda granules, 140
Lamellae, 82–84, 85f
    interstitial, 82–84
Lamellar bodies, 226
Lamellar bone, 82
Lamellar granules, 206
Lamin(s) A, B, and C, 26
Lamina densa, 46, 47f
Lamina lucida, 46, 47f
Lamina propria
    of digestive system lumen, 238
    of gallbladder, 258
    gastric, 240
    large intestinal, 248
    of nasal cavity, 218
    of oviduct, 278
    small intestinal, 244
    of trachea, 222
    vaginal, 284
Lamina reticularis, 46, 47f
Laminae of cardiac muscle, 104
Laminin, 42, 46, 56, 62
    capillary production of, 158
    platelet adhesion and, 140
Langerhans cells, 182, 204, 205f, 208
Lanugo, 214
Large intestine, 248, 249f
    function of, 248
Large pores of capillaries, 158
Laryngeal epithelium
    pseudostratified ciliated columnar, 220
    stratified squamous nonkeratinized, 220
Laryngitis, 221b
Larynx, 220
Late endosomes, 18
Left atrioventricular valve, 164
Left atrium, 164, 165f
Left ventricle, 164, 165f
Leiomyomas, 107b
Leiomyosarcomas, 107b
Lens capsule, 308
Lens fibers, 308
Lens of eye, 308, 309f
    suspensory ligaments of, 308

Leptin, 71b
Leptotene, 38
Leukemia, acute myelogenous, 37b
Leukocyte(s), 70, 132, 136–138, 137t, 144
    basophils as, 137t, 138
    eosinophils as, 137t, 138
    lymphocytes as, 136, 137t
    monocytes as, 136, 137t
    neutrophils as, 137t, 138, 139f
Leukocyte adhesion deficiency I, 139b
Leukocyte function–associated antigen 1
        (LFA-1), 139b
Leukotriene(s), 70b
Leukotriene C4, 68, 69t
Leukotriene D4, 68, 69t
Leukotriene E4, 68, 69t
LFA-1. See Leukocyte function–associated
        antigen 1 (LFA-1).
LH. See Luteinizing hormone (LH).
Ligand(s), 10, 18
Ligand-gated channels, 10
Ligand-gated sodium channels, 100
Light cells
    of inner ear, 320
    of taste buds, 236
Light chains, 170
Light meromyosin, 106
Light microscope, 3f
Light microscopy, 2–4
    advanced visual procedures and, 4, 5f
    interpretation of microscopic sections and,
        4, 5f
    tissue preparation for, 2–4, 3f, 3t
Limbus, 306, 308
Linear movements of head, vestibular
        function and, 322
Lingual papillae, 236
Lingual tonsils, 186, 236
Lining mucosa of oral cavity, 230
Linker DNA, 28
Lip(s), 230, 231b, 231f
Lipid(s), 22
Lipid barrier in stratum granulosum, 206
Lipid deposits of hepatocytes, 256
Lipid rafts, 8, 106
Lipofuscin, 22
Lipomas, 71b
Lipoprotein(s), plasma, 133t
Lipoprotein lipase, 66, 67f
    capillary production of, 158
Liposarcomas, 71b
Lipotropic hormone, 190
Lipotropin, 190
Liver, 254–258, 255f
    bile and, 258
    biliary ducts and, 258
    functions of, 256
    gallbladder and, 258
    hepatic ducts and, 258
    hepatocytes of, 254, 256
    lobules of
        classic, 254
        concepts of, 254, 255f
    regeneration of, 256
    sinusoids of, 256, 257f
Lobar arteries, 266
Lobar bronchi, 224
Lobes of exocrine glands, 60
Lobules of exocrine glands, 60, 61f
Lobuli testis, 286
Lockjaw, 101b
Long bones, 82
Long cortical arteries, 200
Long-chain fatty acids in small intestine,
        246
Long-term weight control, 71b
Loose connective tissue, 72
Low-density lipoproteins, plasma, 133t
L-selectins, 138
    implantation and, 282
Lubricin, 92

Lumen
   of digestive system, 238
   of Schwann tube, 130
Luminal layer of eccrine sweat glands, 212
Luminal spoke ring, 26, 27f
Lung acini, 224
Lung cancer, 229b
Lunula, 216, 217f
Luteal phase of menstrual cycle, 280, 282
Luteinizing hormone (LH), 190
   physiologic effects of, 194t
   receptors for, 274
   testes and, 294
Luteolysis, 276
Lymph, 166
Lymph nodes, 166, 168, 182, 183b, 183f
Lymphatic anchoring filaments, 166
Lymphatic capillaries, 166, 167f
Lymphatic ducts, 166
Lymphatic organs, secondary, 183b
Lymphatic system, 166, 167f
   capillaries and vessels of, 166, 167f
Lymphedema, 167b
Lymphocytes, 70, 136, 137t
Lymphoid cells, interaction among, 176
Lymphoid follicles, 186
Lymphoid nodules, 183b
   in splenic white pulp, 184
   of tonsils, 186
Lymphoid organs, 178–186
   primary (central), 170, 178
   secondary (peripheral), 170, 178
Lymphoid system. *See also* Immune system.
   diffuse, 168
Lymphoma, Burkitt's, 37b
Lymphopoiesis, 150
Lysosomes, 9f, 18, 19f, 138, 140
Lysozyme
   as antimicrobial peptide, 168
   esophageal gland production of, 238
   salivary production of, 230
   small intestinal, 244, 244b
   in tears, 316

M cells, small intestinal, 244
M cells in mucosa-associated lymphoid tissue,
   186
M cyclins, 34
M line, 94, 96, 97f
Mac-1. *See* Macrophage-1 (Mac-1).
Machette, 290
Macrophage(s), 68, 88, 136, 142, 182
   alveolar, 226
   corpus luteum and, 276
   innate immune system and, 168
   in splenic red pulp, 186
   stellate reticular cells and, 182
Macrophage-1 (Mac-1), 139b
Macrophage inhibitory protein-α, 148
Macula
   of saccule, 318–320
   of utricle, 318–320
Macula densa, 262, 264, 268
Macula lutea, 310
Maculae adherentes, 52, 53f, 54, 55f, 57f
Macular degeneration, 315b
Main pancreatic duct, 252
Major basic protein, 138
Major dense line, 114
Major histocompatibility complex antigens II,
   136
Major histocompatibility complex molecules,
   172, 176
   loading, 176
   MHC I, 173b
Male reproductive system, 286–302, 287f. *See
   also specific organs.*
Malignant melanoma, 211b
Malleus, 318
MALT. *See* Mucosa-associated lymphoid tissue
   (MALT).

Maltase, 246
Mammary glands, 284, 285f
Mammotrophs, 190
Mantle of lymph nodes, 182
MAP2, 22
Marfan syndrome, 63b
Marginal fold of capillaries, 156
Marginal sinuses, splenic, 184
Marginal sinusoids, splenic, 186
Marginal zone of spleen, 184
Marrow cavity, 78, 82
Masson trichrome, 3t
Mast cells, 66–68, 67f, 69t
   activation and degranulation of, 66
   inflammatory response and, 68, 69t
   sensitization of, 66
Masticatory mucosa, 230
Matrix granules, 20
Matrix of hair root, 214
Matrix space, 20, 21f
Matrix vesicles, 88
Maturation phase of spermiogenesis, 290
Mature bone, 82
Mature follicles, ovarian, 274
MBP. *See* Major basic protein; Myelin basic
   protein.
M-CSF. *See* Monocyte colony-stimulating
   factor (M-CSF).
M-CSF receptors, 80
Mechanoreceptors, 208, 304, 305f
Median eminence of neurohypophysis, 192,
   193f
Mediastinum testis, 286
Medulla of hair shaft, 214
Medullary cords of lymph nodes, 173,
   183b
Medullary epithelial reticular cells, 180
Medullary sinuses of lymph nodes, 182
Megacolon, congenital, 109b
Megakaryoblasts, 146, 150
Megakaryocytes, 150
Meibomian glands, 316
Meiosis, 38, 288
   equatorial division of, 38, 39f
   nondisjunction and, 39b
   reductional division of, 38, 39f
Meiosis-inducing substance, 276
Meiosis-preventing factor, 272
Meissner's corpuscles, 304, 305f
Meissner's plexus, 124, 244
Meissner's submucosal plexus, 238
Melanin, 22, 209b
   defects of, 23b
Melanocyte(s), 204, 205f
   in epidermis, 208
α-Melanocyte-stimulating hormone (α-MSH),
   190
Melanoma, malignant, 211b
Melatonin, 202, 202b, 203t
Membrana granulosa, 274, 276
Membrana granulosa cells, 274
Membrane attack complexes, 168
Membrane potential, 116
Membrane trafficking, 18, 19f
   endocytosis and, 18
   endosomes and, 18, 19f
   lysosomes and, 18
   peroxisomes and, 18
   proteasomes and, 18
Membrane transport proteins, 10, 11f
Membrane-bound antibodies, 170
Membrane-coating granules, 206
Membranous labyrinth, 318–320, 319f
Memory cells, 170
Memory T cells, 172
Ménière's disease, 323b
Meningeal layer of cranial dura mater, 126
Meninges, 126, 127f
Meningiomas, 127b
Meningitis, 127b
Menopause, 272

Menses, 280
Menstrual cycle, 280, 281f
   luteal phase, 280, 282
   menstrual phase of, 280
   secretory phase of, 280, 282
Menstruation, 276
Merkel cell(s), 204, 205f, 208
Merkel cell–neurite associations, 208
Merkel's disks, 304, 305f
Merocrine glandular secretion, 58, 59f
Merocrine secretory portion of eccrine sweat
   gland, 212
Mesenchymal cells, 62, 70
Mesenchymal connective tissue, 70
Mesenchyme, 62
Mesoblastic phase of hematopoiesis, 144
Mesoderm, 48, 62
Mesovarium, 272, 273f
Messenger ribonucleoprotein (mRNP), 30
Messenger RNA (mRNA), 12, 30
   precursor, 30
Metachromasia, 66
Metaphase, 36, 37f, 276
Metaphase I of meiosis, 38, 39f
Metaphase plate, 36
Metaphase/anaphase checkpoint, 34
Metaphyses, 82
Metaplasia, 57b
   of respiratory epithelium, 222b
   squamous, 57b
Metarterioles, 158
Methotrexate, 35b
MHC. *See* Major histocompatibility complex
   entries.
MHSCs. *See* Multipotential hematopoietic
   stem cells (MHSCs).
Micelles, 246
Microfibrils, 44
Microfilaments, 9f, 24, 25f
Microfold cells, small intestinal, 244
Microglia, 131b
Microglial cells, 112
Microscopic sections, interpretation of, 4, 5f
Microscopy
   confocal, 6, 7f
   electron, 6, 7f
   light, 2–4
      advanced visual procedures and, 4, 5f
      interpretation of microscopic sections
         and, 4, 5f
      tissue preparation for, 2–4, 3f, 3t
Microtubule(s), 9f, 22–24, 23f
Microtubule organizing centers (MTOCs), 22,
   36
Microvilli, 9f, 50, 51f
Midbody, 36
Middle ear, 318, 319f
Migrating dendritic cells of lymph nodes,
   182, 183b
Milk, formation of, 284
Minimal change disease, 262b
Minus end
   of microfilaments, 24
   of microtubule, 22
   of thin filament, 96
Misfolded proteins, 14
MIT. *See* Monoiodinated tyrosine (MIT).
Mitochondria, 9f, 20, 21f
   of hepatocytes, 256
   outer membrane of, 20, 21f
Mitochondrial encephalomyopathy, 21b
Mitochondrial myopathies, 21b
Mitochondrial sheath, 290
Mitosis, 34, 35f, 36, 37f
Mitotic spindle apparatus, 36
Mitotic spindle microtubules, 36
Mitral cells, olfaction and, 220
Mitral valve, 164
Mixed glandular secretions, 58
Mixed saliva, 250
MLCK. See Myosin light chain kinase.

Modified fluid mosaic model, 8
Modiolus, 318
Mole(s), 209b
Molecular layer of cerebellar cortex, 130
Monocyte(s), 68, 70, 136, 137t
  in alveolar septa, 226
Monocyte colony-stimulating factor (M-CSF),
      78, 80, 148, 149t
  receptors for, 80
Monocytopoiesis, 150
Monoglycerides in small intestine, 246
Monoiodinated tyrosine (MIT), 196
Mononuclear-phagocyte system, 68, 80, 136
Morphodifferentiation stage of odontogenesis,
      232
Motor components of peripheral nervous
      system, 108
Motor end plates, 100
Motor nervous system, somatic, 122, 123f
Motor neurons, 112
  α-motoneurons, 100
  τ-motoneurons, 102
  preganglionic, 124
Mouth, 230–236
  lips and, 230, 231b, 231f
  palate and, 234
  teeth and, 230–234, 231b, 231f
  tongue and, 236, 237f
MPZ. See Myelin protein zero (MPZ).
mRNA. See Messenger RNA (mRNA).
mRNP. See Messenger ribonucleoprotein
      (mRNP).
α-MSH. See α-Melanocyte-stimulating
      hormone (α-MSH).
MTOCs. See Microtubule organizing centers
      (MTOCs).
Mucin, 222
Mucinogens, 222, 223f, 250
  small intestinal, 244
Mucoid cells of eccrine sweat glands, 212
Mucoid connective tissue, 70
Mucosa(e)
  as defense, 168
  of digestive system, 238
  esophageal, 238
  masticatory, 230
  oral, 230
    lining, 230
    specialized, 230
  of oviduct, 278
  small intestinal, 244, 245f
  of soft palate, 234
  ureteral, 270
  vaginal, 284
Mucosa-associated lymphoid tissue (MALT),
      186, 187f, 238
Mucous cells of salivary glands, 250
Mucous glandular secretions, 58
Mucous neck cells, 240
Mucus
  esophageal, 250
  of goblet cell, 58
  small intestinal, 244
  tracheal, 222
Müller cells, 314
Müllerian ducts, 273b
Multicellular exocrine glands, 58
Multilaminar primary follicles, 274, 275f, 275t
Multilocular adipose tissue, 72, 73b
Multilocular fat cells, 62
Multiple sclerosis, 115b
Multipolar neurons, 112, 113f
Multipotential hematopoietic stem cells, 146,
      148
Multiunit smooth muscle, 106
Mumps, 251b
  orchitis due to, 291b
Muscle(s), 94–106, 95f
  cardiac, 94, 95f, 105f, 162–164
    cells of, 104
  skeletal. See Skeletal muscle.

Muscle(s) (Continued)
  smooth, 94, 106
    contraction of, 106
    electron microscopy of, 106
    light microscopy of, 106, 107f
  striated, 94
  of tongue, 236
Muscle fibers, 94
  dynamic, 102
  extrafusal, 102
  intrafusal, 102
  nuclear bag, 102
  nuclear chain, 102
  static, 102
Muscle spindles, 102, 103f, 304, 305f
Muscularis
  of oviduct, 278
  vaginal, 284
Muscularis externa
  of appendix, 248
  of digestive system lumen, 238
  esophageal, 238
  gastric, 240, 242
  large intestinal, 248
  small intestinal, 244
Muscularis mucosae
  of appendix, 248
  of digestive system, 238
  gastric, 240, 242
  large intestinal, 248
  small intestinal, 244
Mutations
  myofibrillar organization of skeletal muscle
      and, 99b
  NADPH oxidase and, 139b
Myasthenia crisis, 103b
Myasthenia gravis, 103b
Myelin basic protein, 114
Myelin protein zero (MPZ), 114
Myelinated axons, 100
Myelination, 114
Myeloblasts, 146, 150, 151t
Myelocytes, 150, 151t
Myelofibrosis, 147b
Myeloid phase of hematopoiesis, 144
Myenteric plexus, 238
Myoblasts, 94
Myocardial infarction, 105b
Myocardium, 162–164
Myoclonus epilepsy, 21b
Myoepithelial cells
  of eccrine sweat glands, 60, 212, 213f
  of mammary glands, 284
  of salivary glands, 60, 250
Myofibrils, 94, 97f
  structural organization of, 96–98, 97f
Myofibroblasts, 64, 232, 256
Myofilaments, 94, 104, 106, 140
  thick, 96
  thin, 96
Myoglobin, 94, 96, 104
Myomesin, 96
Myometrium, 278
Myopathies, inflammatory, 95b
Myosin, 140
Myosin II, 96, 98, 106
Myosin light chain kinase (MLCK), 106
Myosin phosphatase, 106
Myositis, 95b
  temporary, 95b
Myotendinous junction, 94
Myotubes, 94
Myxedema, 199b
Myxoid liposarcomas, 71b

Na+ channels, voltage-gated, 116–118
NADH, 20
NADPH oxidase, hereditary deficiency of, 139b
Nail(s) (nail plates), 216, 217f
Nail groove, 216
Nail matrix, 216

Nail root, 216, 217f
Nail walls, 216
Naïve B lymphocytes, 146
Naïve cells, 170
Naïve T cells (lymphocytes), 146, 172, 180
Na+,K+ pumps, 116
Na+,K+-ATPase pumps, 10
  of distal tubule, 264
  of gallbladder, 258
Nares, 218
Nasal cavity, 218
  histophysiology of, 220
Nasal septum, 218
Nasolacrimal duct, 316
Natural immune system, 168, 169t
  cells of, 168, 169t, 172–178
Natural T killer cells, 174
Natural T reg cells, 174
Nebulin, 96
Nerve conduction velocity, 122, 122t
Nerve deafness, 323b
Nerve impulses
  generation and conduction of, 116–118,
      117f, 119f
  synapses and, 118–120, 119f, 119t
  propagation of, 116–118
Nerve regeneration, 130, 131f
  axon reaction and, 130
Nerve supply of skeletal muscle, 100
Nervous system, 108–130
  autonomic, 108
  cells of, 110–114
  central, 108, 126–130
    blood-brain barrier of, 128
    cerebellar cortex of, 130
    cerebral cortex of, 128, 129t
    choroid plexus of, 128
    meninges of, 126, 127f
  development of, 108
  enteric, 238
  ganglia and, 124, 125f
  nerve impulse generation and conduction
      and, 116–118, 117f, 119f
    synapses and, 118–120, 119f, 119t
  nerve impulse propagation and, 116, 118
  nerve regeneration and, 130, 131f
    axon reaction and, 130
  parasympathetic, 124, 125f
    arterial blood pressure and, 154
    enteric nervous system and, 238
    penile erection and, 302
  peripheral, 108, 120–122
    conduction velocity and, 122, 122t
    connective tissue investments and, 120,
        123f
    functional classification of nerves and,
        120
  somatic, 108, 122–124, 123f, 125f
  sympathetic, 124, 125f
    arterial blood pressure and, 154
    ejaculation and, 302
    enteric nervous system and, 238
Network-forming collagens, 42, 44
Neural crest cells, 108
Neural groove, 108
Neural plate, 108
Neural tube, 108
Neuroendocrine tumors, 60b
Neuroepithelial cells of inner ear, 320, 321f
Neuroepithelium, 108
Neuroglia, 108
Neuroglial cells, 108, 112–114, 113f, 115f
Neuroglial processes, 126
Neurohormones, 120
Neurohypophysis, 188, 189f, 189t, 190, 192,
      193f, 195f
Neuromodulators, 120
Neuromuscular junctions, 100, 101f, 103f
Neuron(s), 108, 110
  bipolar, 112, 113f
  motor (efferent), 112

Neuron(s) (Continued)
multipolar, 112, 113f
parasympathetic, 124
postganglionic, 108, 122
preganglionic, 108, 122
sensory (afferent), 112
structure and function of, 110, 111f
sympathetic, 124
unipolar, 112, 113f, 124
Neuronal layer of retina, 310
Neuronal plasticity, 131b
Neuronal stem cells, 131b
Neuropil, 126
Neurotransmitter(s), 118, 120, 121t
Neurotransmitter-gated channels, 10
Neurotrophins, 131b
Neutral proteases, 66, 69t
Neutrophil(s), 70, 137t, 138, 139f
Neutrophil chemotactic factor, 66, 68, 69t
Neutrophilic myelocytes, 150, 151t
Nevi, 209b
Nexin bridge in axonemes, 50
N-glygosylated proteins, 14
Nidi of crystallization, 88
Nidogen, 42
Nitric oxide (NO), 140
    arterial blood pressure and, 154
    gas exchange and, 228
    penile erection and, 302
Nitric oxide synthase, 268
NK cells, 136, 168
NO. See Nitric oxide (NO).
Nociceptors, 304
Node of Ranvier, 114, 115f
Nonalcoholic steatohepatitis, 259b
Nonciliated secretory cells, endometrial, 278
Nondisjunction, 39b
Nonencapsulated mechanoreceptors, 304, 305f
Nonkeratinocytes in epidermis, 208, 209f
Nonpolar, hydrophobic molecules, 10
Non-snRNP splicing factors, 30
Nonsyndromic deafness, 57b
Nontoxic goiter, 195b
Norepinephrine, 66, 121t, 124, 200, 203t
    blood vessels and, 154
Nosebleeds, 221b
Nostrils, 218
Notch-1 receptors, 180
Nuclear bag muscle fibers, 102
Nuclear basket, 26, 27f
Nuclear chain muscle fibers, 102
Nuclear envelope, 8, 9f, 26–28, 27f
Nuclear export signals, 28
Nuclear lamina, 26
Nuclear localization signals, 28
Nuclear matrix, 32
Nuclear membranes, 26, 27f
Nuclear pore(s), 26, 27f
    function of, 28, 29f
Nuclear pore complexes, 26, 27f
Nuclear ring, 26, 27f
Nuclear thyroid receptor protein, 196
Nucleolar matrix, 32
Nucleolar organizing regions, 36
Nucleolus, 9f, 32, 33f
Nucleolus-associated chromatin, 32
Nucleoplasm, 26, 32, 33f
Nucleoplasmic ring, 26, 27f
Nucleotide-gated channels, 10
Nucleus, 8, 26–38
    chromatin of, 28–32, 29f
    nuclear envelope of, 26–28, 27f
Null cells, 136
Nutrient canals, 142
    of alveolar bone, 234

Obesity
    adult, 71b
    hypercellular (hyperplastic), 71b
    hypertrophic, 71b

Objective lenses, 4
Occluding junctions, 288
Occludins, 54
Occlusal trauma, 235b
Ocular lenses, 4
Odontoblast(s), 230, 232, 233f
Odontoblastic layer of dental pulp, 230
Odontoclasts, 230
Odontogenesis, 232, 233f
Odor receptor molecules, 220
Odorants, 220
OEE. See Outer enamel epithelium.
Olfactory bulb, 220
Olfactory cells, 218
Olfactory epithelium, 220, 221f
Olfactory region of nasal cavity, 218
Oligodendrocytes, 112
Oligosaccharidases, 246
    small intestinal, 244
Oncogenes, 37b
Onychomycosis, 217b
Oocytes
    fertilization and, 280
    primary, 272
    secondary, 276
OPG. See Osteoprotegerin (OPG).
OPGL. See Osteoprotegerin ligand (OPGL).
Opisthonos, 101b
Optic cup, 310
Optic nerve, 310
Optic nerve fiber layer of retina, 314
Optic stalk, 310
Optic vesicle, 310
Ora serrata, 310
Oral cavity, 230–236
    lips and, 230, 231b, 231f
    palate and, 234
    teeth and, 230–234, 231b, 231f
    tongue and, 236, 237f
Oral cavity proper, 230
Oral mucosa, 230
Oral pharynx, tonsils and, 186
Orcein elastic stain, 3t
Orchitis, mumps and, 291b
Organ(s), 8
Organ of Corti, 320, 323f
Organ systems, 8
Organelles, 8, 9f
Orthochromatophilic erythroblasts, 150t
Osmotic pressures, gastric, 242
Osseous spiral lamina, 318
Ossicles, 318
Ossification centers, 84, 86, 86t
Osteoarthritis, 93b
Osteoblasts, 78, 79f, 84
    alkaline phosphatase in, 79b
    formation of, 78
Osteocalcin, 78
Osteoclast(s), 68, 78, 79f, 80
Osteoclastogenesis, 80
Osteoclast-stimulating factor, 78, 92, 198
Osteoclast-stimulating factor-1 receptor, 80
Osteocytes, 78, 79f, 80, 82, 84
Osteocytic processes, 80, 82
Osteogenic cells, 78
Osteoid, 78
Osteomalacia, 93b
Osteon(s), 82–84
Osteonectin, 42, 62, 88
Osteopetrosis, 81b
Osteopontin, 42, 78
Osteoporosis, 91b
Osteoprogenitor cells, 76, 78, 88, 90
Osteoprotegerin (OPG), 80, 90, 92
Osteoprotegerin ligand (OPGL), 90, 92
Osterix, 84
Otitis media, 323b
Otoconia, 320
Otolith(s), 320
Otolithic membrane, 320
Outer enamel epithelium, 232

Outer fibrous layer
    of cartilage, 76
    of periosteum, 78, 82
Outer hair cells, 320
Outer limiting membrane of retina, 314
Outer membrane of mitochondrion, 20, 21f
Outer nuclear layer of retina, 314
Outer nuclear membrane, 26, 27f
Outer plexiform layer of retina, 314
Outer segments of retina, 312
Outer table of compact bone, 82
Oval window, 318
Ovaries, 272–276, 273f
    follicles of, 272, 274, 275f, 275t
Oviducts, 276, 278, 279f
Ovulation, 276, 277f
Oxidative phosphorylation, 20
Oxygen
    erythrocyte release of, 134
    erythrocyte transport of, 134
Oxygen delivery, 218
Oxyhemoglobin, 134
Oxyntic cells, 240
Oxyphil cells, 198
Oxytocin, 192, 278
    physiologic effects of, 194t

Pachytene, 38
Pacinian corpuscles, 210, 304, 305f
Pakoglobins, 54
Palate, 234
Palatine tonsils, 186
Pale-staining fibrillar center, 32
Palpebral conjunctiva, 316
PALS. See Periarterial lymphatic sheath (PALS).
Pampiniform plexus of veins, 286
Pancreas, 252, 253f
    endocrine, 252, 253t
    exocrine, 252
Pancreatic duct, 246, 258
    main, 252
Pancreatic lipase, 66
Pancreatic polypeptide, 252, 253t
Paneth cells, 244
Panniculus adiposus, 210
Pap smear, 279b
Papanicolaou smear technique, 279b
Papilla of Vater, 246, 252, 258
Papillary aperture, 308
Papillary collecting tubules, 264
Papillary layer of dermis, 207t, 210
Papillary zone, 308
Paracrine effects, 58
Paracrine hormones, 240
Paraesophageal hiatal hernia, 241b
Paraffin blocks, 2
Parafollicular cells, 196
Parallel bundles, 24
Paramesonephric ducts, 273b
Parasympathetic nervous system, 124, 125f
    arterial blood pressure and, 154
    enteric nervous system and, 238
    penile erection and, 302
Parasympathetic neurons, 124
Parathyroid glands, 196, 197f, 198, 199f, 203t
Parathyroid hormone, 80, 90, 198, 203t
Parathyroid hormone receptors, 78
Paratrabecular sinuses of lymph nodes, 182
Paraventricular nucleus of hypothalamus, 192
Parenchyma, 58
Parietal cells, 240
Parietal pericardium, 164
Parietal pleura, 228
Parkinson's disease, 121b
Parotid gland, 250
Pars ciliaris of retina, 308
Pars convoluta, 262
Pars distalis, 190, 191f
Pars fibrosa, 32

Pars granulosa, 32
Pars intermedia, 190, 191f
Pars nervosa of neurohypophysis, 191t, 192, 193f, 194t
Pars recta, 262
Pars tuberalis, 190, 191f
Passive transport, 10, 11f
Patellar reflex, 103b
P/D1 cells, 71b
PDL. See Periodontal ligament.
Pectinate line, 248
Peg cells, 278
Pemphigus vulgaris, 55b
Penicillar arteries, 184
Penis, 300–302, 301f, 303f
Pepsin, 240
Pepsinogen, 238, 240
Peptide YY, 71b
Perforins, 174
Periarterial lymphatic sheath (PALS), 184
Periaxial space, 102
Peribiliary capillary plexus, 254
Pericardial cavity, 164
Pericarditis, 163b
Pericardium
    parietal, 164
    visceral, 164
Pericellular capsule, 76
Perichondrium, 74, 76
Perichromatin granules, 32
Pericranium, 82
Pericytes
    of blood vessels, 152, 156
    of connective tissue, 64, 65f
Perilymph, 320
Perimysium, 94, 95f
Perineurium, 120, 123f
Periodic acid-Schiff, 3t
Periodontal ligament, 230, 232, 234
Periosteal layer of cranial dura mater, 126
Periosteocytic spaces, 80
Periosteum, 78, 82, 83f, 84
Peripheral lymphoid organs, 170, 178
Peripheral nervous system (PNS), 108, 120–122
    conduction velocity and, 122, 122t
    connective tissue investments and, 120, 123f
    functional classification of nerves and, 120
Peripheral proteins, 8
Perisinusoidal space of Disse, 256
Peristalsis, 238
Peristaltic waves, 246
Peritoneum, 254
Peritrichial nerve endings, 304, 305f
Perivascular glia limitans, 128
Perlacan, 46
Permanent dentition, 230
Peroxisomes, 18
    of hepatocytes, 256
Peyer's patches, 186, 187f, 246
P-face, 8, 9f
Phagocytosis, 18
    by monocytes, 136
    by neutrophils, 138
Phagosomes, 18
Pharyngeal tonsils, 186
Phospholipase A₂, 66
Phospholipoproteins, 20
Photosensory organs. See Eye(s).
PHSCs. See Pluripotential hematopoietic stem cells (PHSCs).
Pia mater, 126, 127f, 202
Pia-glial membrane, 112
Pigment(s), 22
Pigment epithelium of retina, 312, 313f
Pigment layer of retina, 310
Pineal gland (body), 202, 203t
Pinealocytes, 202
Pinocytosis, 18
Pinocytotic vesicles, 18, 156, 158

Pit cells, 256
Pituicytes, 192
Pituitary adenomas, 192b
Pituitary gigantism, 89b
Pituitary gland, 188–192, 189f, 189t, 191t
    anterior, 188, 189f, 189t, 190, 191f
    arterial blood pressure and, 156
    hormones of, physiologic effects of, 194t
    posterior, 188, 189f, 189t, 190, 192, 193f, 195f
Placenta, development of, 282, 282t
Placental barrier, 282, 282t
Plakins, 24
Plaque(s), psoriatic, 207b
Plaque regions of urinary bladder, 270
Plasma, blood, 132, 133t
Plasma cells, 68, 69f, 136, 170, 176, 182, 183b
    in splenic marginal zone, 184
Plasma membrane. See Cell membrane.
Plasma proteins, follicular cell binding to, 196
Plasmalemma. See Cell membrane.
Plasmalogen, 18
Plasmin, 140, 276
Plasminogen, 140
Plasminogen activator, 140
Plasticity, neuronal, 131b
Platelet(s), 140, 141f, 141t
Platelet activating factor, 68, 69t
Platelet activation, 140
Platelet adhesion, 140
Platelet aggregation, 140
Platelet factor 3, 140
Pleats of tonsils, 186
Plectin, 24, 96
Pleural cavity, 228
Plicae circulares, 244
Pluripotential hematopoietic stem cells (PHSCs), 146–148, 147f
Plus end
    of microfilaments, 24
    of microtubule, 22
    of thin filament, 96
Pneumocytes, 226
PNS. See Peripheral nervous system (PNS).
Podocytes, 260, 261f
Polar bodies, first, 276
Polar microtubules, 36
Polar molecules, 10
Polarization of cell membranes, 116
Poly(s), 136, 137t, 138, 139f
Polymorphonuclear leukocytes, 136, 137t, 138, 139f
Polypeptide proteins, 188
Polysomes, 14
Polyubiquinated protein, 18
Pores
    of capillaries, 156
        large, 158
        small, 158
    in rough endoplasmic reticulum, 14
Porins, 20
Porosomes, 16
Porta hepatis, 254
Portal lobule, hepatic, 254
Portal vein, hepatic, 254
Positive feedback, 188
Posterior chamber of eye, 308
Postganglionic motor cell bodies, 124
Postganglionic neurons, 108, 122
Postsynaptic membranes, 100, 118, 119f
Potassium channels, voltage-gated, 116–118
Potassium ion
    gastric, 242
    salivary, 250
Potassium leak channels, 10, 116
Power stroke of muscle contraction, 94
Preameloblasts, 232
Precursor cells, 144, 145t, 146
Precursor messenger RNA (pre-mRNA), 30

Preformed mediators, 66
Preganglionic motoneurons, 124
Preganglionic neurons, 108, 122
Pregnancy, corpus luteum of, 276
Pre-mRNA. See Precursor messenger RNA (pre-mRNA).
Preosteoclasts, 78
Preprocollagen chains, 44
Preproparathyroid hormone, 198
Prepuce, 300
Presbyopia, 309b
Presynaptic membranes, 100, 118, 119f
Pre-T cell receptors, 180
Primary bile, 256
Primary bone, 82
Primary bronchi, 224
Primary capillary plexus, 190
Primary cilia, 52
Primary follicles, ovarian, 274, 275f, 275t
Primary hyperparathyroidism, 198b
Primary immune response, 170
Primary lymphoid nodules, 182, 183b
Primary lymphoid organs, 170, 178
Primary mediators, 66
Primary oocytes, 272
Primary ossification centers, 84, 86, 86t
Primary saliva, 250
Primary spermatocytes, 288
Primary synaptic clefts, 100
Primary villi, 282
Primitive germ cells, 272
Primitive sex cords, 272
Primordial follicles, 272, 274, 275t
Principal cells, 264
    of epididymis, 296
Principal fiber groups
    gingival, 234
    of periodontal ligament, 234
Procapsaces, 38
Procentriole organizers, 52
Prochromatophylic erythroblasts, 150t
Procollagen, 44, 45f
Procollagen peptidase, 44
Proenzymes, 252
Proerythroblasts, 146, 150, 150t
Progenitor cells, 144, 145t, 146
Progesterone, 274, 276
    mammary gland development and, 284
    syncytiotrophoblast secretion of, 282
Programmed cell death, 38, 170, 174, 178, 180, 183b
Prolactin, 190
    decidual cell synthesis of, 282
    physiologic effects of, 194t
Prolactin-releasing factor, 190
Proliferative phase of menstrual cycle, 280
Proline, 62
Prometaphase, 36, 37f
Promonocytes, 146
Promyelocytes, 150, 151t
Pro-opiomelanocortin, 190
Proparathyroid hormone, 198
Prophase, 36, 37f
Prophase I of meiosis, 38, 39f
Propionibacterium acnes, 215b
Proprioceptors, 304
Propulsive contractions, 246
Prostacyclins, 140
    capillary production of, 158
Prostaglandins, 278
    decidual cell synthesis of, 282
    gastric, 242
    prostaglandin D₂, 68, 69t
    prostaglandin E₂, 268
Prostate gland, 298, 299f
Prostatic concretions, 298
Prostatic urethra, 296
Proteasomes, 18, 176
Protein(s). See also specific proteins.
    in plasma, 133t
    in ribosomes, 12

Protein hormones, 188
Protein kinases, 34
Protein synthesis, 12, 13f
  Golgi apparatus and, 16, 17f
  of nonpackaged proteins, 14, 15f
  of proteins that are to be packaged, 14, 15f
Protein trafficking, 16, 17f
Proteoglycans, 40, 41f, 62, 74, 88, 100
Prothrombin, 140
Protofilaments, 22
Proton motive force, 20
Proto-oncogenes, 34, 37b
Protoplasm, 8
Protoplasmic astrocytes, 112
Proximal convoluted tubule, 262
Proximal nail fold, 216
Proximal tubule, 260, 262, 263f, 268
Pseudostratified ciliated columnar laryngeal
  epithelium, 220
Pseudostratified epithelium, columnar, 49f,
  49t
P-site, 12, 14, 15f
Psoriasis, 207b
Psoriatic arthritis, 207b
Psoriatic plaques, 207b
PTH. See Parathyroid hormone entries.
PTH-related protein, 88
Pulmonary lobules, 224
Pulmonary neuroepithelial bodies, 222
Pulmonary surfactant, 226
Pulmonary trunk, 164
Pulp cavity of tooth, 230
Pulp chamber of tooth, 230
Pulp of tooth, 230, 232
  radicular, 232
Pupil of eye, 308
Purines, 30
Purkinje cell(s), inhibitory output of, 130
Purkinje cell layer of cerebellar cortex, 130
Purkinje fibers, 162
Pus, 138
Pyloric region of stomach, 240
Pyloric sphincter, 240
Pyrimidine, 30
Pyruvate, 20

Quanta, 100

Rab(s), 16
Rab3A, 118
Radial spoke in axonemes, 50
Radiation therapy, 115b
Radicular dentin, 232
Radicular pulp, 232
RANK, 80
RANK receptors, 80
RANKL, 78, 80
Raschkow's plexus, 230
Raynaud's phenomenon, 163b
RBCs. See Red blood cells (RBCs).
Receptor(s), 108
Receptor coupling factors, 66
Receptor-associated ion channels, 118
Receptor-mediated endocytosis, 282
Receptor-mediated transport, 28, 128
Rectum, 248
Recycling endosomes, 18
Red blood cells (RBCs), 134, 144, 150t
  carbon dioxide and oxygen transport by,
    134, 135t
  cell membrane of, 134, 135f, 135t
Red fibers, 94
Red marrow, 82, 142
Red pulp
  of spleen, 184
  splenic, 186
Reflexes
  cough, 221b
  jaw-jerk, 235b
  patellar, 103b

Reflexes (Continued)
  simple reflex arcs and, 103b
  somatic and autonomic, 109f
  stretch, 102
Refractory period, 116–118
Regenerative cells, 240
  of capillaries, 156
  gastric, 240
  small intestinal, 244
Regulated pathway of secretory proteins, 16
Regurgitation, 239b
Rehydration for light microscopy, 2
Releasing hormones, pituitary, 190
Renal artery, 260, 266, 267f
Renal calyces, 270
Renal corpuscle, 260
Renal failure, 265b
Renal infarcts, 266b
Renal interstitium, 266
Renal pelvis, 260, 270
Renal pyramids, 260
Renal vein, 260
Renin, 104, 268
Rennin, 240
Repolarization, 116–118
RER. See Rough endoplasmic reticulum (RER).
Rescue, 22
Resident macrophages, 68
Residual bodies, 18
Resolution of microscopes, 6
Resorption cavities, 90
Respiration
  cellular, 228, 229f
  external, 218
  internal, 218
Respiratory bronchioles, 226, 227f
Respiratory burst, 138
Respiratory epithelium, 222, 223f
Respiratory portion of respiratory system,
  218, 226–228, 227f
Respiratory system, 218–228
  conducting portion of, 218–224, 219t,
    221f
  respiratory portion of, 218, 226–228, 227f
Resting potential, 116, 117f
Rete apparatus, 204
Rete testis, 286, 296, 297t
Reticular cells
  adventitial, 142
  of lymph nodes, 182
  of spleen, 184
Reticular fibers, 44, 70, 106
  in splenic red pulp, 184
Reticular layer of dermis, 207t, 210
Reticular tissue, 72
Reticulocytes, 150t
Reticulum of clot, 140
Retina, 310–314, 311f
  detached, 311b
  layers of, 312–314, 313f, 315f
  pars ciliaris of, 308
Retina proper, 310
Retrograde propagation, 116–118
Retrograde transport, 16
Rh antigens, 134, 135b
Rheumatic heart disease, 163b
Rheumatoid arthritis, 93b
Rhodopsin, 312
Ribophorins, 12
Ribosomal RNA, 12, 30
Ribosomes, 12
  A-site of, 12, 14
  E-site of, 12
  formation of, 32, 33f
  of hepatocytes, 256
  P-site of, 12, 14, 15f
Ribozymes, 12
Rickets, 93b
Right atrioventricular valve, 164
Right atrium of heart, 164, 165f
Right lymphatic duct, 166

Right ventricle, 164, 165f
Rigor mortis, 99b
Rima glottidis, 220
RNA molecule, 30
Rods, retinal, 312, 313f
Romanovsky-type stain, 132
Root canal, 230
Root of tongue, 236
Rotor of ATP synthase, 20
Rough endoplasmic reticulum (RER), 9f, 12
  of hepatocytes, 256
Round cell liposarcomas, 71b
Round window, 318
rRNA. See Ribosomal RNA.
Ruffini's corpuscles, 210
Ruffini's endings, 304, 305f
Ruffled border of osteoclasts, 80
Rugae, 240
Rumination, 239b
Ryanodine receptors, 96

S cyclins, 34
S (synthetic) phase, 34, 35f
S phase of meiosis, 38, 39f
SA node. See Sinoatrial node.
Saccule, 318
Saliva, 230
  flow of, 251b
  mixed, 250
  primary, 250
  secondary, 250
Salivary amylase, 230, 250
Salivary glands
  major, 250, 251f
  minor, 230
    mucous, 234
    mucous, posterior, 186
Salivary lipase, 250
Salivon, 250
Salpingitis, 279b
Saltatory conduction, 122
Sarcolemma, 94
Sarcomeres, 94, 97f
Sarcoplasmic reticulum, 94, 104
Sarcosomes, 94
Satellite cells, 94
Satellite oligodendrocytes, 112
Scala tympani, 320
Scala vestibuli, 320
Scanning electron microscope, 3f, 7f
Schmidt-Lanterman incisures, 114
Schwann cells, 100, 114, 115f
Schwann tube, 130
  lumen of, 130
Sclera, 306
Scurvy, 45b, 93b
Sealing zone of osteoclasts, 80
Sebaceous glands, 212, 213f
Sebum, 212
Second messenger(s), 188
Second messenger system, 10, 240
Secondary active transport, 10
Secondary bone, 82
Secondary bronchi, 224
Secondary capillary bed, 190
Secondary electrons, 6
Secondary follicles, ovarian, 275f, 275t
Secondary immune response, 170
Secondary lymphatic organs, 183b
Secondary lymphoid nodules, 182, 183b
Secondary lymphoid organs, 170, 178
Secondary mediators, 66
Secondary oocytes, 276
Secondary ossification centers, 86, 86t
Secondary saliva, 250
Secondary spermatocytes, 288
Secondary synaptic clefts, 100
Secondary villi, 282
Secretin, 240
Secretion granules, 9f
Secretory granules, 58

Secretory lobules of mammary glands, 284, 285f
Secretory phase of menstrual cycle, 280, 282
Secretory proteins
  constitutive pathway of, 16
  regulated pathway of, 16
Sections for light microscopy, 2
Segmental arteries, 266
Segmental bronchi, 224
Self-MHC–self-epitope complexes, 180
Semicircular canals, 318
Semicircular ducts, 318, 320, 321f, 322
Semilunar valve, 164
Seminal vesicles, 298
Seminiferous epithelium, 286, 288
  cycle of, 292–294, 293f
Seminiferous tubules, 286, 288–290, 289f
Sensorineural hearing loss, 323b
Sensory components of peripheral nervous system, 108
Sensory ganglia, 124
Sensory neurons, 112
Septa of exocrine glands, 60
Septal cells, 226, 227f
SER. See Smooth endoplasmic reticulum (SER).
Serosa
  of appendix, 248
  of digestive system, 238
  esophageal, 238
  large intestinal, 248
  small intestinal, 244
  uterine, 278
Serotonin, 121t
Serous cells
  of respiratory epithelium, 222
  of salivary glands, 250
Serous demilunes, 250
Serous glandular secretions, 58
Sertoli cells, 288, 289f
Sesamoid bones, 82
Sex chromosomes, 28
Shaft of ATP synthase, 20
Sharpey's fibers, 82, 83f, 234
Sheath cells, 154
Shock, anaphylactic, 70b
Short bones, 82
Short-term weight control, 71b
Sialoproteins, bone, 78
Sickle cell anemia, 15b
Signal peptidase, 12
Signal peptides, 14
Signal recognition particle(s) (SRP[s]), 14, 15f
Signal recognition particle receptors, 12, 14, 15f
Signal transduction, 188
Signaling cells, 10, 58
Signaling molecules, 10
  monocyte release of, 136
sIgs. See Surface immunoglobulins (sIgs).
Sildenafil, 303b
Silver stain, 3t
Simple coiled tubular glands, 212
Simple columnar epithelium, cervical, 278
Simple epithelium, 48, 49t
Simple goiter, 199b
Simple multicellular exocrine glands, 60
Simple reflex arcs, 103b
Single positive thymocytes, 180
Singlet microtubules in axoneme, 50
Single-unit smooth muscle, 106
Sinoatrial node, 162
Sinusoid(s), 156
  in bone marrow, 142
  hepatic, 256
  in splenic red pulp, 184
Sinusoidal capillaries, 156, 200
Sinusoidal domains, 256, 257f
Sinusoidal lining cells, 256
Sister chromatids, 36
Sjögren syndrome, 58b

Skeletal muscle, 94–102, 95f
  contraction of, 98
  electron microscopy of, 96, 97f
  innervation of, 100
  light microscopy of, 94
  myofibrillar organization of, mutations and, 99b
  relaxation of, 100
  sensory system of, 102
  of soft palate, 234
  structural organization of myofibrils in, 96–98, 97f
Skin, 204–210, 205f
  dermis of, 204
  disorders affecting, 209b, 211b
  epidermis of, 204–208, 205t
  glands of, 212, 213f
  thick, 204, 205f, 205t, 206, 207t, 209f
  thin, 204, 205f, 205t, 206
Skull cap, 82
Sliding hiatal hernia, 241b
Slow sodium channels, 104
Small granule cells of respiratory epithelium, 222
Small intestine, 242–246, 243f
  common histologic features of, 244
  histology of, 244–246, 245f
  histopathology of, 246, 247f, 247t
  motility of, 246
Small nuclear ribonucleoprotein particles, 30
Small pores of capillaries, 158
Smooth endoplasmic reticulum (SER), 9f, 12
  of hepatocytes, 256
Smooth muscle, 94, 106
  contraction of, 106
  electron microscopy of, 106
  of epididymis, 296
  light microscopy of, 106, 107f
  multiunit, 106
  unitary (single-unit, vascular), 106
Smooth muscle cells, arterial, 152
Smooth muscle coat of gallbladder, 258
SNAP-25 (soluble N-ethylmaleimide-sensitive fusion protein attachment protein-25), 118
SNARE proteins, 16
snRNPs. See Small nuclear ribonucleoprotein particles.
Sodium channels
  fast, 104
  ligand-gated, 100
  slow, 104
  voltage-gated, 116–118
Sodium ion
  extracellular concentration of, 10
  salivary, 250
Soft palate, 234
Solar elastosis, 45b
Soluble N-ethylmaleimide-sensitive fusion protein attachment protein-25, 118
Somatic motor innervation, 122
Somatic motor nervous system, 122, 123f
Somatic nervous system, 108, 122–124, 123f, 125f
Somatic reflexes, autonomic reflexes compared with, 109f
Somatomedins, 92
Somatostatin, 242, 253t
Somatotrophs, 190
Somatotropin, 92, 190
  physiologic effects of, 194t
Sonic Hedgehog, 232
Sox9, 76
Space of Moll, 254
Specialized mucosa of oral cavity, 230
Specific granules, 138
Spectrin tetramers, 134
Speech, 220
Spermatids, 288
Spermatocytes, 288
Spermatocytogenesis, 288

Spermatogenesis, 292, 293f
Spermatogenic cells, 288–290, 289f
Spermatozoa, 290, 291f
  capacitation of, 278
  tail of, 290, 291f
Spermiation, 288
Spermiogenesis, 290
Spherocytosis, hereditary, 135b
Sphincter, vaginal, 284
Sphincter of Oddi, 258
Sphincter pupillae muscle, 308
Sphingomyelin, 114
Spicules, 82
Spike trigger zone, 116–118
Spina bifida, 109b
Spina bifida anterior, 109b
Spinal dura mater, 126
Spinal motor nerves, 122
Spleen, 168, 184–186, 185f
  functions of, 184, 185f
  marginal zone of, 184, 185f
  red pulp of, 184, 185f
  vascular supply of, 184, 185f, 186
  white pulp of, 184, 185f
Splenic artery, 184, 185f
Splenic cords, 184
Splenic phase of hematopoiesis, 144
Spliceosomes, 30
Spongiocytes, 200
Spongiosa, 234
Spongy bone, 82
Squames, 206
Squamous cell carcinoma
  of oral cavity, 231b
  of skin, 211b
Squamous epithelium, 49f, 49t
  stratified, of oral cavity, 230
Squamous metaplasia, 57b
SRP(s). See Signal recognition particle(s) (SRP[s]).
SRP receptors, 12, 14, 15f
SRY gene, 272
Staining for light microscopy, 2, 3t
Stapedius muscle, 318
Stapes, 318
Staphylococcus aureus, endometritis due to, 279b
Start/restriction point, 34
Static τ-motoneurons, 102
Static muscle fibers, 102
Static nerve fibers, 102, 103f
Stator of ATP synthase, 20
Steatohepatitis, 259b
Steel factor, 148, 149t
Stellate reticular cells
  of lymph nodes, 182
  splenic, 184
Stellate reticulum, 232
Stem cell(s), 136, 144, 145t, 146–148, 147f
  neuronal, 131b
Stem cell factor, 148, 149t
Stem of goblet cell, 58, 59f
Stereocilia, 50, 320, 322
Sterility, male, 301b
Steroid hormones, 188
Stigma of ovarian capsule, 276
Stomach, 240–242, 241f
  fundic glands of, cellular composition of, 240–242, 241f
  histopathology of, 242, 243f
Stop codons, 14
Straight arteries, 278
Stratified epithelium, 48, 49t
Stratified squamous nonkeratinized laryngeal epithelium, 220
Stratum basale, 206, 207t
Stratum corneum, 206, 207t
Stratum germinativum, 206, 207t
Stratum granulosum, 206, 207t
Stratum intermedium, 232
Stratum lucidum, 206, 207t

Stratum spinosum, 206, 207t
Stratum vasculare, 278
Streptococcus, endometritis due to, 279b
Stretch reflex, 102
Striated ducts of salivary glands, 250
Striated muscle, 94
Stroma, 58, 306
  salivary, 250
Stromal cells, ovarian, 272
Structure, function related to, 2
Subarachnoid space, 126
Subcapsular epithelium of lens, 308
Subcapsular plexus, adrenal, 200
Subcapsular sinus of lymph nodes, 182
Subdural hemorrhage, 127b
Subdural space, 127b
Subendocardial layer, 162
Subendothelial connective tissue, 152
Sublingual gland, 250
Sublobular vein, 254, 255f
Submandibular gland, 250
Submucosa
  of appendix, 248
  of digestive system, 238
  esophageal, 238
  gastric, 240
  large intestinal, 248
  small intestinal, 244
  of tracheal lamina propria, 222
Subosteoclastic compartment, 80
Subperiosteal intramembranous bone
      formation, 88
Subunit A
  in axoneme, 50
  of cilium, 52
Subunit B
  in axoneme, 50
  of cilium, 52
Subunit C of cilium, 52
Succedaneous laminae, 232
Sucrase, 246
Sulci, 128
Sulcus terminalis, 236
Superficial fascia, 204
Superoxides, 138
Supraoptic nucleus of hypothalamus, 192
Suprarenal cortex, 200, 201f, 203t
Suprarenal glands, 200, 201f
Suprarenal medulla, 200, 201f, 203t
Suprarenal vein, 200
Surface absorptive cells, small intestinal, 244
Surface immunoglobulins (sIgs), 170
Surface lining cells, gastric, 240
Surface opening tubular system, 140
Surface remodeling, 90
Suspensory ligaments of lens, 308
Sustentacular cells of olfactory epithelium,
      218
Sweat glands
  apocrine, 212
  eccrine, 212, 213f
Swell bodies, 221b
Sympathetic ganglion cells, 200
Sympathetic nervous system, 124, 125f
  arterial blood pressure and, 154
  ejaculation and, 302
  enteric nervous system and, 238
Sympathetic neurons, 124
Symport transport, 10
Synapses, 116, 118–120, 119f, 119t
  chemical, 118
  electric, 118
Synapsin-I, 118
Synapsin-II, 118
Synaptic clefts, 100, 118, 119f
Synaptic ribbons, 202, 314
Synaptic vesicles, 100, 118
Synaptobrevin, 118
Synaptonemal complexes, 38
Synaptophysin, 118
Synaptotagmin, 118

Synarthrosis joints, 92, 93f
Synchondrosis, 92
Syncytiotrophoblasts, 282
Syndesmosis, 92
Synemin, 24
Synostosis, 92
Synovial fluid, 92
Synovial layer (membrane), 92
Syntaxin, 118
Systemic anaphylaxis, 70b

T3. *See* Triiodothyronine.
T4. *See* Thyroxine.
T cell(s) (lymphocytes), 136, 172–174,
      173t
  luteolysis and, 276
  in splenic marginal zone, 184
T cell lineage, 180
T cell markers, 180
T cell precursors, 180
T cell receptors (TCR[s]), 170, 172
T killer cells, 174
T reg cells, 170, 174
T tubules, 96, 97f, 104
Taeniae coli, 248
Talins, 46
Target cells, 10, 58
Target proteins, 38
Tarsal plates, 316
Taste buds, 236, 237f
Taste hairs, 236
Taste pores, 236
TATA box, 273b
Tau, 22
Taurocholic acid, 258
TCM(s). *See* Central memory T cells (TCM[s]).
TCR(s). *See* T cell receptors (TCR[s]).
TCR complex, 172
Tectorial membrane, 320
Teeth, 230–234, 231f
  age-related changes in, 231b
  deciduous, 230
  odontogenesis before bell stage and, 232,
      233f
  permanent, 230
  structures associated with, 234, 235f
Telogen phase of hair growth, 214
Telophase, 36, 37f
Telophase I of meiosis, 38, 39f
TEM(s). *See* Effector memory T cells (TEM[s]).
Temporary myositis, 95b
Tenascin, 42
Tendons, 94
Tensor tympani muscle, 318
Terminal bars, 52
Terminal bronchioles, 224, 225f
Terminal cisternae, 96, 97f
Terminal ductules, 284
Terminal hairs, 214
Territorial matrix, 76
Tertiary bronchi, 224
Tertiary granules, 138
Testes, 286–290, 287f
  histophysiology of, 294, 295f
Testicular arteries, 286
Testicular cancer, 294b
Testis-determining factor, 272
Testosterone, 292, 294
Tetanus, 101b
Tetraiodothyronine, 196, 203t
TGF-β. *See* Transforming growth factor-β
      (TGF-β); Tumor growth factor β (TGF-β).
TGN. *See* trans-Golgi network (TGN).
T$_H$ cell(s), 174, 175t
  T$_H$1, 170
  T$_H$2, 170
  T$_H$17, 170
T$_H$1 cell-mediated immune response, 178,
      179f
T$_H$2 cell-mediated immune response, 176,
      177f

Theca, 222, 223f
  of goblet cell, 58, 59f
Theca externa, 274, 275f, 275t
Theca lutein cells, 276
Thermogenins, 20, 73b
Thermoreceptors, 304
Thick filaments, 98, 99f
  of smooth muscle, 106
Thick myofilaments, 96
Thick skin, 204, 205f, 205t, 206, 207t, 209f
Thin filaments, 22–24, 23f, 25f, 98, 99f
  of smooth muscle, 106
Thin myofilaments, 96
Thin skin, 204, 205f, 205t, 206
Thoracic duct, 166
Thoroughfare channels, 158
Thrombi, 140
Thrombin, 140
Thrombomodulin, 140
Thromboplastin, platelets and, 140
Thrombopoietin, 148, 149t
Thromboxane A$_2$, 68, 69t
  platelets and, 140
Thymic corpuscles, 180
Thymic cortex, 170
Thymic stromal lymphopoietin, 180
Thymocytes, 180
Thymus, 168, 180, 181f
Thymus-independent antigens, 186
Thyrocalcitonin, 203t
Thyroglobulin, 196
Thyroid gland, 196, 197f, 203t
Thyroid peroxidase, 196
Thyroid-stimulating hormone
  binding of, 196
  physiologic effects of, 194t
Thyrotrophs, 190
Thyrotropin, 190
Thyroxine, 196, 203t
Tight junctions, 52, 53f, 54, 55f, 114, 156
Tissue(s), 8
Tissue preparation, 2–4, 3f, 3t
Tissue thromboplastin, 140
Titin, 96
TnC. *See* Troponins.
TNF. *See* Tumor necrosis factor *entries*.
TnI. *See* Troponins.
TnT. *See* Troponins.
Toll-like receptors, 168, 169t
Tongue, 236, 237f
  lingual papillae of, 236
  root of, 236
  taste buds and, 236, 237f
Tonofibrils, 206
Tonofilaments, 56, 206
Tonsils, 168, 186
  lingual, 186, 236
  palatine, 186
  pharyngeal, 186
Tooth germ, 232
Trabeculae, 82, 84, 126
  of lymph nodes, 182
  of spleen, 184
Trabecular arteries, 184
Trabecular meshwork, 306
Trachea, 222, 223f
Trachealis muscle, 222
Transcription, 30, 31f
Transcription factor Cbfa1, 84, 88
Transcription factor Runx2, 84, 88
Transcytosis, 158
Transduction, 10
trans-face of Golgi apparatus, 16
Transfer RNA (tRNA), 30
Transfer vesicles, 14
Transferrin, testicular, 288
Transferrin receptors, 127b
Transforming growth factor, 204
Transforming growth factor-β (TGF-β), 78, 90,
      92
trans-Golgi network (TGN), 16

Transient macrophages, 68
Transitional cell carcinomas, renal, 270b
Transitional endoplasmic reticulum, 16, 17f
Transitional epithelium, 49f, 49t
  of renal calyces, 270
  ureteral, 270
Translation, 12
Translocator proteins, 12, 14
Transmembrane linker proteins, 54, 56
Transmembrane proteins, 8
Transmission electron microscopy, 3f, 7f
Transneuronal degeneration, 130
Transport
  active, 10, 11f
  passive, 10, 11f
  receptor-mediated, 28
Transport vesicles, 16
Transporter, 26
Transporter proteins, 176
Trauma, occlusal, 235b
Triads, 96, 97f
  retinal, 314
Tricellulin, 54
Trichohyalin, 214
Tricuspid valve, 164
Trigone of urinary bladder, 270
Triiodothyronine, 196, 203t
Trimerization, 80
Triplet microtubules, 52, 53f
Trisomy 21, 39b
tRNA, 14. See also Transfer RNA (tRNA).
Trophoblasts, 276, 282
Tropocollagen, 42, 43f, 44, 45f
Tropomodulin, 96
Tropomyosin molecules, 98
Troponins, 98
  troponin C, 98
  troponin I, 98
  troponin T, 98
Trypsin inhibitor, 252
TSH. See Thyroid-stimulating hormone.
Tubular exocrine glands, 60, 61f
Tubular necrosis, acute, 265b
Tubuli recti, 286, 296, 297t
α Tubulin, 22, 23f
β Tubulin, 22, 23f
τ Tubulin, 22
Tubuloalveolar glands
  exocrine, 60, 61f
  mammary gland as, 284
Tubulovesicular system, 240
Tuftelins, 230
Tumor(s). See also Cancer; specific tumors.
  neuroendocrine, 60b
Tumor growth factor β (TGF-β), 256
Tumor necrosis factor, 90, 92, 138
Tumor necrosis factor-α (TNF-α), 68
  corpus luteum and, 276
  origin and functions of, 175t
  small intestinal, 244
Tunica adventitia, 152–154, 153f, 155f
  arterial, 155t
  venous, 161t
Tunica albuginea
  ovaries and, 272
  of penile erectile bodies, 300
  testes and, 286
Tunica fibrosa of eye, 306
Tunica intima, 152–154, 153f, 155f
  arterial, 155t
Tunica lamina, venous, 161t
Tunica media, 152–154, 153f, 155f
  arterial, 155t
  venous, 161t
Tunica propria, 288
Tunica vaginalis, 286
Tunica vasculosa
  of eye, 308, 309f
  testicular, 286
Tympanic cavity, 318, 319f

Tympanic membrane, 316
  pressure equalization and, 317b
Type 1 diabetes mellitus, 253b
Type 2 diabetes mellitus, 253b
Type A cells
  of collecting tubules, 264
  in synovial layer of diathrosis joints, 92
Type A fibers, 122t
Type B cells
  of collecting tubules, 264
  in synovial layer of diathrosis joints, 92
Type B fibers, 122t
Type C fibers, 122t
Type I cells
  of carotid body, 154
  of taste buds, 236
Type I pneumocytes, 226
Type Ib axons, 102
Type II cells
  of carotid body, 154
  of taste buds, 236
Type II pneumocytes, 226, 227f
Type III cells of taste buds, 236
Type IV cells of taste buds, 236

Ubiquinone, 18
Ugastrone, 242
UI1, origin and functions of, 175t
Ultraviolet (UV) rays, 209b
Uncoupling protein-1 (UPC-1), 73b
Ungated channels, 10
Unicellular exocrine glands, 58, 59f
Unilaminar primary follicles, 274, 275t
Unilocular adipose tissue, 72, 73f
Unilocular fat cells, 62
Unipolar neurons, 112, 113f, 124
Uniport transport, 10
Unit membranes, 8
Unitary smooth muscle, 106
UPC-1. See Uncoupling protein-1 (UPC-1).
Uracil, 30
Ureters, 270, 271f
Urethra
  male, 300
  prostatic, 296
Urinary bladder, 270
Urinary space, 260
Urinary system, 260–270
  Bowman's capsule and, 260–262, 261f
  collecting tubules of, 264
  distal tubule of, 260, 262–264, 265f
  excretory passages of, 270
  Henle's loop of, 260, 262
  juxtaglomerular apparatus of, 264, 265f
  proximal tubule of, 260, 262, 263f
  renal circulation and, 266, 267f
  renal interstitium and, 266
  urine formation and, mechanism of, 266–268, 269f
  vasa recta of, 268, 269f
Urinary tract infections (UTIs), 270b
Urine, formation of, mechanism of, 266–268, 269f
Uriniferous tubule, 260, 261f
Urogastrone, 246
Uronic sugars, 40–42
Uterine endometrium, implantation and, 282
Uterine glands, 278
Uterus, 278, 279f
Uterus bicornis, 273b
Uterus didelphys, 273b
UTIs. See Urinary tract infections (UTIs).
Utricle, 318
UV rays. See Ultraviolet (UV) rays.
Uvula, 234

α,β³ integrins, 80
Vagus nerve, 258

Valves
  cardiac, 164
  of Kerckring, 244
  venous, 160
Varicose veins, 161b
Vas deferens, 286, 296, 297t
Vasa recta, 266, 268, 269f
Vasa vasorum, 154
Vascular endothelial growth factor, 88
Vascular smooth muscle, 106
Vasectomy, 296b
Vasoactive intestin peptide, 253t
Vasomotor center, 154–156
Vasopressin, 192
  arterial blood pressure and, 156
  physiologic effects of, 194t
Veins, 152, 160, 161t. See also specific veins.
  in bone marrow, 142
  of splenic pulp, 184, 185f
  varicose, 161b
Vellus, 214
Venae rectae, 266, 268
Ventilation, 218
  mechanism of, 228
Ventral horns, 126
Ventricles of heart, 164, 165f
Venules, 160, 200
Vermiform granules, 208
Vermis, 130
Very low density lipoproteins (VLDL)
  of hepatocytes, 256
  plasma, 133t
Vesicle coat protein AP-2, 118
Vesicular zone of osteoclasts, 80
Vesicular-tubular cluster (VTC), 16
Vestibular division of vestibulocochlear nerve, 320, 321f
Vestibular folds of larynx, 220
Vestibular function of ear, 322
Vestibular mechanism, 318
Vestibular membrane, 320
Vestibule
  of bony labyrinth, 318
  between labia minora, 284, 285f
  of oral cavity, 230
Viagra, 303b
Villi of small intestine, 244
Villin, 24, 50
Vimentin, 106, 156
  binding of, 24
Vincristine, 35b
Vinculin, 104
Virally transformed cells, T$_H$ cell-mediated killing of, 178, 179f
Virgin cells, 170
Visceral pericardium, 164
Visceral pleura, 228
Visual purple, 312
Vitamin(s)
  affecting hyaline cartilage, 77t
  bone development and, 93t
Vitamin A, bone development and, 93t
Vitamin B$_{12}$, 240
Vitamin C, bone development and, 93t
Vitamin D, 198
  bone development and, 93t
Vitiligo, 209b
Vitreous body, 310
VLDL. See Very low density lipoproteins (VLDL).
Vocal folds, 220
Vocal ligament, 220
Vocalis muscle, 220
Volkmann's canals, 82–84
Voltage-gated Ca⁺ channels, 100
Voltage-gated channels, 10
Voltage-gated K⁺ channels, 116–118
Voltage-gated Na⁺ channels, 116–118
Volume transmission of neurotransmitters, 120
von Willebrand factor, 140, 153b
VTC. See Vesicular-tubular cluster (VTC).

Wallerian degeneration, 130
Water
    flow into parietal cell, 242
    resorption of, bone calcification and, 88
Wave of depolarization, 116–118
WBCs. *See* White blood cells (WBCs).
Weigert's elastic stain, 3t
Weight control, short- and long-term, 71b
Well-differentiated liposarcomas, 71b
Wharton's jelly, 70
White adipose tissue, 72, 73f
White blood cells (WBCs), 136–138, 137t,
    144
    basophils as, 137t, 138
    eosinophils as, 137t, 138
    lymphocytes as, 136, 137t
    monocytes as, 136, 137t
    neutrophils as, 137t, 138, 139f

White fibers, 42, 94
White matter, 126
White pulp of spleen, 184
Woven bone, 82
Wright stain, 3t, 132

X chromosomes, second, 138

Yellow fibers, 44, 45f
Yellow marrow, 82, 142

Z disk (line), 94, 97f
Zellweger syndrome, 19b
Zollinger-Ellison syndrome, 241b
Zona fasciculata, adrenal, 200
Zona glomerulosa, adrenal, 200
Zona intermedia, 190, 191f
Zona occludens, 114

Zona pellucida, 274, 275f
Zona reaction, 280
Zona reticularis, adrenal, 200
Zone of calcification, 88, 89f
Zone of maturation and hypertrophy, 88, 89f
Zone of ossification, 88, 89f
Zone of proliferation, 88, 89f
Zone of reserve cartilage, 88, 89f
Zonula adherens, 52, 53f, 54, 55f, 57f
Zonula occludens, 52, 53f, 54, 55f, 57f
Zonule fibers, 308
ZP_1, 274
ZP_2, 274
$ZP_{2,3}$, 274
Zygote, 280, 281f
Zygotene, 38
Zymogen granules, 250
Zymogenic cells, 240